Precision Nursing Science:

Integrative Holistic Nursing with the Elements of Care®

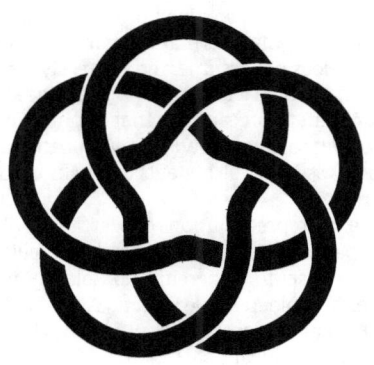

Martha Mathews Libster,
PhD, MSN, APRN-PMHCNS, APHN-BC, FAAN

Content Copyright© 2022 Golden Apple Publications
Cover Copyright© 2022 Golden Apple Publications

All rights reserved. No part of this publication may be reproduced, translated, stored in a retrieval system, or transmitted in any form or by any means, electronic, mechanical, photocopy, recording, Web distribution, information storage and retrieval systems or otherwise, without the prior written consent of the Publisher, except by a reviewer who may quote brief passages in a review.

Cover/Book Design and Artwork: Mark Gelotte www.markgelotte.com

Copy Edit: Graphic World, Inc.
Printed in the United States

Library of Congress Control Number: 2022937748

Includes bibliographical references and Index ISBN 979-8-9860801-0-9
Libster, Martha Mathews 1960-

1. Holistic/Integrative Health 2. Nursing Science 3. Nursing Practice
4. Herbalism/Herbalist 5. Body Mind & Spirit Hermeticism

I. Libster, Martha Mathews author

Golden Apple Healing Arts does not warrant or guarantee any of the products, recipes, or remedies described or discussed on its website, or in a seminar, webinar, or publication; nor has it performed any independent analysis in connection with any of the information shared in good faith with attendees, readers, and guests. Golden Apple Healing Arts does not assume, and expressly disclaims, any obligation to obtain and include information other than that which it deems important. The attendee, reader, or guest is expressly warned to consider and adopt all safety precautions that might be indicated by the activities described herein and to avoid all potential hazards. By following any educational instructions contained herein, the attendee, reader, or guest willingly assumes all benefits and risks in connection with such education.

Golden Apple Healing Arts makes no representations or warranties of any kind, including but not limited to, the warranties of fitness for particular purpose or merchantability, nor are any such representations implied with respect to the material set forth herein, and Golden Apple Healing Arts takes no responsibility with respect to such material. Golden Apple Healing Arts and its subsidiaries shall not be liable for any special, consequential, or exemplary damages resulting, in whole or part, from the attendee, reader, or guest's use of, or reliance upon, this educational material.

Information presented by Golden Apple Healing Arts and Golden Apple Publications is not intended to be a substitute for the services of a health care professional nor is it meant to authorize or endorse the use of herbs or other therapeutic modalities by the professional reader in the care of patients. Neither Dr. Martha Libster nor Golden Apple Healing Arts are responsible for any consequences incurred by those employing remedies. Botanical and other therapeutic knowledge is constantly changing. Different opinions by experts, continued research and clinical results, individual circumstances and possible error in preparing educational content requires the attendee, reader, and guest to use their own judgment and other information when making decisions based on the material contained in or derived from Golden Apple Healing Arts resources and publications. Although Dr. Martha, contributor(s), and Golden Apple Healing Arts have, as is humanly possible, taken care to ensure that the information is accurate and up-to-date at the time of inclusion on this web site and in events and services, people are strongly advised to confirm that the information meets their unique needs and health patterns and complies with the latest legislation and health care standards where they reside in the world. Dr. Martha Libster and Golden Apple Healing Arts cannot accept any legal responsibility or liability for an attendee's, reader's, or guest's use of botanicals or any other therapeutic modality discussed during an educational service or event in the care of themselves or others.

CONTENTS

Table of Contents 3
Figures and Tables 10
Introduction 11
Purpose 12

PART I Introduction to Precision Nursing Science: Integrative Holistic Nursing Practice 13

Chapter 1: Integrative Holistic Nursing: An Enduring Philosophy 14
Learning Outcome 14
Chapter Objectives 14
The Concept of Holism 14
   What are Holism, Energetic Patterns, and Precision? 15
   Roots of Integrative Holistic Nursing 16
The Elements of Care® 17
   Holistic Nursing as a Specialty 18
Complementary Therapies 19
   Complementary Therapies and Nursing 20
      Natural Products 20
      Mind and Body Practices 21
   Clarifying Terms Used in Integrative Holistic Nursing 21
Summary 23
Resources 23
References 24

Chapter 2: Precision Nursing Science With the Five Elements of Care 26
Learning Outcome 29
Chapter Objectives 26
Introduction 26
The Five Elements of Care® in Comfort and Care 27
   Change, Transition, and Transformation 29
   Nursing Theory and Process 30
Focus on the Five Elements 33
   Fire (Hot, Dry) 33
   Air (Hot, Moist) 33
   Water (Cold, Moist) 34
   Earth (Cold, Dry) 35
   Ether (Pneuma) 35
Case Study: Elements of Care® Questions 36
   Nurse's Answers 36
Holistic Transformation 37
Summary 38
References 39

Chapter 3: Health Cultures and Healing Systems 41

Learning Outcome 41
Chapter Objectives 41
Introduction 41
Professional Formation 41
Health Culture Diplomacy and Integrative Holistic Nursing 42
Traditional/Indigenous Healing Systems 45
    Alaska Native American Indian Healing 46
    European-American "Old Way" 47
    African Healing Traditions 50
    Classical Traditional Chinese Medicine 51
    Ayurveda 55
Professional Considerations Related to Traditional/Indigenous Healing Systems 56
Case Study: Refining the Elements of Cultural Skill 57
    Questions 57
    Nurse's Answers 57
Holistic Transformation 58
Summary 59
Resources 59
References 60

Part II
Precision Nursing Science: Integrative Holistic Nursing Interventions 63

Chapter 4: Overview of Interventions 64

Learning Outcome 64
Chapter Objectives 64
Introduction 64
Precision Nursing Science and Integrative Holistic Nursing 66
    Welcoming Integrative Insights 66
    Accents to the Nursing Process 67
        Assessment 67
        Clinical Vignette #1 67
        Diagnosis 68
        Planning and Implementation 69
            Clinical Vignette #2 70
        Evaluation 71
        Clinical Vignette #3 71
Choosing Modalities 72
    Discernment 72
        Clinical Vignette #4 73
    Safety Considerations 73
Holistic Transformation 75
Summary 75
References 76

Chapter 5: Pain Relief and Comfort: Non-Pharmacological Interventions 77

Learning Outcome 77
Chapter Objectives 77
Introduction 77
A Path Beyond Disease and Cure 78
    Placebo Effect 80
Stress Relief 81
Elements and Remedies 84
    Earth Element – Physical Pain and Suffering 85
    Pain Measures 86
    Remedy to Alleviate Physical Pain and Suffering 86
    Air Element – Psychological Pain and Perception 88
    Biofeedback 88
    Water Element – Emotional Pain 89
    Hot-Water Bottles to Hug 89
    Clinical Vignette – School Nurse– Hug the Bear Therapy 91
    Fire Element – Religious and Spiritual Pain 91
    Heartfelt Appreciation Experiment 92
    Ether Element – Multi-Dimensional Pain and the Elements 93
Conscious Breathing 94
Case Study: Refining the Elements of Comfort Skill 94
    Questions 94
    Nurse's Answers 95
Holistic Transformation 96
Summary 97
Resources 97
References 98

Chapter 6: Mindfulness Practice Interventions 100

Learning Outcome 100
Chapter Objectives 100
Introduction 100
Background 100
    Mindfulness versus Mindlessness 101
    Transforming Mindless Habits 102
    Consciousness and the Mechanism of Mindfulness 103
Mindfulness in Practice 105
    Breath and Present Moment 105
    Mindfulness Experiments 106
    The Orange 106
    Ringing the Bell 106
    Research 107

> Obesity 108
> Low Back Pain 108

Case Study: Refining the Elements of Observation Skill 109
> Questions 109
> Nurse's Answers 109

Holistic Transformation 110
Summary 111
Resources 111
References 112

Chapter 7: Touch Therapies and Bodywork Interventions 114

Learning Outcome 114
Chapter Objectives 114
Introduction 114
Background 115
Touch Therapies and Bodywork in Practice 116
> Massage and Bodywork Techniques 116
> Research 117
> Professional Notes ` 119
> Infant Massage: An Educational Approach 119
> Research 121
> Professional Notes 122
> Foot Reflexology: Adding a Dimension to Touch 122
> Science of Energy Flow® 123
> Research 125
> Dysmenorrhea 126
> Sleep 126
> Blood Pressure 126
> Labor 126
> Stress, Fatigue, and Depression 127
> Professional Notes 127
> Case Study: Refining the Elements of Touch Skills 128
> Questions 126
> Nurse's Answers 128
> Holistic Transformation 129
> Summary 130

Resources 130
References 131

Chapter 8: Communication Interventions 134

Learning Outcome 134
Chapter Objectives 134
Introduction 134
Background 135

Cultivating Therapeutic Relationships 135
Empathy 136
Self-Awareness 137
Counseling and Coaching Techniques 139
Communication Interventions in Practice 141
    Expressive Arts Therapies: Music Therapy 141
        Research 142
        Professional Notes 143
    Animal-Assisted Therapies 144
        Research 145
        Professional Notes 146
Case Study: Refining the Elements of Communication Skills 146
    Questions 146
    Nurse's Answers 146
Holistic Transformation 147
Summary 148
Resources 148
References 149

Chapter 9: Water Element: Hydrotherapy 152

Learning Outcome 152
Chapter Objectives 152
Introduction 152
Background 153
Hydrotherapy in Practice 157
    Research 158
        Immersion Baths 158
        Footbaths 159
    Sitz Baths 161
    Packs and Wraps 161
    Water Irrigations 161
    Aquatic Exercise, Aqua or Water Therapy 162
    Balneotherapy 163
    Saunas and Steam Baths 163
        Water Immersion During Labor and Water Birth 164
    Professional Notes 165
Holistic Transformation 166
Summary 167
Resources 167
References 168

Chapter 10: Air Element: Essential Oils and Aromatherapy 171

Learning Outcome 171
Chapter Objectives 171

Introduction 171
Background 172
    Methods of Extracting Essential Oils 173
        Steam Distillation 173
        Maceration 173
        Expression 174
        Enfleurage 174
        Solvent Extraction 174
        Synthetics 174
Essential Oils and Aromatherapy in Practice 174
    Methods of Administering Essential Oils 176
        Bath Therapy 176
        Inhalation Therapy 177
        Aerial Dispersion via Aerial Diffusers 177
        Hot or Cold Compress Therapy 177
    Research 178
    Professional Notes 180
Holistic Transformation 182
Summary 183
Resources 183
References 184

Chapter 11: Fire Element: Religious and Spiritual Interventions 186

Learning Outcome 186
Chapter Objectives 186
Introduction 186
Background 187
Religious and Spiritual Interventions in Practice 190
    Prayer and Faith Healing 190
    Imagery 191
    Effort-Shape Movement 194
Professional Notes 195
Holistic Transformation 197
Summary 198
Resources 198
References 199

Chapter 12: Earth Element: Nutrition Interventions 202

Learning Outcome 202
Chapter Objectives 202
Introduction 202
Background 203

  Energetics First with Eight Principle Patterns 204
  Nutrition Interventions in Practice 207
  Broth and Porridge 207
  The Macrobiotic Diet 209
    Macrobiotics Research 210
Professional Notes 211
Holistic Transformation 212
Summary 213
Resources 213
References 214

Chapter 13: Ether Element:
Herbal Interventions 216

Learning Outcome 216
Chapter Objectives 216
Introduction 216
Background 218
  Approaches to Nurse-Herbalism 218
  Herbs Versus Drugs 219
  Herb Safety 220
  Herbs as Dietary Supplements 221
Herbal Interventions in Practice 222
  Oral Intervention : Tea 222
  Topical Intervention: Compress 223
  Environmental Intervention – Herbal Baths 224
Professional Notes 224
Holistic Transformation 226
Summary 227
Resources 228
References 229

Conclusion 231
Next Steps 232
Publications by Dr. Martha 233
Index 237

FIGURES AND TABLES

Table 3-1:   Five Elements in Classical Traditional Chinese Medicine
Figure 3-1: The Cultural Diplomacy Model©
Figure 3-2: Going Green: Sprouting
Figure 4-1: How to Prepare a Rosemary Footbath
Figure 5-1: Healing Relationship Model©
Figure 5-2: Recipe for Ginger Compress for Pain
Figure 5-3: Simple Biofeedback Device
Figure 7-1: Science of Energy Flow® Foot Reflexology Chart
Figure 9-1: Water Course
Figure 12-1: Five Seasons and Tastes in Classical Traditional Chinese Medicine
Figure 12-2: Yin-Yang

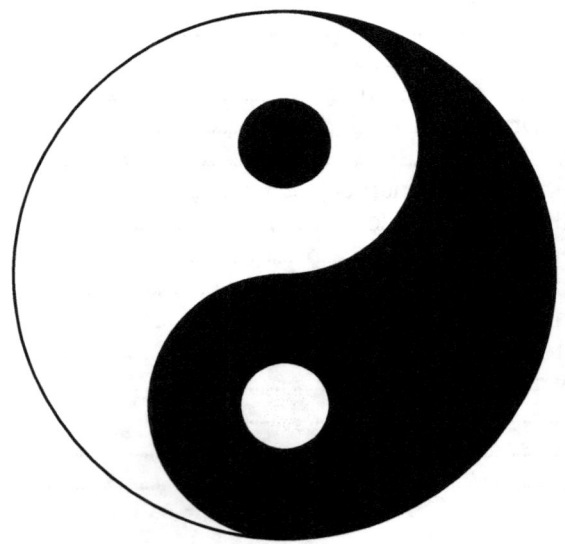

INTRODUCTION

Holism defines a philosophical approach to care in nursing that is centuries old. Today, integrative holistic nursing is a specialty practice, which has a defined focus on nursing care that incorporates complementary therapies, natural products, mind and body practices, and aspects of traditional healing systems. The actions of every nurse are defined by a holistic philosophical approach that has endured the centuries to include physical, emotional, mental, and spiritual care. How that nursing care is applied, not simply what is done to a patient, is an enduring theme that defines the Elements of Care® that are foundational to integrative holistic nursing.

For centuries, the five Elements of Care® – Fire, Air, Water, Earth, and Ether, (defined as a vital energy or infinite substance which encompasses all of the elements), have provided a structural focus for nature cure and sickroom management, creating healing environments, and the nursing care of the whole patient, be they individuals, families, or communities. When in balance, the five elements are considered a full measure of health. The structure of this text around the Elements of Care® may seem familiar to nurses as nature cure and sickroom management. This text incorporates the same five elements that appear throughout the history of medicine and science as well as in the traditional and indigenous systems of health belief and healing in which nurses frequently engage. In today's culturally diverse healthcare environment, nurses will gain a broad understanding of how the five Elements of Care® are relevant today. This in-depth understanding provides a new perspective on clinical care, practice management, and quality of life for both the patient and the nurse. It is also the foundation for precision nursing science referred to in this text that places energetics first.

The 13 chapters of this text are divided into two parts. Part I introduces and defines the elements of integrative holistic nursing practice. Separate chapters address the philosophy of holism and the five elements as well as the traditional and indigenous healing systems that continue to inform precision nursing science and the health culture diplomacy of the integrative holistic nurse. Part II focuses on the ways a nurse can apply the knowledge gained from part I in integrative holistic nursing interventions and plans of care that demonstrate precision nursing science. Chapters 4 – 8 are general chapters that provide an overview of integrative holistic nursing interventions, pain relief and comfort, mindfulness practice, touch therapies, and communication interventions. This is followed by specific chapters exemplifying the application of the knowledge of each of the five elements to integrative holistic nursing practice: Water (Hydrotherapy); Air (Essential Oils and Aromatherapy); Fire (Religious and Spiritual Interventions); Earth (Nutrition Interventions); and Ether (Herbal Interventions).

Applying integrative holistic nursing philosophy and the five Elements of Care® in nursing practice is a highly creative process that is precision nursing science. This text includes time for self-discovery with the intent that you will take the time to reflect upon and transform your own creative expression of integrative holistic care as precision nursing science so as to be more authentically congruent with your personal and professional purpose.

PURPOSE

After reading this text, the learner will be able to:

1. Explain integrative holistic nursing philosophy, precision nursing science, and the concept of holism.
2. List the five Elements of Care® that guide healing traditions, self-care, and holistic nursing practice.
3. Discuss the difference between complementary therapies and traditional/indigenous healing.
4. Explore ways to demonstrate holistic nursing philosophy in the practice of integrative nursing.
5. Promote pain relief and comfort with non-pharmacological interventions.
6. Demonstrate mindfulness practice interventions in integrative holistic nursing care.
7. Describe one way to integrate touch therapies and body work interventions into your nursing practice.
8. Utilize integrative holistic nursing communication interventions with patients.
9. Include hydrotherapy interventions in integrative holistic nursing practice.
10. Apply essential oils and aromatherapy interventions in integrative holistic nursing practice.
11. Incorporate religious and spiritual interventions in integrative holistic nursing practice.
12. Select nutrition interventions for use in integrative holistic nursing practice.
13. Analyze the essential nature of herbal interventions (ether element) applied in integrative holistic nursing practice.

PART I:
INTRODUCTION TO PRECISION NURSING SCIENCE:

INTEGRATIVE HOLISTIC NURSING PRACTICE

CHAPTER 1

INTEGRATIVE HOLISTIC NURSING: AN ENDURING PHILOSOPHY

LEARNING OUTCOME

After completing this chapter, the learner will be able to explain integrative holistic nursing philosophy and the concepts of holism and integrative care.

CHAPTER OBJECTIVES

After completing this chapter, the learner will be able to:

1. Define the concept of holism.
2. Discuss integrative holistic nursing philosophy.
3. Explain the history of holistic nursing.
4. List the five Elements of Care®.
5. Define and evaluate the state of precision nursing science.
6. Analyze the role of complementary therapies in nursing practice.

THE CONCEPT OF HOLISM

Biomedicine, or conventional medicine, is the dominant healthcare culture in the United States. It is a rich culture of health beliefs and practices backed by considerable social, economic, and political power. Nursing has developed within this culture; however, the history of nursing demonstrates the unique and distinct relationship that nurses have with their patients and the public. Nurses focus on caring science as well as the biological, cure-based science of the medical profession. "Nurses have developed a professional culture in which the focus is caring, comfort, and the development of a healing relationship in which the patient is valued as a whole person" (Libster, 2001, p. 11).

The mechanistic and reductionist Newtonian model of the universe that has been the foundation for biomedicine is changing. Biomedical practices that engage Newtonian values in the reduction of the human body, health, and disease to that of a machine and its parts are being replaced. Other beliefs and paradigms or worldviews about health care, medicine, and nursing culture have been evolving alongside the development of the new order of thought in physics.

For example, we have in Einstein's *relativity* and Bohm's *implicate order*, a movement toward the notion of "undivided wholeness" (Bohm, 1980, p. 170). (See Bohm speaking in the YouTube link in the Resources section.)

It is known that Aristotle compared the universe to a living organism, exemplifying the philosophy of wholeness as that which is above is also below and that which is without is also within. The ocean is an example of this view of the inseparability between the whole and the parts. Each drop removed from the ocean is still biologically, constitutionally, and energetically "ocean." The concept of wholeness is reflected throughout time: from the ancient cultures to the beliefs of those engaged in the medieval science of alchemy, or self-transformation, to the enduring health beliefs and healing practices of traditional and indigenous peoples throughout the world today. As will be discussed here, although people may have never stopped holding their traditional health beliefs and practicing self-care according to their heritage, the public demand for greater integration of biomedical approaches and those traditional and self-care beliefs and practices is growing. Emerging public health crises suggest that fragmented and disparate solutions are not sufficient to solve tough problems, thus pushing the trend toward holism.

What are Holism, Energetic Patterns, and Precision?

Holism is a term used to define a philosophy in which the "whole" is greater than the sum of the parts and whose parts can only be understood "in relation to their functions in the complete and ongoing whole" (Flew, 1979, p. 152). The word "holism" is derived from the Greek word holos, which means "whole." Those engaged in holistic care therefore view a patient (whether the patient is an individual, a family, a community, or a nation), as a whole being with physical, psychological, emotional, and spiritual needs that cannot be reduced or distinguished as separate parts. All patients are but patterns of organization, relationship, interaction, and processes when framing health not as the absence of disease but as a "dynamic, evolving pattern of the whole" (Newman, 1994, p. 134) in which caregivers, with patients as partners, find deep meaning in relationships. Patterns, as they are defined in holistic philosophy, are energetic information that depicts the whole. They allow us to perceive and understand the meaning of all relationships at once. For example, each person is a unique energetic pattern that is more than their genetic code or fingerprints. An energetic pattern is relatedness and is "self-organizing over time, i.e., it becomes more highly organized with more information" (Newman, 1994, p. 72). The energetic patterns, which are the focus of this text, are inclusive of but not limited to the often-recognized types of human energy: thermal (temperature), mechanical (movement), electrical (nerve impulse), and chemical (metabolism of food). The patient's underlying energetic pattern(s) and a nurse's "energetics first" approach applying the Elements of Care® as described in this text are a foundation for precision nursing science. As will be demonstrated in this text, nurses have a history of centuries of practice in precision health and therefore are well positioned to lead its development in "shifting the fundamental change from disease-focused care to one that uses precision medicine to avoid serious clinical diseases from emerging before they take place" (Fawaz, 2021, p. 938). The energetics first approach with the Elements of Care® integrative holistic nursing practice, defined here as "precision nursing science" complements the works of those nurses' who are seeking to define precision nursing science in terms of omics (health status at the molecular level) combined with "lifestyle, social, economic, cultural and environmental factors" (Fu et al, 2021).

ROOTS OF INTEGRATIVE HOLISTIC NURSING

The emergence of machines, advancement of technologies, and reductionism have entered into many societal domains (including nursing) over the past 150 years. Early American professional nursing was first formed in religious communities, where the notion of addressing a patient's holistic, that is, spiritual, emotional, and mental health as well as bodily needs, was foundational to the trainings and preparation for administering to the sick (Libster & McNeil, 2009). The model of nurse training not affiliated with organized religion was advanced by British nurse, Florence Nightingale. The adoption of this model, first at Bellevue Hospital in New York in 1873, was a major shift in nursing history that was initiated in support of the advancement of science and hospitals. American nurses often cite Nightingale's work and the severing of religious ties as the beginning of "professional" nursing in America (Libster & McNeil, 2009, p. 327). This development is exemplified in Nutting and Dock's 1907 history of nursing in which they stated, "Gone forever, ... was the conception of nursing as a charity ... The self-sacrifice remained but under her sway nursing shone forth as part of the invincible and glorious advance of science" (p. 168). However, the roots of professional nursing in America run deeper than the period of the advancement of science and are linked to enduring healing traditions in which nurses were renowned for their holistic care.

Professional nursing in the United States began with the Sisters of Charity of Vincent de Paul in 1827. The religious women's community was founded by Elizabeth Ann Seton. who transported the centuries-old policies and procedures for instituting the original educational and healing missions of the Daughters of Charity in France founded by Louise de Marillac and Vincent de Paul in 1633. de Marillac's charitable service to humanity suggested the possibility that "a deep spiritual experience of God, often referred to as 'consolation,' could be found in the simple, humble acts of nursing the sick poor. Nursing was charity, the spiritual essence encompassed in the name of a Company of sisters deeply devoted to its physical expression" (Libster & McNeil, 2009, p. 17). The Sisters followed the *Common Rules* (dating back to 17th-century France) and their training manual, *Instruction on the Care of the Sick* by Sister Mary Xavier Clark (1846). These works encouraged those involved in nursing care to administer corporal care and comfort first (Libster & McNeil, 2009, p. 47), and then prayer and spiritual care as requested. The *Rules* forbade them to proselytize their religion to the sick. The American Sisters and those who merged with the French in the 1850s to become Daughters of Charity were recognized experts in the holistic care of the mentally ill in particular (Libster & McNeil, 2009). They attended to the physical, emotional, mental, and spiritual needs of the ill, for whom they created healing environments in their hospitals that endured into the 20th century, most notably the Mount Hope Retreat in Maryland. Their successful approach to care was acknowledged by the 19th-century healthcare reformer, Dorothea Dix, and Nightingale, who studied with the Daughters in Paris twice before she led her nursing operation in the Crimea in Turkey.

In 19th-century Europe, the Careful Nursing model was developed by Catherine McAuley in Ireland, who founded the Dublin Institute of Our Lady of Mercy home and hospital nursing service in 1828. The nurses were Catholics and Protestants who in 1831 became the Religious Sisters of Mercy. In 1843, Frances Warde led the first Sisters of Mercy to the United States from Ireland at the invitation of the Bishop of Pittsburgh, Pennsylvania, and the order spread across the United States of America. "Their nursing work consisted of physical care and emotional consolation provided from a spiritual perspective ... She stressed that gentleness, kindness, and patience must characterize all interactions with patients (Meehan, 2003, p. 100). Teaching people to care for and help themselves was considered essential to the development and well-being of the whole person and the health of the community. McAuley's original Guide to the Visitation of the Sick (1832) contains many assumptions and principles that are shared by Christians and non-Christians alike. The major themes of careful nursing include "disinterested love," "contagious calmness" nourished by practice of meditation and prayer, and an "enduring trust in the sustaining love of the Supreme Being" and the "creation of a restorative environment" (Meehan, 2003, p. 102). The Sisters of Charity in America and the Religious Sisters of Mercy in Ireland were deeply engaged in professional nursing as the creation of healing and restorative environments decades before Nightingale was asked to write Notes on Nursing in 1859.

The Elements of Care®

Nursing care in the 19th century was focused on the creation of healing environments. This approach was used at the time of the Sisters of Charity and Mercy nurses in America and, on the other side of the ocean, with the Daughters of Charity in Paris, Florence Nightingale in England, and others. The science and art of integrative holistic nursing in the 19th century was demonstrated in what was referred to as "sickroom management," in which the nurse partnered with nature to create a healing environment (Libster, 2008). Elements of the natural environment, such as water and medicinal plants, were highly valued therapeutics that were thought to assist nature in her ability to cure. Nightingale is best known for her statement, "Nature alone cures ... and what nursing has to do in either case, is to put the patient in the best condition for nature to act upon him" (Nightingale, 1980, p. 110). This nature cure *philosophy* of care was commonly practiced and often written about by physicians, nurses, midwives, and health reformers in

America throughout the early and mid-19th century (Libster, 2004).

Nature cure and sickroom management included attention to the five elements that appear throughout the history of medicine and science around the world. The five elements thought to be the elements of all creation according to the ancients, including the Greeks, were fire, air, water, earth, and ether (defined as a vital energy that the Greeks called "pneuma"). When in balance, the five elements are considered a full measure of health. All of the elements are understood and utilized according to their essential qualities: Fire is hot and dry; air is hot and moist; water is cold and moist; and earth is cold and dry. Sickroom management and nature cure meant the creative utilization of these elements to secure changes that promoted greater balance in health and life. For example, if a person had a headache and felt heat in their head, the nurse might seek to cool the head with cool-water compresses and sips and inhalations of mint *(Mentha piperita)* tea known for its cooling energetic action to the head. The sickroom was the "laboratory for the invention and application of remedies and the creation of a healing environment in which nature could affect a cure" (Libster, 2008, p. 163). Nurses practiced the science and art of regulating the warmth of a space, opening and closing windows, and preparing the proper sick diet for the patient that would help to establish balance in body, mind, and spirit. The ether element, the "pneuma" that encompassed all four elements (fire, air, water, and earth), is represented in the essence of an environment, such as in the quality of presence of the nurse and their approach to care, such as "offering respect" (Coskery, p. 26, as cited in Libster & McNeil, 2009). The focus on how nursing care is applied, not simply what is done to a patient, is an enduring theme that defined nursing centuries ago and now defines integrative holistic nursing today. The nurse and the patient, as human beings, are made from the same elements that are applied in sickroom management. Precision nursing science, as the application of these five Elements of Care® in the design of person-centered relationship-centered care and healing environments, is discussed in greater detail in Chapter 2.

Holistic Nursing as a Specialty

As nursing has progressed in its pursuit of science, holistic nursing as a philosophy of care has endured. Definitions of nursing found in state practice acts as well as the definition of nursing from the American Nurses Association (ANA) include the use of the term "holistic" as a required element of practice. "The common thread uniting different types of nurses who work in varied areas is the nursing process – the essential core of practice for the registered nurse to deliver *holistic,* (italics added) patient-focused care" in which the assessment includes "not only physiological data, but also psychological, sociocultural, spiritual, economic, and life-style factors as well" (ANA, n.d.).

Although the actions of every nurse are defined by a holistic, philosophical approach that has endured the centuries to include physical, emotional, mental, and spiritual care, there are some nurses who specialize in holistic nursing. Just as a school nurse might specialize in school/public health after basic education in child development and pediatric nursing care, the holistic nurse specializes in holistic care of individuals, families, and communities beyond what is required of all nurses implementing the nursing process. Holistic nursing is currently recognized by the ANA as a nursing "specialty."

The American Holistic Nurses Association (AHNA) has partnered with the ANA to produce Holistic Nursing: Scope and Standards of Practice, now in its third edition (AHNA, 2018). AHNA's definition of holistic nursing is "all nursing practice that has healing the whole person as its goal" (AHNA, 1998, p. 1). Holistic nursing often includes the integration of complementary therapies (CT). Nurses who incorporate CT in care must be educated and competent in the CT they use. Practicing within a holistic nursing framework does not fundamentally imply competency or expertise in the effective and safe application of a CT. A nurse practicing a specific CT is required, typically by state statute, to have the education, skills, and credentials required for that modality. Nurses also must operate within the legal scope of practice of their licensure and scope of practice. If the nurse is employed, he or she is also subject to the policies and procedures regarding CT for that institution. Certifications in holistic nursing available through the American Holistic Nurses Credentialing Corporation (a separate organization from the AHNA) include basic, advanced, and advanced practice nurse credentials. AHNCC certification examinations are accredited by the Accreditation Board for Specialty Nursing Certification [ABSNC] and are recognized by the American Nurses Credentialing Center [ANCC] Magnet Program.

COMPLEMENTARY THERAPIES

In 1992, the U.S. Congress mandated the creation of the Office of Alternative Medicine (OAM) at the National Institutes of Health. In 1998, the OAM was renamed the National Center for Complementary and Alternative Medicine (NCCAM), a federal government agency to investigate and evaluate "promising unconventional medical practices" (National Center for Complementary and Integrative Health [NCCIH], 2017a). At the time of the establishment of the OAM, the term "alternative medicine" was popularized primarily among physicians. Subsequent use of the term complementary and alternative medicine (CAM) still focused on the biomedical paradigm.

In a seminal survey of the U.S. population's use of CAM, Harvard physician David Eisenberg and colleagues documented the working definition of CAM as "any medical intervention not taught widely at U.S. medical schools or generally available at U.S. hospitals" (1993, p. 246.) In that study, 34% of the 1,539 adults surveyed reported using at least one "unconventional" therapy in the past year, and one third saw "alternative therapy practitioners." In a follow-up survey in 1998, Eisenberg's team reported increased use of CAM by the public.

When the first list of "alternative medicines" was published on the OAM website in the late 1990s, I remember seeing "science-based nursing" on the list. It was peculiar to think of nursing – which for so many centuries had been complementary to the practice of medicine – as being "alternative" to it. Like nursing, many traditional, indigenous, and healing practices were relegated to the list of alternatives to medicine. Nursing was subsequently removed.

After the Eisenberg studies demonstrated that 1 of 3 Americans surveyed who visited a medical physician also sought care from complementary therapies practitioners, the movement toward more inclusive language took hold. The NCCAM title was changed in 2014, during the Obama administration, to the National Center for Complementary and Integrative Health (NCCIH). The name was changed to more "accurately reflect the Center's research commitment to studying promising health approaches already in use by the American public" (NCCIH, 2017a). Nonpharmacological complementary and integrative health interventions for chronic pain have become a stated focus for NCCIH research funding in light of the current opioid crisis in America. The general term used to describe techniques and modalities that fall outside the specific realm of the practice of medicine, dentistry, and podiatry is "complementary therapies" (CT).

The public and their federal and state representatives have been the impetus for much of the change toward the recognition of the complementary community-based care that is prevalent in what has been referred to as "the hidden health care system" in America (Levin & Idler, 2010). Nurses' understanding of patient health behaviors and choices related to a broad range of CT are best understood in relation to the sociocultural context that shapes their meaning. Nurses are often bridge walkers between those providing care from within the structures of the biomedical culture and the broader public experience in which many are willing to pay out of pocket for the care that they value. The public uses an integrative approach to care that nurses are well positioned to support and lead – whether nurses specialize in holistic nursing or not.

Complementary Therapies and Nursing

Many modalities more recently identified as CT have been historically analyzed as foundations of nursing practice. These foundations include five areas of therapies: engaging in touch, energy flow, and communication; providing counsel in diet and nutrition; and creating a healing environment (Libster, 2001). The NCCIH currently uses the term "complementary health approaches" when discussing the practices and products it studies, and it separates the approaches into two subgroups: "natural products" *and* "mind and body practices." These terms are new terms for the modalities that have been fundamental in nursing care and comfort of patients for centuries (Libster, 2001).

Natural Products

The natural products group includes a variety of products, such as vitamins, minerals, herbs, and probiotics. These products are widely marketed, readily available to consumers, and often marketed as *dietary supplements*. The U.S. Food & Drug Administration (FDA) regulates both finished dietary supplement products and dietary ingredients. Manufacturers of dietary supplements must comply with the FDA-issued Good Manufacturing Practice, which provides federal regulations for all domestic and foreign dietary supplement companies regarding their products and their distribution within the United States. Today, it is known as the "Dietary Supplement Current Good Manufacturing Practices" (FDA, 2018). According to the 2012 National Health Interview Survey, which included a comprehensive survey on the use of complementary health approaches by Americans, "17.7 percent of American adults had used a dietary supplement other than vitamins and minerals in the past year. These products were the most popular complementary health approach in the survey" (NCCIH, 2017b).

Mind and Body Practices

The second NCCIH group is large and diverse, encompassing techniques, therapies, and systems of care. The mind and body group is sorted into five categories, although many therapies could actually be listed in several categories: biologically based therapies, mind-body therapies, manipulative and body-based therapies, energy therapies, healing systems of traditional and indigenous healers, and other ancient healing traditions, such as Ayurveda and traditional Chinese medicine (NCCIH, 2017a). The 2012 national study showed that yoga, chiropractic and osteopathic manipulation, meditation, and massage therapy are among the most popular mind and body practices used by adults (NCCIH, 2017b). The popularity of yoga has grown dramatically in recent years. Other mind and body practices include acupuncture, relaxation techniques (such as breathing exercises, guided imagery, and progressive muscle relaxation), tai chi, Qi Gong, healing touch, hypnotherapy, and movement therapies, such as the Feldenkrais method, the Alexander technique, Pilates, Rolfing Structural Integration, and Trager psycho-physical integration (NCCIH, 2017a).

The use of the term CT in nursing is indicative of the integrative nature of practice. Nurses do not practice "alternative medicine" because that would still be the practice of medicine rather than nursing. A comprehensive study of the State Boards of Nursing's approach to incorporating CT language was published by Sparber in 2001. The paper described the responsibilities customarily referenced in Practice Acts related to the incorporation of CT in practice, such as continuing education and additional licensure as required. At the time of publication, the Louisiana Board of Nursing was specifically cited as stating that, "The Law Governing the Practice of Nursing authorizes registered nurses to provide care in supportive to or restorative to life and well-being," which Sparber's 2001 study concluded was the premise "underlying much of the thinking and support throughout the states for the justification of practice of CT." The website for the AHNA also provides current information on state practice acts' references and position papers on CT and holistic nursing.

Clarifying Terms Used in Precision Nursing Science: Integrative Holistic Nursing with the Elements of Care®

- **Nursing**. According to the ANA (n.d.), "Nursing is the protection, promotion, and optimization of health and abilities, prevention of illness and injury, facilitation of healing, alleviation of suffering through the diagnosis and treatment of human response, and advocacy in the care of individuals, families, groups, communities, and populations."

- **Conventional medicine or biomedicine** should be used rather than "Western" or "traditional" medicine when referring to orthodox medicine.
- **Integrative Nursing** is the "creation of evolving healing relationships with patients. The nurse observes the patient's needs for greater harmony and balance in their life and then addresses those needs by offering care that is a holistic blend of biomedical and caring modalities" (Libster, 2001, p. 26). The integrative holistic nurse embodies a personal professional identity rooted in holism. "Integration is a quality of heart – a welcoming heart" (Libster, 2012, p. 51) that invites consideration of a variety of ways of knowing about health and healing and the associated health beliefs, thoughts, feelings, and practices exemplified by patients and practitioners alike that is expressed in design of care that meets the unique and precise needs of the individual, family, group, or community.
- **Precision Nursing Science** incorporates traditional healing philosophies including hermeticism as represented in the five Elements of Care® – ether, fire, air, water, and earth – and the body energetic with emerging science related to human nature, physiology, and the environment. The goal of precision nursing science is to provide care and comfort that addresses the unique energetic needs for healing the whole person. This person-centered, relationship-centered approach is the ethical and clinical foundation for precision nursing science.
- **Traditional medicine** or **Traditional Healing** is the term used to describe systems of care that have endured for generations (World Health Organization, 2013). Nurses have held relationships with traditional healers for centuries. Today, traditional healers may also be licensed nurses. When nurses are able to incorporate both the beliefs and practices of their cultural traditions and that which they have learned in the biomedical culture when providing care, they are practicing integrative holistic nursing.
- **Spirituality** is not the same as religiosity. Spirituality as it is used here (as in the Careful Nursing system) refers to a transcendent reality of the Supreme Being/ Consciousness/ Creator. The spiritual is in connection with the body mind as a means of connecting with the Supreme Being / Consciousness/ Creator. His Holiness, the 14th Dalai Lama of Tibet and 1989 winner of the Nobel Peace prize, differentiates spirituality from religion:

Religion I take to be concerned with belief in the claims of one faith tradition or another connected with this are the religious teachings or dogma, ritual prayer and so on. Spirituality I take to be concerned with those qualities of the human spirit – such as love and compassion, patience, tolerance, forgiveness, contentment, a sense of responsibility, a sense of harmony, which bring happiness to both self and others (Dalai Lama, 1999, p. 22).

- **Therapeutic modalities** are those therapeutic interventions employed by integrative holistic nurses in the care of patients, families, and communities. Integrative holistic nurses recognize the important role the patient holds in directing nursing care and therefore, integrative holistic nurses, although educated to intervene with a specific modality, do not employ their skill without the consent of the patient.

SUMMARY

Holism is an enduring philosophy that embraces the notion that there is unity between all life forms. Holism defines a philosophical approach to care in nursing that is centuries old. Today, holism is foundational to the nursing process of all professional nurses and also is a specialty practice, which focuses on the integration of conventional nursing care with complementary therapies that include natural products, mind and body practices, and aspects of traditional healing systems. For centuries, the five Elements of Care® – ether, fire, air, water, and earth – have provided a structural focus for sickroom management, creating healing environments, and the holistic care of patients, be they individuals, families, or communities. Precision nursing science and person-centered, relationship-centered integrative holistic nursing practice address the unique energetic needs for healing the whole person.

RESOURCES

American Holistic Nurses Credentialing Corporation. http://www.ahncc.org

Bohm, D. (1990). Excerpt from *Art meets science and spirituality in a changing economy – From Fragmentation to wholeness [Documentary].*
Available from: https://www.youtube.com/watch?v=mDKB7GcHNac

REFERENCES

American Holistic Nurses Association. (2018). Holistic nursing: Scope and standards of practice (3rd ed.). Silver Spring, MD: American Nurses Association Press.

American Nurses Association. (n.d.) The nursing process. Retrieved 2022 from https://www.nursingworld.orpractice-policy/scope-of-practice/

Bohm, D. (1980). Wholeness and the implicate order. New York, NY: Routledge.

Dalai Lama (1999). Ethics for the new millennium. New York, NY: Riverhead Books.

Eisenberg, D. M., Davis, R. B., Ettner, S. L., Appel, S., Wilkey, S., Van Rompay, M., & Kessler, R. C. (1998). Trends in alternative medicine use in the United States, 1990-1997. JAMA, 280(18), 1569-1575.

Eisenberg, D. M., Kessler, R. C., Foster, C., Norlock, F. E., Calkins, D. R., & Delbanco, T. L. (1993). Unconventional medicine in the United States – Prevalence, costs, and patterns of use. *New England Journal of Medicine*, 328(4), 246-252.

Fawaz, M. (2021). Role of nurses in precision health. *Nursing Outlook*, 69, 937 – 940.

Flew, A. G. (1979). A dictionary of philosophy (Rev. 2nd ed.). New York, NY: St. Martin's Press.

Fu, M., Kurnat-Thoma, E., Starkweather, A., Henderson, W., Cashion, A, Williams, J., & Calzone, K. (2020). Precision health: A nursing perspective. *International Journal of Nursing Sciences*, 7(1), 5-12.

Levin, L. S., & Idler, E. L. (2010). *The hidden health care system: Social resources in health care*. Wauwatosa, WI: Golden Apple Publications.

Libster, M. (2001). *Demonstrating care: The art of integrative nursing.* Albany, NY: Delmar Cengage Learning.

Libster, M. M. (2004). *Herbal diplomats: The contribution of early American nurses (1830-1860) to 19th century health care reform and the Botanical Medical Movement.* Wauwatosa, WI: Golden Apple Publications.

Libster, M. M. (2008). Elements of care: Nursing environmental theory in historical context. *Holistic Nursing Practice*, 22(3), 160-170.

Libster, M. M., & McNeil, B. A. (2009). *Enlightened charity: The holistic nursing care, education, and "Advices Concerning the Sick" of Sister Matilda Coskery, (1799-1870).* Wauwatosa, WI: Golden Apple Publications.

Libster, M. (2012). *The Nurse-herbalist: integrative insights for holistic practice.* Wauwatosa, WI: Golden Apple Publications.

Meehan, T. C. (2003). Careful nursing: A model for contemporary nursing practice. *Journal of Advanced Nursing*, 44(1), 99-107.

National Center for Complementary and Integrative Health. *Important events in NCCIH history*. (2017a). Retrieved from https://www.nih.gov/about-nih/what-we-do/nih-almanac/national-center-complementary-integrative-health-nccih

National Center for Complementary and Integrative Health. *Types of complementary health approaches.* (2017b). Retrieved from https://nccih.nih.gov/health/integrative-health.

Newman, M. (1994). *Health as expanding consciousness.* New York, NY: National League for Nursing Press.

Nightingale, F. (1980). *Notes on nursing: What it is, and what it is not.* New York, NY: Churchill Livingstone. First published 1859.

Nutting, M. A., & Dock, L. L. (1907). *A history of nursing: The evolution of nursing systems from the earliest times to the foundation of the first English and American training schools for nurses.* New York, NY, and London, England: G. P. Putnam's Sons.

Sparber, A. (2001). State boards of nursing and scope of practice of registered nurses performing complementary therapies. *Online Journal of Issues in Nursing, 6*(3), 1-7.

U.S. Food & Drug Administration (2018). Dietary Supplements. https://www.fda.gov/food/guidanceregulation/cgmp/default.htm

World Health Organization. (2013). *WHO traditional medicine strategy: 2014-2023.* Geneva, Switzerland: Retrieved from: https://www.who.int/publications/i/item/9789241506096

CHAPTER 2

PRECISION NURSING SCIENCE WITH THE FIVE ELEMENTS OF CARE®

LEARNING OUTCOME

After completing this chapter, the learner will be able to begin to develop a plan for applying precision nursing science with the five Elements of Care® in integrative holistic nursing practice.

CHAPTER OBJECTIVES

After completing this chapter, the learner will be able to:
1. Discuss the history of nurses' partnership with the environment.
2. Describe the differences between change, transition, and transformation.
3. Explain how the five elements of all matter are rooted in precision integrative holistic nursing care.
4. Identify nursing theories used in guiding precision integrative holistic nursing practice.

INTRODUCTION

Through the ages, an element of mystery has surrounded the healing arts. Questions about the nature of health and disease persist despite the ever-expanding body of knowledge of anatomy, physiology, chemistry, and pathology. The ancients relied on their relationship with nature to define and understand health and disease as well as to formulate cures. The dance between humans and nature continues, at times with nature leading and, at other times, with humans leading. There have even been periods in the history of medicine and science when humans have become disillusioned by their creations for cure. The renowned physician and healthcare reformer, Oliver Wendell Holmes (1809 – 1894), criticized errors in thought about medical science, both homeopathic and allopathic (conventional medicine with the use of remedies to suppress symptoms). Holmes wrote:

"Throw out opium, throw out a few specifics ... throw out wine ... and the vapors which produce the miracle of anesthesia, and I firmly believe that if the whole materia medica, as now used, could be sunk to the bottom of the sea, it would be all the better for mankind – and all the worse for the fishes" (as cited in Porter, 1997, p. 680).

He was not alone. From time to time, since the burgeoning of industry, people and their health community leaders have had mixed feelings about moving away from nature's remedies to those produced by industry. For example, a cultural shift to health and self-care in the 19th century embraced nature and the "natural" state. A contemporary of Holmes, physician Jacob Bigelow, read his essay before the Massachusetts Medical Society in 1835, "Discourse on self-limited disease." He suggested that physicians rethink their practice of prescribing medicines for all diseases because "some diseases are controlled by nature alone" and the role of the physician was but the "minister and servant of nature" who would remove obstacles from her path" (p. 34-35). This message is similar to what Florence Nightingale wrote in 1859 about putting a person "in the best condition for nature to work upon them." She also wrote "We must consult nature and experience as to how best we can animate and elevate the spirit in which we live" (Nightingale, Calabria, & Macrae, 1994, p. 96). There is a power, wisdom, and a presence in nature that philosophers and scientists alike have agreed is evidenced within all creation. Nurses – in their expertise in sickroom management and creating healing environments – have partnered with nature in care of others. Yet the lure of technology has posed challenges for those in nursing who would focus on caregiving that specializes in consultation with nature. This text seeks to support the nurse who would harmonize technology with the tradition of providing nature care.

It is the consultation with five elements of nature within each person and permeating the environment without that has been the foundation of the healing arts and nursing for centuries. The goal of precision integrative holistic nursing is providing care in consultation with nature that addresses the unique energetic needs for healing the whole person and the environment. This person-centered, relationship-centered approach is the ethical and clinical foundation for precision nursing science. The following chapters provide the structure for demonstrating precision nursing science. The nursing process, supported by nursing science and the *science of energetics as the application of the five elements* is first used in the assessment of the unique energetic health patterns and needs of a patient or client, (individual, family, or group). The nursing process is then used in designing and providing nursing care that applies modalities precisely matched to address those identified needs that consider energetic patterns first.

THE FIVE ELEMENTS IN COMFORT AND CARE

Nature care has often been relegated to the "nurturing" side of nursing practice as if there were opposition at stake. During the 1970s, Jerome Lysaught's report on nursing education in America stated that caregiving practices were "noninstrumental 'niceties' that somehow did not really count as knowledge and skill at all compared to medicine's therapeutic and curative enterprise" (Benner, Sutphen, Leonard, & Day, 2010, p. 23). But he had not done his homework. Those "niceties" had already stood the test of time. In 1840, for example, Sister Matilda Coskery, considered an "oracle" in the holistic care of the mentally ill by her physician colleagues, wrote in her advice book to nurses that the "curative point" in the care of the ill "mostly rests in the hands of the nurse" (as cited in Libster & McNeil, 2009, p. 187). A watchful eye, attendance upon the comfort needs of the ill, and judicious thinking about time and place of interventions are skills well documented as responsible for securing the lives of many. In his report, Lysaught offered "an oversimplified choice: nurses had to represent themselves either as highly effective interventionists who were knowledgeable and skillful in science and technology or as nonskilled nurturers ... two mutually exclusive options, neither of which accurately represents the complexity of nursing care" (Benner et al., 2010, p. 24). Current studies, such as the Carnegie Foundation Report by Benner et al., recognize the need for nurses to continue their healing tradition, as complex and challenging as it may be, to fully integrate all of the "niceties" and nurturing skill historically developed as the science, art, and skill of nature care with emerging science and technologies. Integrative holistic nursing seeks to *integrate* rather than dismiss the biomedical science and technologies. Integrative holistic nursing activates and, in some cases, reactivates, interest in nature care with all of its associated science, technologies, and art in which all elements are represented. The elements of integrative holistic nursing practice are the "agency that nurses have used historically, consciously or unconsciously, to create a healing environment. Partnership with 'environment' is fundamental to holistic nursing care; it is an essential component of nursing identity" (Libster, 2008). Integrative holistic care designs and practices include comfort measures that consider all five elements of creation.

The art and science of comfort and care are the heart of demonstrating holism in nursing practice. Caring is the affect or feeling of moral responsibility that motivates nursing actions (Morse, 1992, p. 92). It is the "essence of and unifying intellectual and practical dimension of professional nursing" (Leininger, 1984, p. 5). *Caring* science is informed by science and the humanities and "grounded on a set of universal values such as kindness, concern and the love of self and others" (Watson, 1985, p. 10). "Caritas" is identified in nursing as the spiritual motivation for nursing care and comfort (Levy-Malmberg, Eriksson, & Lindholm, 2008). Although agreement has been seen over the decades among nurse theorists about the definition of caring as an affect, there is less agreement that caring encompasses all nursing actions. Early on, scholars acknowledged that the "inadequacies of the caring paradigm as nursing theory" tend to "ignore the body and its associated physical care" (Morse, 1992, p. 92). One might argue that this is the case today. Some nurses do focus only on the bodily needs of patients; others are so spiritually focused that they may neglect the physical needs. Comfort, as the endeavor to create positive change that is person centered, requires a holistic approach in which the nurse employs the nursing process, from assessment to evaluation, in a manner that addresses physical, emotional, psychological, and spiritual needs: in other words, the whole needs of patients. Comfort is the "end state of therapeutic nursing actions" resulting in a "state of well-being that may occur during any stage of the illness-health continuum" (Morse, 1982, p. 93). Caring and comfort, together, address the what, why, and how nurses demonstrate care (Libster, 2001).

Change, Transition, and Transformation

Some people perceive caring actions from nurses differently than other people do. For example, they may feel a difference between touch that is procedural as opposed to comforting (Mulaik et al., 1991). Because nursing exists to care and comfort others, caring actions must be perceived by their recipients as positive change that moves them toward healing. All healing requires change. Care and comfort in integrative holistic nursing focuses on the person-centered (person meaning individual, family, or community) and relationship-centered needs for care and comfort related to life changes from birth to death. Herodotus, a Greek historian in the 5th century, is quoted as saying, "Diseases always attack men when they are exposed to change." People are often very fearful of change. But William Bridges, author of the bestselling book *Managing Transitions: Making the Most of Change*, says that it is transition rather than change that really causes people problems. "Change is situational, the move to the new site … Transition, on the other hand, is "psychological" (Bridges & Bridges, 2017, p. 3); that is, a process people go through as they internalize the change. People instigate change in their lives perhaps inviting an attack by disease. Integrative holistic nursing offers support for people as they adapt to change and move through the process of transition when they ultimately let go of the old way of being and doing. Transitions "start with an ending and finish with a beginning" (Bridges & Bridges, 2017, p. 5).

The focus of change is on an outcome, such as a life change (i.e., the birth of a child). Change is often viewed as a negative life event in which something must be relinquished, such as a personal habit, an object, or a belief. Stress mounts as people identify change with the responsibility of giving up something as a result of decisions made. However, change can also be a result of decisions made to add something or shift something in one's life, such as entering into a marriage. *Transition*, a central concept in nursing, is a process of adaptation to any change whether or not it is perceived as stressful or welcomed. "Clients' daily lives, environments, and interactions are shaped by the nature, conditions, meanings, and processes of transition experiences" (Meleis et al., 2000, p. 12).

During periods of change and transition, people and their caregivers often seek sources of comfort that seem to restore their sense of balance in body, mind, emotion, and spirit. People can experience change and transition and even the process of reestablishing balance as "stress." During periods of high stress, the fight-or-flight response may be triggered. How stressful a change is for a person is related to their perception of the change that they have experienced. People naturally seek stability when experiencing the discomforts of the stress associated with change. That process of achieving a new sense of stability, known as *allostasis*, occurs as a result of a dynamic shift in adjustment to environmental demands and management of individual tolerance of stress—termed *resilience* (Tonhajzerova & Mestanik, 2017, p. S174).

Nurses are often the most accessible professional supporters for many individuals' life transitions resulting from personal, family, and community changes. Nurses even have a history of leading large social change, such as healthcare reform movements in their communities (Libster, 2004). They are sought out to help people and communities during times of great personal transition. Integrative holistic nursing skills that nurses use in supporting people in transition include employing the structure of a nursing theory and following the nursing process informed by the five Elements of Care® so as to assist the patient in the re-creation of internal and external environments.

Nursing Theory and Process

All scientific theories in nursing address four major concepts: person, health, nursing, and environment (Fawcett, 1984). The environment is under-stood as that which is within and around the person and the relationship between the two. The external environment is the space where health and healing are promoted and varies greatly in nursing, from a more controlled hospital space to community centers and pharmacies to parish houses and beyond. Nurses adapt their caring work to the person's space, more so when they are actually in the person's living or community space. As the earliest of nursing textbooks stresses, the nurse's job is to create an environment that does not "tax the strength or vital power the patient needs for healing" (Libster, 2001). Familiarity decreases the stress response. Creating an external environment with the patient that is familiar to them decreases stress and increases the patient's ability to manage transitions. The internal environment – organ systems, neuropeptides, hormones – is also affected by lifestyle choices and change. Lifestyle includes sleep and rest, food choices, relationships, spiritual connections, activity, housing, and work, to name a few. Achieving the old adage of "everything in balance" is not always as easy as it may sound for people. Moving to the center from deficiency and excess is an ongoing process of adaptation.

According to Roy's Adaptation Model, a systems theory focused on adaptation response, the changing environment (within and without) "stimulates the person to make adaptive responses" (Andrews & Roy, 1986, p. 7). Theories, such as Roy's Model, provide structure for integrative holistic nursing care, particularly assessment. Adaptation theory focuses on four modes (physiological, self-concept, role function, and interdependence), which can be used by the nurse to guide his or her assessment and subsequent choices of support in patient care. The person and the environment are held to be "mutually enhancing instead of in opposition" so that the nurse can assist persons to interact positively with the world around them" (Andrews & Roy, 1986, p. 5). The theories of Eriksson and Morse cited previously provide a rich understanding of how nurses mobilize the four nursing concepts in care and comfort that are intrinsic to nursing practice. The unitary-transformative philosophies and theories of Watson, Newman, and Parse, who drew upon the scholarly works of Martha Rogers and her nursing interpretation of the principles of helicy, energy fields, pandimensionality, and patterns (Rogers, 1992), each address holism or wholism as "flowing motion" in which person and environment are unitary; that is, the "person transforms with the environment and the environment transforms with the person" (as cited in Newman, 1994, p. 83). Parse's theory of simultaneity suggests that change is a transforming process that involves the whole person, all at once, as they integrate the familiar and unfamiliar (Parse, 2012). Health is the evolving pattern of the whole (Newman, 1994, p. 82). One way to tell whether you are engaging a holistic paradigm is to ask the following questions (adapted from Newman, 1994):

1. Am I seeking to understand health patterns or trying to treat symptoms?
2. Are pain and disease informative to care, or are they viewed as something negative that should be removed?
3. Is the body an energy field within other fields or a machine in good or bad repair?
4. Is disease an evolutionary process or an entity?
5. Am I trying to relate to another person's pattern or fix something that I think is wrong?

Be sure to operationalize the nursing process within a holistic approach that uses the four major concepts, nursing theory, and nursing process that starts with assessment, then health pattern diagnosis (discussed further in Chapter 4), plan, intervention, and evaluation. The focus on integration and holism in nursing does not require deviation from conventional nursing standards, such as the nursing process. If anything, applying an integrative holistic approach to the nursing process strengthens the associated skills.

The link between the five elements and integrative holistic nursing is the art and science of comfort that is the center of nursing care wherever and whenever it is practiced. An oral history study of how skilled nurses care and comfort others discovered that the modalities used by the nurses were very similar. Caring modalities are the "instruments" nurses use in demonstrating comfort and care. The modalities mentioned by the skilled nurses were also similar to those mentioned in historical nursing texts (Libster, 2001). However, the stories of how the skilled, older nurses demonstrated care and comfort with those modalities were very unique. *How* nurses demonstrate care and comfort with a person depends on the following:

- The person's cultural beliefs, rituals, learned health practices, experience
- The perception of change and stress response as it is related to illness, birth, death, etc.
- Familiarity with what the nurse offers in terms of modalities and the nurse's familiarity with the patient's self-care modalities

People's cultural beliefs will be addressed further in Chapter 3. For a person to be able to perceive nurses' acts of comfort and care as helpful, such acts must connect in some way to the patient's own healing beliefs, memories, and experiences. When a modality or approach to care and comfort is perceived as "new" or a change from someone's sense of what is normal, it can create a stress response. Therefore, choosing a modality with a patient that is familiar can be a very helpful person-centered action that reduces a negative stress response and promotes healing. An example is providing a food that a patient perceives to be a comfort food and is helpful when a person is sick with the common cold.

In preparation for reviewing modalities in Part II, the next section on the Elements of Care® provides examples and brief explanations of the unique qualities of the five elements. The five elements are "archetypes of first matter according to the Greeks" (Hauck, 1999, p. 71) used in the design and practice of integrative holistic care as the nurse partners with patients to create a healing environment within and without. The five elements – fire, air, water, earth, and ether – are discussed in the ancient philosophy, *The Emerald Tablet*. The text of *The Emerald Tablet* was translated by Hermes Trismegistus, whom the Greeks considered a "messenger of the Gods." These Hermetic texts have been read by scientists, philosophers, and healers from Socrates to Paracelsus to Nightingale (Calabria, 1997). Hermetic texts, the oldest spiritual tradition in the West, have inspired Judaism, Christianity, Islam, Gnosticism, and Eastern religions such as Buddhism, Taoism, and Hinduism. Foundational to hermeticism is the emphasis on the understanding of self and all matter as a manifestation of the elements of creation: ether, fire, air, water, and earth. Ancient systems of medicine from the East and the West, such as traditional Chinese medicine and Alaska Native American Indian healing, continue to utilize knowledge of the five elements as a foundational understanding of how to affect health, disease, and long life. (See Chapter 3.) The foundation of conventional biomedicine is also rooted in the five elements in the Greek philosophy of medicine known as humoral medicine. Employing knowledge of the five elements is foundational to care and cure throughout the world. Nursing theory and knowledge of the five elements can be used in integrative holistic nursing practice as a framework to guide the nurse following each step of the nursing process toward the purposes of stress reduction, care, and comfort.

FOCUS ON THE FIVE ELEMENTS

Being the assistant of nature and placing patients in the best condition for nature to work upon them begins with focus on the five elements: fire, air, water, earth, and ether. Ether is the essence of all matter, and the other four elements, according to ancient Greeks such as Aristotle, are archetypal or foundational. The descriptions provided here are simple examples used historically, scientifically, and aesthetically to describe the different energetic qualities of the five elements. Nurses employ these five elements found in all matter in the universe and within themselves so as to foster balance and allostasis. Integrative holistic nursing care and comfort includes the actual presence or representation of all five elements during the nursing process. Examples will be given throughout the chapters in Part II of how this can be accomplished. As you read through this description of the elements, consider the possibility that some of the care plans you are already implementing in your practice may instinctively include an energetic balance of all five elements.

Fire (Hot, Dry)

The fire element is related to the spiritual domain of being as inspiration, ideas, and creation. The fire element is associated with beliefs and the spiritual and religious practices that demonstrate those beliefs. As Roerich (1933) stated:

> One cannot define Fire by any other term than splendor ... The inexhaustibility of giving is found in varying degrees in all of nature. But Fire is the element in which giving is most apparent. The very principle of Fire is transmutation and constant giving. (p. 299)

The fire element manifests energetically as giving of self in service to humanity, as warmth, light and power, and as matters of the heart and of consciousness. Caring from the heart without judgment is expression of the fire element. Some other examples of engaging the fire element in integrative holistic care are:

- Offering warm blankets to a postoperative patient
- Suggesting steamed vegetables versus salads for older adults
- Adding Epsom salt to a bath
- Praying with a patient

Air (Hot, Moist)

The air element is related to the mental domain of the mind, thoughts, ideas, images, memory, reflection, perception, and intuition. "The mind is a trickster, often casting illusion into the field of human perception. Ideas and mental impressions come and go like the wind" (Libster, 2012, p. 161). Just relying on knowledge and what one holds in one's mind is insufficient to support and manifest precision integrative holistic nursing practice. Bohm wrote that thought as a system not only includes thoughts, "felts and feelings, but it includes the state of the body; it includes the whole of society – as thought is passing back and forth between people in a process by which thought evolved from ancient times" (1994, p. 19). Thus, we are reminded that air and all of the five elements do not exist in a vacuum but are energetically interrelated and inseparable, as are body-mind-emotion-and-spirit. Air element is breath and movement of air in ventilation. Air is thought that is embodied and demonstrated through communication, teaching, listening, study, and touch. In cultivating the science mind, "We will be compelled to distinguish, differentiate, and resynthesize, a process which finally leads to an order we can survey with some degree of satisfaction" (Goethe, 1996, p. 32). There is beauty in that order and even in the chaos that is perceived when one does not yet have order and understanding. Examples of engaging the air element in integrative holistic care are:

- Rubbing the back of a newborn baby as he or she is taking the first breaths
- Showing pictures of the anatomy of the leg to a child with a femur fracture
- Dancing to the favorite piece of music of an older adult patient with dementia
- Closing the windows in the home of a family living near a forest fire

Water (Cold, Moist)

The water element is related to the domain of emotion as energy-in-motion. Without the *flow* of pure, clean water, there is no life. The water element includes feelings, flow, and beauty. The definition of beauty for the Greeks was *symmetria*, the harmonious flowing relationship of one part of the body to another. There is no expenditure of vital energy when the emotions flow smoothly. A bath, according to Bertha Harmer and Virginia Henderson's *Principles and Practice of Nursing* (1939), is "soothing and quieting in its effects and gives a chance for repair and the storage of vital energy" (p. 475). The flow of vital energy is the definition of health in ancient systems of healing such as classic traditional Chinese medicine. Emotions must also flow. Blockages in the domain of the emotions can lead to illness. To understand the emotional patterns of each unique patient and prevent disease by assisting nature to move emotions, remove blocks to flow, and preserve vital energy, the holistic nurse begins by "modeling" or entering the environment of the patient to understand their world. The world of the patient includes feelings, perspectives, thoughts, and desires. This step is followed by "role-modeling" or purposeful interventions. The *Modeling and Role-Modeling* theory (Erickson, Tomlin, & Swain, 1983) provides a structure for implementing integrative holistic nursing practice utilizing the Elements of Care®. Examples of engaging the water element in integrative holistic care are:
- Providing a hot-water bottle or foot bath for the cold feet of an older adult

- Starting intravenous fluids in a patient who is dehydrated
- Preparing broth for a patient receiving home care
- Applying a ginger decoction compress to the kidneys of a patient with chronic joint pain

Earth (Cold, Dry)

The earth element is related to the physical domain and the intrinsic connection between persons and the environment. The physical domain includes space and the substance of which all things are made: animal, vegetable, and mineral. The nurses who work in the Anthroposophical hospitals in Switzerland and Germany that provide care according to the holistic philosophy of Rudolf Steiner incorporate all aspects of nature in the creation of their nursing units. For example, there may be large amethyst geodes in the front hallway to the hospital and a rose at every nurse's station. The hospitals are designed to harmonize with the energetic patterns and rhythms that occur in the natural environment. For example, the walls are painted certain muted colors found in nature. The nurse, the patient, and nature are the healing environment within and without. Designing physical spaces as well as creating interventions that actively engage the physical senses and body in healing and promoting health is the object of the earth element. Examples of engaging the earth element in integrative holistic care are:

- Changing the linens on a sick bed
- Making and applying an herbal oil
- Emptying a bed pan
- Taking a walk in the woods with a patient

Ether (Pneuma)

The ether element integrates all four elements and domains. Paracelsus and the alchemists of old knew of this element as being the "One Thing" or "pneuma" that is the source of all life. Ether as essence or life force is associated with consciousness and the transformation of Self with a capital S, referring to one's true nature. Nursing is a "spiritual path of Self-discovery" (Libster, 2012, p. 321). That Self is the five elements of the person. Hildegarde von Bingen, one of the earliest of holistic healers, described the task of personhood as "building of the house of wisdom in ourselves as individuals and community with other humans and all other creatures of our earth" (von Bingen, 1986, p. xxi). All elements engaged in holistic care hold the potential to *create or catalyze* change in addition to supporting adaptation responses and transition related to changes, which have already occurred. That change begins with a shift in awareness or consciousness. Families, friends, and teachers can instigate such shifts. Healing crises often compel such shifts. Demonstrating care that is mindful of the five elements is kind and compassionate, two essential qualities of being human and humane. The formulation for precision integrative holistic design of care begins with modeling the patient's world. This then is followed with caring interventions that incorporate the five elements in a way that is meaningful for the patient. Examples of engaging the ether element in integrative holistic care are:

- Timing interventions to match the timing and pace of the patient
- Describing the patient's behaviors instead of drawing conclusions and passing judgment
- Picking up litter
- Helping a hospitalized patient connect with his or her family and favorite plants and pets

CASE STUDY: ELEMENTS OF CARE®

Nurse Johns is assigned to insert a new nasogastric tube for Mrs. Smith, who lives alone with her paid caregivers in a large home overlooking a lake. When you arrive, you notice that Mrs. Smith is comatose and quietly lying in her bed, which has an ornate headboard facing a large picture window with a view of the lake. There is nothing in the room or on the headboard except a small statue of Quan Yin, Bodhisattva of compassion. Quan Yin's hand, symbolizing the hand of mercy and compassion, is lightly attached, as is customary, because it can be removed. Answer the following questions about integrative holistic nursing and then compare your responses to the "nurse's answers" that follow.

Questions

1. What approach to the care of Mrs. Smith would differentiate that nursing care as "integrative and holistic"?
2. Give examples for employing each of the five Elements of Care® that complement the assigned task of nasogastric tube insertion.
3. Using an integrative holistic approach to assessment and diagnosis of Mrs. Smith's environment and your knowledge of nursing theories mentioned here, would you consider any interventions related to that assessment?

Nurse's Answers

1. Entering a person's home compels a nurse to begin to model the world of the patient. Integrative holistic nursing suggests conducting an assessment of the person, which in this case requires observation of the environment and Mrs. Smith's staff's stories about their patient (emotional). Before inserting the nasogastric tube, the nurse assesses Mrs. Smith for any requirements for comfort, using the five elements as a guide. Mrs. Smith is unconscious, and therefore the nurse will use her knowledge of health care (mental / physical), combined with observation skills, to perceive any needs beyond the task of placing a new tube. The nurse also seeks to make the task as comfortable as

possible for the patient and is respectful of her body and person as though she were conscious (spiritual).

2. Nurses understand that the boundaries between elements are blurred. The five elements are related, and some interventions could be associated with more than one element. Fire element: The nurse washes her hands with warm water and examines the thermal nature of Mrs. Smith's extremities (fire). Upon finding Mrs. Smith's feet and hands to be very cold to the touch, the nurse places socks on the patient's feet (earth) and applies a hot-water bottle (water) while she does a gentle hand massage (air). The nurse talks with Mrs. Smith about the comfort measures and the nasogastric tube (ether).

3. Applying modeling and role-modeling theory by Erickson et al., the nurse notices that there is only one object other than the bed and medical equipment in the patient's bedroom. She infers that the object must have some meaning for the patient. Using health as expanding consciousness theory by Newman, the nurse asks the staff about the meaning of the Quan Yin statue for Mrs. Smith. The nurse waits for an answer and then seeks further information about Quan Yin on the Internet so that she can talk with Mrs. Smith about the statue at the next visit. In this way, the nurse can provide Mrs. Smith with an association that is familiar, thus incorporating it into her nursing care.

HOLISTIC TRANSFORMATION

Each chapter's holistic transformation section prompts reflection upon the application of content discussed in the chapter to personal and professional situations. Consider these questions:

- *What is the first step for incorporating what I have learned about integrative holistic nursing practice in my work with patients?*

- *Using the five Elements of Care® as a reference point, what have I learned about care and comfort from this chapter's content? What elements do I favor? What elements do I want to work on?*

SUMMARY

Integrative holistic nurses are mindful that healing crises and illnesses are evolutionary in that they are a period of change, transition, and transformation for the patient. Numerous nurse scholars have explained the concept of holism and its application in caring and comfort. Design of person-centered, relationship-centered care begins with modeling the patient's world and then is followed with caring interventions that incorporate the five elements in a way that is familiar and meaningful for the patient. The five elements that historically are found in religious, cultural, and scientific records across cultures are ether, fire, air, water, and earth. Because they are in so many healing traditions from the East and West, these Five Elements of Care® can be applied as an easily accessible and familiar guide to the practice of precision integrative holistic nursing science.

REFERENCES

Andrews, H. A., & Roy, C. (1986). Essentials of the *Roy Adaptation Model*. Norwalk, CT: Appleton-Century-Crofts.

Benner, P., Sutphen, M., Leonard, V., & Day, L. (2010). *Educating nurses: A call for radical transformation. In The Carnegie Foundation for the Advancement of Teaching: Preparation for the Professions Series*. San Francisco, CA: Jossey-Bass.

Bigelow J. (1835). Discourse on self-limited diseases. Delivered before the Massachusetts

Medical Society. Boston, MA: Nathan Hale Water Street.

Bohm, D. (1994). *Thought as a system*. London, England: Routledge.

Bridges, W., & Bridges, S. (2017). *Managing transitions: Making the most of change*. Philadelphia, PA: Perseus Books.

Calabria, M. D. (1997). *Florence Nightingale in Egypt and Greece: Her diary and "visions."* Albany, NY: State University of New York Press.

Erickson, H. C., Tomlin, E. M., & Swain, M. A. P. (1983). *Modeling and role-modeling*. Englewood Cliffs, NJ: Prentice-Hall.

Fawcett, J. (1984). The metaparadigm of nursing: Present status and future refinements. *Image: The Journal of Nursing Scholarship, 16*(3), 84-87.

Goethe, J. (1996). *Goethe on science: An anthology of Goethe's scientific writings* (J. Naydler, compiler). Edinburgh, Scotland: Floris Books.

Harmer, B., & Henderson, V. (1939). *Textbook of the principles and practice of nursing* (4th ed.). New York, NY: Macmillan.

Hauck, D. W. (1999). *The Emerald Tablet: Alchemy for personal transformation*. New York, NY: Penguin Putnam.

Leininger, M. M. (Ed.) (1984). *Care: The essence of nursing and health*. Detroit, MI: Wayne State University Press.

Levy-Malmberg, R., Eriksson, K., & Lindholm, L. (2008). Caritas – Caring as an ethical conduct. *Scandinavian Journal of Caring Sciences, 22*(4), 662-667.

Libster, M. (2001). *Demonstrating care: The art of integrative nursing*. Albany, NY: Delmar Cengage Learning.

Libster, M. M. (2004). *Herbal diplomats: The contribution of early American nurses (1830-1860) to 19th century health care reform and the Botanical Medical Movement*. Wauwatosa, WI: Golden Apple Publications.

Libster, M. M. (2008). Elements of Care: Nursing environmental theory in historical context. *Holistic Nursing Practice, 22*(3), 160-170.

Libster, M. M., & McNeil, B. A. (2009). *Enlightened charity: The holistic nursing care, education, and "Advices Concerning the Sick" of Sister Matilda Coskery (1799-1870)*. Wauwatosa, WI: Golden Apple Publications.

Libster, M. (2012). *The nurse-herbalist: Integrative insights for holistic practice*. Wauwatosa, WI: Golden Apple Publications.

Meleis, A. I., Sawyer, L. M., Im, E.-O., Hilfinger Messias, D. K., & Schumacher, K. (2000). Experiencing transitions: An emerging middle-range theory. *Advances in Nursing Science*, 23(1), 12-28.

Morse, J. M. (1992). Comfort: The refocusing of nursing care. *Clinical Nursing Research*, 1(1), 91-106.

Mulaik, J. S., Megenity, J. S., Cannon, R. B., Chance, K. S., Cannella, K. S., Garland, L. M., ... Massey, J. A. (1991). Patients' perceptions of nurses' use of touch. *Western Journal of Nursing Research*, 13(3), 306-323.

Newman, M. (1994). *Health as expanding consciousness*. New York, NY: National League for Nursing Press.

Nightingale, F. (1994). In Calabria, M. D., & Macrae, J. A. (Eds.) *Suggestions for thought by Florence Nightingale*. Philadelphia, PA: University of Pennsylvania Press.

Parse, R. R. (2012). New human becoming conceptualizations and the human becoming community model: Expansions with science and living the art. *Nursing Science Quarterly*, 25(1), 44-52.

Porter, R. (1997). *The greatest benefit to mankind: A medical history of humanity*. New York, NY: W. W. Norton.

Roerich, H. (1933). *Fiery world Part I*, 1933. New York, NY: Agni Yoga Society. Retrieved from http://agniyoga.oray_en/Fiery-World-I.php

Rogers, M. E. (1992). Nursing science and the space age. *Nursing Science Quarterly*, 5(1), 27-34.

Tonhajzerova, I., & Mestanik, M. (2017). New perspectives in the model of stress response. *Physiological Research*, 66(Suppl. 2), S173-S185.

von Bingen, H. (1986). *Hildegarde von Bingen's mystical visions*. (B. Hozeski, Trans.). Santa Fe, NM: Bear & Co.

Watson, J. (1985). *Nursing: The philosophy and science of caring*. Niwot, CO: University Press of Colorado.

CHAPTER 3

HEALTH CULTURES AND HEALING SYSTEMS

LEARNING OUTCOME

After completing this chapter, the learner will be able to discuss the difference between complementary therapies and traditional/indigenous healing.

CHAPTER OBJECTIVES

After completing this chapter, the learner will be able to:
1. Discuss formation in nursing and health culture diplomacy.
2. Describe the health beliefs of at least one traditional/indigenous healing system.
3. List some of the professional considerations related to traditional/indigenous healing systems.

INTRODUCTION

As is the case with all disciplines in the healing arts and sciences, nursing is a cultural construction. Every country, every nursing school, and every nurse interprets the practice of nursing within the circle of their own culture. Although a consensus definition from the International Council of Nurses and the American Nurses Association had been reached many years ago, nursing practice is still permeated with beliefs about health, illness, birth, dying, medicine, and life. Some of those beliefs and associated cultural values and customs are taught to nurses in their educational programs.

PROFESSIONAL FORMATION

The process that complements the learning process, which occurs as a result of a person or a group of persons preparing another to be a nurse, is referred to historically as "formation" (Libster, 2017). Benner, Sutphen, Leonard, & Day (2010) expanded on this concept:

Formation occurs over time with the transformation from the well-meaning layperson to the nurse who is prepared to respond with respect and skill to people that are vulnerable and suffering ... students develop notions of good from their practice that transform their understanding of nursing's social contract to care for vulnerable patients (p. 166).

Nurse educators often use dance as a metaphor for the formation process. Dance is "relational and changes appropriately and knowingly according to the context, partner, and music" (Benner et al., 2010, p. 167). In nursing, the context, partner, and "music" are the cultural construction of space, time, and effort that holds the idea of "nursing." In other words, a nurse appropriately considers the sociocultural context for care. There is a general global definition of nursing, but each nurse individually and collectively – when working in teams or in an institution such as a hospital – forms his or her own expression of demonstrating nursing care that is nuanced with culture.

To return to the dance metaphor, Kabuki-style Japanese dance has its own flavor, as do bharata natyam dance of India and flamenco dance in Spain. They are all dance forms that express the five elements (described in this chapter under classical Traditional Chinese Medicine) in different ways. The essence, spirit, thought processes, and emotional, physical, and energetic expression of the dance from Japan to India to Spain is completely different, and yet each dance is beautiful in its own way and communicates a partnership. The science as well as the art and spirit of the dance is a cultural construction. So, too, is the science, art, and spirit of nursing and the healing arts in general. Dr. Madeleine Leininger (1925-2012), a nurse theorist and anthropologist, conducted studies of 30 cultures, "clearly indicating that differences are more prevalent than universals" in terms of how people demonstrate caring (1984, p. 9). Cultural diplomacy and other transcultural nursing skills, such as being able to communicate with and adapt to others' beliefs and practices, are central to formation of holistic nurses.

HEALTH CULTURE DIPLOMACY
AND INTEGRATIVE HOLISTIC NURSING

Health culture diplomacy and transcultural nursing are highly inclusive skills that include keen observation, communication, negotiation, mindfulness, and transcultural person-centered, relationship-centered care (Libster, 2015). Health culture diplomacy differs from global health diplomacy, advocacy, culture brokering, and mediation. According to Libster (2015), the following defines cultural diplomacy in health care and nursing:

> ... activation of the internalized qualities and motivations identified in cultural awareness, sensitivity, and competence work ... comprises acts that demonstrate the knowledge and insight gained as a result of nurses' internal exercises that seek to address a unique patient or client's cultural care needs. Cultural diplomacy is foundational to the cultivation of person-centered care and coaching. (p. 3)

Nurses routinely encounter opportunities to adapt to and respond diplomatically to different patients' and communities' cultural constructions and paradigms related to health care and nursing. As is shown in Figure 3-1, the Cultural Diplomacy Model© (Libster, 2015) references four cultural paradigms in health care: biomedical, traditional, and complementary therapies, and self-care.

FIGURE 3-1: CULTURAL DIPLOMACY MODEL©

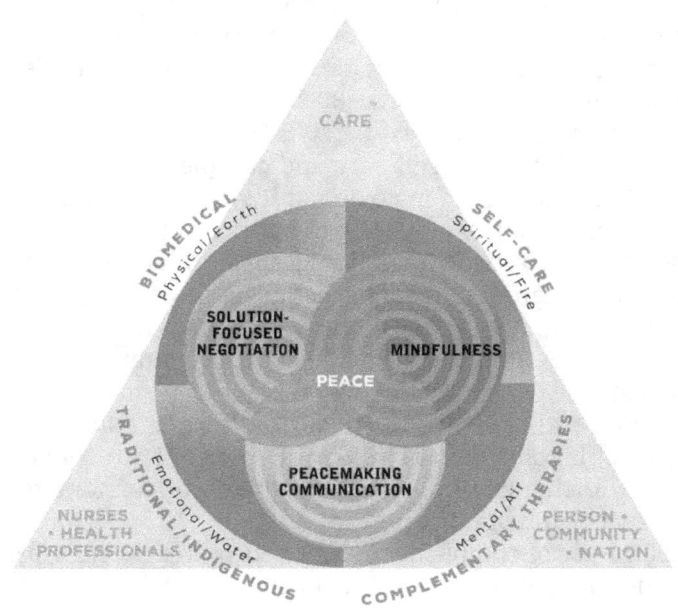

Those who specialize in integrative holistic nursing, like the transcultural nurse, often move beyond the beliefs and nursing care expressions that are taught as part of conventional contemporary formation in nursing programs focused on biomedical values. A diplomatic person-centered, relationship-centered approach coupled with a desire to incorporate what they learn from patients and communities often leads nurses into new dimensions of caring and healing modalities that "work" for others. For example, nurses practice self-care and also learn new self-care remedies from their patients. This practice is common in nursing culture.

Research demonstrates that self-care, also known as home remedies or domestic medicine, is an American tradition (Libster, 2004). Over the centuries, the relationship between people's self-care and the emergence of nursing as a discipline was so refined that nursing science identifies knowledge of self-care and the differentiation from dependent care as an expertise in nursing (Orem, 2001).

The culturally constructed term *complementary therapies* references healing modalities that are outside the biomedical mainstream. These modalities are termed "alternative" by those of the biomedical culture when a patient chooses a path of care that is not within the biomedical culture. Complementary therapies can be the same modalities as alternative therapies, but with different names. The difference is in the cultural expression. The patient, family, or community typically chooses biomedical care, cure, and therapies not offered in the mainstream. The boundaries between the practices can actually be quite blurred. Some sociological research suggests that this inclusive practice has functioned very well for decades within a "hidden health care system" of American culture (Levin & Idler, 2010). It provides the public ready access to care for self-care support, complementary therapies practitioners, and traditional and indigenous healing systems. There is a very high prevalence of complementary therapies use, particularly herbal remedies, among Hispanic (88.8%) and non-Hispanic (81.3%) white women (Green, Santoro, Allhouse, Neal-Perry, & Derby, 2017).

Studies also have found that self-care and complementary therapies use is prevalent in the United States among older adults, and these therapies are more heavily used by ethnic minority groups than by those who are white (Grzywacz et al., 2006, p. 40). Although the 2002 National Health Interview Survey indicated that individuals with greater financial hardship are more likely to seek self-care and complementary therapies, the Grzywacz research team results concluded that the reason elders used self-care and complementary therapies was not because biomedical care was unaffordable or they had no access to it, which is a common assumption of those in the biomedical culture. The study suggested that ethnic elders use home remedies to *stretch* the money that they do have (2006). The team called for further cultural research to better understand these nuances of elders' health beliefs and practices.

Disclosure of the use of complementary health approaches (CHA) is an important yet understudied health behavior with important implications for patient care. Yet research into disclosure of CHA has been atheoretical and has neglected the role of health beliefs (Sirois, Riess, & Upchurch, 2017). A seminal study before the 2002 study also had found that nonorthodox medicine practices are not used by people who are "poor, uneducated, or socially isolated, and perpetrated by practitioners who are either fraudulent or simply ignorant of the great, though relatively recent, accomplishments of 'scientific medicine" (Clouser & Hufford, 1993, p. 101). These views are simply unsubstantiated beliefs within the biomedical culture, which in the United States is the politically and legally dominant culture (Thorne, 1993).

The most common challenge nurses encounter when they transition to a specialized focus in integrative holistic nursing from conventional nursing is this very issue of biomedical cultural dominance. This challenge occurs even though integrative holistic nursing includes a holistic framework for the nursing process within the biomedical culture. Until they work closely with people such as traditional and indigenous healers and people who are helped by them, nurses may not realize just how much biomedical cultural values and beliefs have been part of the formation of their automatic responses to care. In a crisis or emergency situation, there is no doubt that people want and expect immediate biomedical intervention, which typically involves the suppression of symptoms that are life threatening. The biomedical culture may not be the first choice of peoples in any other health scenario. They may rely on their family self-care recipes or their traditional remedies, or they may seek help from the traditional healers within their culture or the help of therapies that complement their biomedical treatments. Some nurses may not realize that there is a vast cultural difference between traditional healing and complementary therapies paradigms.

The World Health Organization (WHO) Traditional Medicine Program states that "Traditional and complementary medicine (T&CM) is an important and often underestimated part of health care. T&CM is found in almost every country in the world and the demand for its services is increasing" (WHO, 2014). Traditional medicine is defined as the

> ... sum total of the knowledge, skill, and practices based on the theories, beliefs, and experiences indigenous to different cultures, whether explicable or not, used in the maintenance of health as well as in the prevention, diagnosis, improvement or treatment of physical and mental illness. (WHO, 2014)

The terms "complementary medicine" or "alternative medicine" are medical terms for what is referred to in this text as "complementary therapies." They are a "broad set of health care practices that are not part of that country's own tradition or conventional medicine and are not fully integrated into the dominant healthcare system" (WHO, 2014). Self-care practices often cross over into the complementary therapies and traditional medicine (called healing here) paradigms. For example, a person may visit a massage therapist who teaches how to massage an injured knee. The person might see the massage therapist for a full-body massage (which will affect posture and therefore stress on the knees) and leave with some knowledge of the self-care practice that can be used to care for the person's knees when knee pain is experienced.

Traditional healers are recognized by their communities as holding special healing knowledge, wisdom, and spiritual gifts that may be taught only to those chosen to succeed them in the community. Traditional healers, like complementary therapists, may also teach self-care to individuals and families. Therefore, a cultural diplomacy approach suggests that the best cultural practice and education in person-centered, relationship-centered care and coaching in formation of integrative holistic nursing focuses on the balance of the five elements of creation and the complementarity of all four paradigms: biomedicine, self-care, complementary therapies, and traditional healing (Libster, Phillips, Smith-Taylor, Southard, & Bryant, 2015).

TRADITIONAL/INDIGENOUS HEALING SYSTEMS

The remainder of this chapter highlights some prominent enduring traditional healing systems from around the world. It is beyond the scope of this text to provide a complete overview of each and every system. Although we wish that every culture could be represented, the intention is to provide a few examples that may spark interest in further cultural education that cultivates more understanding and appreciation for integrative holistic nursing within a society with deep richness in terms of cultural health beliefs and practices. It is also not possible to provide a sense of all of the subcultures or tribes within the traditions discussed here. Writing about people as a cultural group and seeking to define their ways of healing quickly becomes stereotypical. In the spirit of cultural diplomacy, we ask forgiveness. Our intention for these highlights is to light a fire of interest about the diversity of healing traditions. However, one theme unifies all of the traditions: At their center, they have actual or symbolic representation of all five elements of creation.

Alaska Native American Indian Healing

Alaska Native American Indian (AI), or First Nation, refers to the indigenous peoples of Turtle Island (North America):

> Although the impact of European expansion and colonization has changed the world and lifestyles of Indigenous North Americans, Indigenous peoples' cultural knowledge and practices, though endangered by historical efforts to eradicate Native cultures and traditions, have persisted into the 21st century. (Greymorning, 2016)

This text, as stated earlier, provides only a sampling of the diverse health beliefs and traditional practices of the hundreds of recognized and unrecognized tribes in America. The five nations of the Iroquois Confederacy – Mohawks, Onondagas, Oneidas, Cayugas, and Senecas – were united in peace by the Peacemaker in about 1710 (Wallace, 1946). The Peacemaker said:

> The word that I bring is that all peoples shall love one another and live together in peace. This message has three parts: Righteousness and Health and Power – Gaiwoh, Skenon, and Gashasden-shaa. Righteousness means justice practiced between men and between nations; it means also a desire to see justice prevail. Health means soundness of mind and body; it also means peace, for that is what comes when minds are sane and bodies cared for. Power means authority, the authority of law and custom, backed by such force as is necessary to make justice prevail; it means also religion, for justice enforced is the will of the Holder of the Heavens and has his sanction. (Wallace, 1946, p. 13)

The Peacemaker gave specific teachings that are followed to this day. For example, when fetching water, one was to dip with the current. The Peacemaker said, "One must never go against the forces of nature" (Wallace, 1946, p. 16). The Great Creator is the source of health and life – water, foods and herbal medicines from the earth, the winds and sun, and the "messengers of the Creator who reveal his wishes" (Wallace, 1946, p. 36).

The Iroquois peoples believe the "three sisters" – corn, beans, and squash – to be their "life." It is believed that corn "sprouted from the breast of the mother of the Great Spirit when she died" (Bunson, 1992, p. 38). Sacred dances, such as the Feather Dance, are part of the celebrations to boost morale and "join people to the earth" (Bunson, 1992) so as to promote peace and balance. Healing philosophy is articulated by Navajo physician Lori Alvord: "Navajos make every effort to live in harmony and balance with everyone. Sickness is a "result of things falling out of balance, of losing one's way on the path of beauty ... religion and medicine are one and the same" (Alvord & Van Pelt, 1999, p. 14). Navajos believe in *hózho or hózhoni*, "Walking in Beauty," a belief that everything in life is connected and influences everything else.

For AI peoples, medicine is who a person is, what they carry in their spirit. Peace and balance are symbolized in the medicine wheel (Sun Bear & Wabun, 1980). The medicine wheel offers a path for restoring connection with nature, where all beings are connected: minerals, plants, animals, birds, and human beings. The human body is a transmitter between sky and earth. As people dance in a circle and make music on round drums, they celebrate life as a circle representing movement and change. As people travel the circle of life and live in a way that is open to the Creator's lessons, "the proper lesson will always come at the right time, no matter who the necessary teacher is (Sun Bear & Wabun, 1980). According to tradition, a person's birth moon or month indicates their starting place on the medicine wheel. According to Sun Bear & Wabun (1980):

> The only way you can stop your own growth is to cling to the strengths of one position and refuse to let go of them. When you do this, you block your own energies, 194)

We all travel the medicine wheel, learning its lessons at our own speed and in our own way.

People find the path of healing when they connect with nature rather than seek to conquer her. Chief Leon Shenandoah says that people who are "running in the woods" are those who have forgotten the Creator. As cited in Wall (2001), here is what happens when people are running in the woods:

> [They] personally suffer and even turn on each other ... I never call on the Creator for anything. I don't have to. Nobody does either. The Creator gives us all we need in this life ... He instructed Mother Earth to provide all the necessities to sustain our lives ... She gives us food and she replenishes the waters. She causes the plants to grow for our medicines. So our lives are taken care of (p. 16).

When people begin the journey of the medicine wheel and "take their place in a good manner, all things come to you" (Sun Bear & Wabun, 1980, p. 195). See the Resources for a link to the website for the National Alaska Native American Indian Nurses Association.

European American "Old Way"

European American (EA) healing tradition, or the "old way" of believing about God and healing that predates Christianity, is founded on humanity's relationship to nature. It is perhaps best expressed in the term *viriditas*, or *greenness*, described in the mystical visions of Hildegarde of Bingen, a 12th-century German theologian and healer who wrote of Jesus the Christ as "Greenness Incarnate" and Mary, the Mother of Jesus, as the Viridissima Virga, "the greenest of all branches in God's orchard" (as cited in Metzner, 1999, p. 140). Greenness is associated with life and God's creative power manifest in the natural world. Hildegarde wrote that the elements of the green world made by God (fire, air, water, and earth) are also in man. Man works with the elements that "maintain themselves so tightly together that man calls them the firmament" (Hildegard of Bingen, 1994, p. 2). The image of the green man is carved into the architecture of churches throughout

Europe (Anderson, 1998). The green man, a composite of a man's face emerging from leaves, symbolizes this belief in the connection between humanity and the natural world and the spiritual power of nature in all things, including healing (Metzner, 1999).

Many of those who migrated from Europe to the North American continent sought religious freedom. However, the EA settlements during the colonial period, with its extensive congregation building, were fraught with religious rivalry (Bonomi, 2003). During the latter part of the colonial period and into the 1800s, there were major sociocultural changes and shifts from agrarian to industrial work. With rapid industrialization came a period of great stress because of the rapid growth of science and technology. The early boon of the pharmaceutical industry, credited to the Shaker community's herbal medicine business (Libster, 2004), ultimately morphed into a synthetic drug empire. Families and communities of EA were not making their own medicines and being their own doctors, as they had been during their immigration to America.

Populism in the 19th century, however, included a resurgence in the belief in common sense and resisting the claims of professionals and progressives who believed that "science provided the means of moral as well as political reform" (Starr, 1982, p. 19). As discussed in Chapter 1, the 19th century was a period in which EA physicians, nurses, community healers, and the public valued nature cure. Popular traditional healing of the period once again included domestic remedies with herbs and water cure and being one's own doctor (Beecher & Stowe, 2002). Religious groups, such as the Shakers, Quakers, and Mormons (now Church of Jesus Christ of Latter-day Saints), often interacted with AI peoples and shared knowledge of botanical remedies and other cures (Libster, 2004).

In the 19th century, the rise of American sectarianism prevailed in the emergence of nature once again in the experimental communities, such as Fruitlands in Massachusetts, and in new healing systems such as Thomsonianism that focused on the use of plant medicines (Libster, 2004). However, "progress" in the public sector of the practice of medicine and nursing care over the centuries has become inextricably bound to technology (Sandelowski, 2000, p. 2). The objectification and then subsequent "death" of nature in human endeavors, such as in the healing arts, is correlated with the birth of science (Merchant, 1980).

The remnants of the "old way" and deep connection with nature and a belief in balance and harmony as the foundation for health is still prevalent in the self-care culture of EA people. The desire to be or "go green" reawakens the archetype of the green man and green woman. This desire challenges the underlying beliefs that technology is the healer and that the healing arts require its scientific culture to be separated from nature and God/Creator.

Advice books on home remedies continue to exist, although they are now joined on the Internet with numerous blogs and videos for recipe and remedy exchange. Domesticity and self-help gurus, such as Polish American Martha Stewart and Lithuanian American Dr. Ann Wigmore (1909-1993), have been remarkably successful in sustaining the belief that Americans can and should take care of themselves and partner with the green world. One example of this partnering is taking part in simple healing activities, such as growing sprouts in a jar on the kitchen counter (Wigmore, 1982; see Figure 3-2). Diversity of health beliefs and practices among EA subcultures is easily observed in food choices deemed healthy and in the variety of herbal applications.

FIGURE 3-2: GOING GREEN: SPROUTING

"When you eat a sprout you are eating a tiny, easy-to-digest plant that is at its peak of nutritional value." – Dr. Ann Wigmore

Equipment:
Quart-sized Mason jar with sprouting lids
Sprouting seeds
The amount of seeds used will expand 8x their present state.
Ex.: 3 tablespoons of alfalfa seeds will fill the entire quart jar when sprouted.

Steps:
Soaking – Fill jar halfway with pure water. Soak small seeds for 5 hours, medium seeds for 8 hours, and larger beans or grains for 15 hours.

Draining – After soaking, drain off water. Rinse the sprouts twice a day for 3-7 days with cool water, and drain. Place the jars in an area away from direct sunlight until they start to grow leaves. Alfalfa sprouts need to be put out in indirect light to manufacture chlorophyll in their leaves.

Rinsing – The purpose of rinsing is to keep the seeds moist, but do not let them sit in water, as they could become moldy.

Harvesting – When ready to eat, some sprouts, such as alfalfa sprouts, need to be harvested. This is the process of removing the tiny brown hulls. Swish the sprouts that you plan to eat in a bowl of water and let the hulls rise to the surface. Scoop out the hulls and drain the harvested sprouts in the sprouting jar to remove excess water.

Note. Adapted from Wigmore, A. (1982). *Be your own doctor: A positive guide to natural living.* Wayne, NJ: Avery Publishing Group, p. 50.

African Healing Traditions

To understand African healing traditions, it is important to have an appreciation of the size of the continent of Africa. It is a large continent that comprises 54 countries, each with its own culture and traditions. However, African countries are similar in that traditional and indigenous healing is a prominent part of each country's culture. Egypt, for example, a country in the northeast corner of Africa, has documented traditional healing practices for more than 5,000 years. The predominant healthcare practice of most Africans involves folk healers, native doctors, or cultural, magical, and religious ethnic healers. Traditional and indigenous knowledge is transmitted orally. African folk healers are often referred to as *shamans* or *shamanic practitioners*. However, these practitioners are viewed by Africans as herbal, spiritual, and ritualistic healers.

Folk healers in Africa have special areas of expertise. Folk therapies or remedies include massage, herbal remedies, and dermabrasive practices, such as cupping, pinching, rubbing, and burning of the skin. Dermabrasive therapies and practices are believed to restore health by releasing "bad energy" or "evil spirits" through the skin. In addition, amulets, worn on a bracelet or necklace or pinned to clothing, are believed to provide protection against evil spirits and certain illnesses. The amulets are typically inscribed with verses of the Koran or the Bible, decorated with turquoise stones or charms, and worn on the hand or fingers. They are thought to enhance protective powers or energy against the "evil eye."

In many African countries, specifically in South Africa, folk medicine has been integrated with elements from traditional Africans and immigrant Europeans (Du Toit, 1998). Lock et al. (2001) note that, since the colonial and missionary eras of African history, the mixing of Islamic and Christian religions with African traditional folk healing practices has formed a new medico-religious practice called *syncretic faith healing*. This practice has led to the creation of the celestial churches, which are well known for helping with the healing of illnesses, particularly mental illness. Healing practices and rituals may involve dance, prayers, fasting, bathing, massage, holy water, imagery, and herbal medicines (de Smet, 1999).

Spiritual, faith, and imaginary healing has to do with the relationship of the mind and spirit to the body. Prophets of celestial or syncretic churches are classified as traditional healers or shamans. However, spiritual, faith, and imaginary healers have their roots in ancient spiritual practices as well as in Christian churches. In some religious practices, such as Islam, which dictates health promotion practices, citizens take a passive role. In Christianity, prayers and the healing power of God are used for protection against misfortune, and holy water is used as a symbol of communion with the healer. Christian healing churches, such as the Celestial, "Aladura," or faith healing churches, are common in Africa. Spiritual healing is done by praying for or with someone, by the "laying on of hands," by distance healing, and by symbolic rituals, such as using the cross or rosary. Personal prayers can instill hope and reduce the anxiety associated with many illnesses and stressors.

Many African countries have roots in the traditions of their ancient cultures, and these traditions are passed down from generation to generation or are learned or acquired as a spiritual encounter or calling. Many people seek traditional healers because they have the ability to communicate with a higher being, such as God or Allah or the ancestors. Such powers are used to either save an entire community, as in the case of "town criers," or used to treat simple or complex physical and mental illnesses, stress, and injuries. Traditional faith healers typically attribute illness or misfortune to the anger of indigenous deities or ancestral spirits (de Smet, 1999). Spirit mediums are inducted into a "possessed" state of consciousness through music and rhythmic movements and psychoactive herbs, such as *Datura metel*, called *babba jiji* by the Hausa (an African tribe; de Smet, 1999, p. 51).

Drumming, dancing, and birth rituals are among the spiritual healing rituals that are used in Africa. For example, many babies are still delivered at home, with the mother squatting in a semiseated position or tied to an object as a traditional healer chants and drums. Some traditional midwives, also known as traditional birth attendants (TBAs), recommend the use of bellybands after delivery to assist with expulsion of the placenta and to decrease the size of the abdomen. In some African traditions, newborns are believed to be susceptible to evil influences during the first week of life, and caution is taken to limit the number and type of visitors who come close to the baby. TBAs usually perform circumcision practices for male infants in the first 2 weeks of life. TBAs and midwives are often used for deliveries outside the hospital. Most African countries rely heavily on the birth practices and skills of TBAs and midwives.

African Americans, who are descended from slaves, were brought to the United States as part of the slave trade, some of which originated from West Africa. Healing in West African culture is concerned with the restoration or preservation of human vitality and wholeness (Iwu, 1993). Community healers called "grannies" were described as female elders in the community who had nursed family members through serious illness, brought up a large number of children, or acquired their knowledge regarding health and illness from previous generations in their family. According to Iwu (1993), the word "midwife" in many African languages is synonymous with being a spiritual healer. Grannies held much power in their communities and therefore posed a challenge to slaveholders. "The active engagement of respected older women with the health of slave communities directly contradicted the scorn for ignorant 'old women' so prevalent in antebellum medical journals" (Fett, 2002, p. 55). Traditional medicine of Africa is preserved in the American healing tradition of slave grannie midwives.

Classical Traditional Chinese Medicine

The classical traditional Chinese medicine (TCM) system is thought to have originated around 2900 B.C. with three legendary rulers: u Xi (the Ox-tamer), Shen Nong (the Divine husbandman), and Huang Di (the Yellow Emperor). Shen Nong is considered the father of traditional Chinese herbal medicine. Chinese history is organized into dynasties. It is the Han dynasty, the era of Confucius, that is credited with some of the greatest development in the TCM system that are still practiced today in China as well as around the world.

Taoist philosophy was also founded during the Han dynasty. The great book of Taoism is the *Tao Te Ching*, authored by Lao Tsu. The *Tao Te Ching* teaches that the "fundamental forces of the cosmos itself are mirrored in our own individual, inner structure. And it invites us to try to live in direct relationship to all these forces" (Lao Tsu, 1989, pp. 34-37). A reader of the *Tao Te Ching* works on the inner self as well as the outer life. *Tao Te Ching* is not an instruction book on reflection or meditation per se, for according to Taoist thought, the essence of meditation practice cannot be taught in a book. However, the flow of energy as consciousness is taught in *Tao Te Ching* to be an expression of love. The practice of Taoism is discussed as nonwork or "nonpractice." *Tao Te Ching* speaks equally of "struggle and discipline as it does of nondoing and letting go" (Lao Tsu, 1989, p. xxviii). Disease is defined in TCM as blockage of flow. The goals of TCM care are harmony or balance of energy flow and longevity (Flaws, 1994). The word *qi* means breath, or essential life force. The key to health and longevity and maintaining it is harmonious balance between all vital energies within the body (Reid, 1986).

TCM uses a language of function and perception, and not one of substance and objects (Wicke, 1992, p. 63). Qi is one of five *fundamental processes in TCM*. The others are Blood, Fluids, Jing, and Shen. Qi, as energy, flows through meridians or pathways throughout the body that connect the internal organs and limbs, head and exterior surface of the body. The function of blood is to moisten the tissues of the body. Blood is believed to flow through meridians as well as blood vessels. TCM theory states that "Blood is the mother of Qi and Qi is the commander of Blood" (Wicke, 1992, p. 66). Fluids moisten and nourish body tissues. They are yin as is Blood, but more superficial. *Jing* is essence related to conception and heredity. Jing governs individual health at a deep level. "Jing changes more slowly than Qi" and "represents the gradually changing potential for activity and function as the years pass" (Wicke, 1992, p. 68).

A foundational belief to TCM is that the Eight Principle Patterns describe a patient's energetic qualities: heat/cold, excess/deficiency, interior/exterior, and yin/yang. The qualities are typically grouped together, such as in the diagnosis of *Damp* (excess – interior) *Heat*. The interventions for patients are then assigned that will harmonize or balance the pattern. The two principle patterns called "yin" and "yang" are central concepts to Taoist philosophy. They are relative concepts that are explained in relationship rather than as absolutes. In TCM, the term *yin* is used in reference to the female, negative, passive force and the ability of the body to calm and cool itself. *Yang* is the male, positive, active force and the ability of the body to warm and energize itself. "The interplay between yin and yang sparks all change and movement in the universe" (Reid, 1986, p. 30).

"Many common ailments are simply due to insufficient levels and inferior quality of vital energy in the system. This is why astute Chinese doctors first look to their patients' general lifestyles and daily habits for clues" (Reid, 1986, p. 28). The assessment of lifestyle and diet in TCM includes a holistic review of a person's habits and how they spend their vital energy each day. TCM clinicians first address change in lifestyle, make dietary adjustments, and then introduce herbal formulas when a person is out of balance or ill. This energetic pattern assessment and treatment approach using the eight principle patterns and the "threefold focus for clearing the picture," provides detailed structure for precision nursing science (Libster, in press). If these initial changes are not sufficient to create greater balance in body, mind and spirit, other modalities are then added, such as acupuncture and moxibustion (described later in this section).

This philosophy is exemplified in the case of a person who cannot sleep. In Western biomedicine, a person might report the problem and be prescribed a medication, herbal remedy, or intervention that is known through research to help promote sleep. In TCM, the patient would first be asked about his or her lifestyle. In doing so, the TCM practitioner finds that the person cannot sleep because of worries about their child, who just went to college and has not been seen or heard from for 3 months. The solution is not to medicate the sleeplessness and worry – but to find the child and communicate with the child. This approach, although somewhat simplistic here, is scientifically precise and helpful in the care of clients with multiple and complex health patterns.

Since ancient times, the Chinese have viewed the universe as being created of the five elements. The Five-Element theory in Chinese medicine was established approximately 500 years after the establishment of the Eight Principle Patterns and fundamental processes. Each element is symbolically related to a specific organ, taste, color, direction, and emotion. (See Table 3-1.)

TABLE 3-1: FIVE ELEMENTS IN CLASSICAL TRADITONAL CHINESE MEDICINE

Note: See The Yellow Emperor's Classic of Medicine (Ni, 2011) for a complete list of qualities for each element.

	Fire	Wood (Ether)	Earth	Metal (Air)	Water
Organ	Heart	Liver	Spleen	Lungs	Kidneys
Taste	Bitter	Sour	Sweet	Pungent	Salty
Color	Red	Green	Yellow	White	Black
Direction	South	East	Center	West	North
Emotion	Joy	Anger	Desire	Worry	Fear

In TCM, a comprehensive diagnosis includes lifestyle and diet history, pulse diagnosis of nine pulse positions on the wrists related to the organs, and tongue diagnosis of the tongue tissue and coating. The tongue also shows the state of health of the major organs and the body as a whole in terms of the fundamental processes. Herbal medicine formulations used in TCM are centuries old in some cases. Each herbal remedy prescribed is given to create balance. For example, *Four Gentleman Decoction* is a basic formula prescribed for anyone with a specific pattern related to Qi Deficiency. This ancient formula tonifies Spleen Qi. The four herbs, given together, are: Ren Shen *(Panax ginseng)*, Bai Zhu *(Atractylodis macrocephalae)*, Fu Ling *(Poria cocos)*, a fungus, and Zhi Gan Cao or licorice root

(*Glycyrrhizae uralensis*). They have a synergistic effect on body, mind, and spirit.

Acupuncture and moxibustion are two clinical techniques that are some of the most recognized of the TCM system. Both are used to stimulate points along the meridians. There are 12 major meridians that move qi over the entire body and numerous other smaller channels. More than 800 points have been identified, but only 50 are commonly used (Reid, 1986). The goal of acupuncture is to regulate or move qi in the body. Lifestyle and dietary changes as well as herbal remedies can do the same and provide a foundation for the successful application of acupuncture, should it be necessary. Stimulation of the acupuncture point is achieved through rotating the needles until a tight, twisting sensation is felt by the patient. Acupuncture should not be confused with acupressure, which is a type of touch therapy in which no needles are used. In acupuncture, specially shaped needles that are round or blunt, three-edged, swordlike, sharp, and round or filiform are used to balance body energy. Several clinical studies have been done on acupuncture treatment, particularly for pain relief. For example, a meta-analysis by Xiang, Cheng, Shen, Xu, & Liu (2017) found that acupuncture is effective for immediate analgesic relief of pain.

Moxibustion is also used for pain relief, but more generally, as with acupuncture, to move qi in the channels. *Moxibustion* differs from acupuncture in that instead of needles, the practitioner burns a small mound of dried, crumbled or powdered ai ye *(Artemisia vulgaris)* leaf on or directly over the acupuncture point. Right before the heat touches the skin, the herb is flicked away so as not to burn the skin.

In the United States, "medical acupuncture" is a popular biomedical adaptation of the ancient TCM system, particularly among physicians and advanced practice nurses who study and employ it. Although traditional acupuncture and TCM as a whole system are rooted in the philosophy documented here, medical acupuncture uses a "scientific prescriptive theory" instead. One article by a nurse practitioner who is also a licensed acupuncturist states that traditional acupuncture is "outdated," particularly because it has "never been demonstrated that a meridian system actually exists in the body" (Walling, 2006, p. 141). Some people would argue that medical acupuncture is an incomplete representation of TCM and that the training is very limited, so it may not hold the same record of efficacy and safety as the centuries-old traditional practice.

When a system of healing has been practiced safely for centuries and its underlying philosophy is altered, that safety record is in jeopardy until a new paradigm is developed and tested. Medical acupuncture is not the practice of TCM, nor is it TCM acupuncture. It may, as the Walling study suggests, be effective. However, medical acupuncture is very different in scope, training, and practice and licensure requirements (discussed in the next section). Clinical trials on the effects of medical acupuncture may be easier to conduct than those on traditional acupuncture (American Academy of Medical Acupuncture, n.d.). This is because of medical acupuncture's prescriptive and streamlined approach, which contrasts with the traditional Eight Principle Patterns and Five Elements approach used in traditional acupuncture that is highly person-centered and relationship-centered

(American Academy of Medical Acupuncture, n.d.).

Acupuncture needles received the approval of the U.S. Food & Drug Administration (FDA) for use by licensed practitioners in 1996. The biggest risks associated with acupuncture treatment for patients are the use of needles and the risk for infection or organ injury. Needle manufacturers must label needles for "single use only." Although millions of people are treated with acupuncture each year, few adverse events have been reported to the FDA (National Center for Complementary and Integrative Health, 2017).

Ayurveda

Like TCM, Ayurveda is one of the oldest traditional healing systems on the planet. It originated in India but is now practiced all over the world. The word *Ayurveda* means the "science of life." Ayurveda is more than 3,000 years old and is rooted in Hinduism and the traditions of the Brahmanic and Vedic religion of the Aryan people. The *Vedas*, sacred scriptures and poetry that are sung and read, contain many references to healing and medicine. The *Caraka Samhita* (medical) and *Susruta Samhita* (surgical) are the sacred medical texts of India that represent the first codification of the Ayurvedic system. Underlying the healing system of the Samhitas and the practice of Ayurveda is the Samkhya philosophy of creation. It is believed that the source of all existence is "cosmic consciousness, which manifests as male and female energy – *Shiva and Shakti*" (Lad, 1984). "Ayurveda regards the human body and its sensory experiences as manifestations of cosmic energy expressed in the five basic elements. The ancient rishis perceived that these elements sprang from pure Cosmic Consciousness" (Lad, 1984, p. 25). The Ayurvedic path is followed to bring the body into harmony with that Consciousness.

The five elements are foundational to Ayurveda. They manifest in combination in the human body as three humors referred to as the "tridosha." Ether and air manifest *vata* dosha. Fire and water manifest as pitta dosha. Earth and water manifest as *kapha dosha*. The tridosha are an organizing structure for describing that which governs all functions of the body, mind, and consciousness. Each person is thought to manifest a specific constitutional dosha at conception. There are seven possible constitutions, or prakruti in Sanskrit, meaning "nature": vata, pitta, kapha, vata-pitta, pitta-kapha, vata-kapha, and vata-pitta-kapha. According to the Caraka Samhita, the understanding of the doshas is foundational to healing oneself and others.

Vata manifests as movement. It governs breathing, blinking, heartbeat, movement of muscles, and movement of nerve cells. Vata governs fear, anxiety, pain, and nervousness. Pitta manifests as metabolism. It governs digestions, absorption, nutrition, skin color, luster of the eyes, intelligence, and understanding. Pitta governs anger, hate, and jealousy. Kapha maintains body resistance. It lubricates joints, moisturizes the skin, heals wounds, gives strength, and supports memory and immunity. Kapha governs attachment, greed, and envy as well as calmness, forgiveness, and love.

Metabolism is a function of *agn*i, or fire. The root of all disease is believed to be *ama*. When agni is impaired and the tridosha are out of balance, ama results.

Ama is similar to the biomedical definition of clogging the arteries, waste stagnation in the excretory organs, and circulatory stagnation. Diagnosis of the doshas is performed through pulse, tongue, face, and physical assessment, also known as "reading the patient as a living book" (Lad, 1984, p. 52).

Ayurvedic medicines are of two types. Some of them "tone up the health of a healthy person and some others remove the ailments of a patient" (Caraka Samhita, Vol. III, p. 6). Ayurvedic treatments include dietary changes; medicated ghee (clarified butter); herbal applications, such as inhalations, enemas, and topical oils; various types of massage; and rejuvenation therapies with Amalaki fruit (*Phyllanthus emblica*), which is used in people of all three doshas (Caraka Samhita, 1988). Ayurveda also includes several purification therapies, such as therapeutic vomiting (vamana), mild laxatives (virechana), and nasal washing and herbal applications (neti pot and nasya). Both Carakas require that patients have knowledge of their own condition, be attentive to it, and exercise courage and self-control.

PROFESSIONAL CONSIDERATIONS RELATED TO TRADITIONAL/ INDIGENOUS HEALING SYSTEMS

Nurses who come from the traditions discussed here are excellent resources for others who may not be familiar with beliefs and practices of their patient's culture. Practicing traditional healing in any society carries with it requirements for preparation and practice (offering), in much the way the profession of nursing requires training and passing the NCLEX (nursing licensure) examination. However, people who practice the traditions discussed here may have been in training since they were very young or may be practicing because of a spiritual gift or vision recognized in their communities. Transcultural nursing skill and primary health care include demonstrating deep respect for these healers and their roles in the community so that nursing and traditional healing can exist in harmony. Countries such as India, China, and Peru have systems that fully integrate biomedical care and conventional nursing with Ayurveda, TCM, and Peruvian traditional healing (WHO, 2014).

Nurses who wish to practice the systems discussed in this chapter will require education and sociocultural-spiritual preparation. Nurses who practice according to these traditional healing systems may be required to hold additional licensure. Integrative holistic nursing and the legal and ethical considerations for practice are discussed further in Chapter 5. Many states in the United States do license practitioners of TCM, Doctors of Oriental Medicine, and acupuncturists. Educational programs in TCM are typically between 4 and 5 years long. Graduates are awarded either a diploma or master's degree, depending on the scope of the program. Graduates of these programs are referred to as Doctors of Oriental Medicine or Acupuncturists. Programs can be accredited by The Accreditation Commission for Acupuncture and Oriental Medicine (ACAOM), which is the national accrediting agency recognized by the U.S. Department of Education. The National Certification Commission for Acupuncture and Oriental Medicine (NCCAOM) is the only national organization that validates entry-level competency in the practice of acupuncture and Oriental medicine (AOM) through professional certification. The education and certification necessary to be able to perform acupuncture varies from state to state. Only a person fully trained in the practice of Chinese medicine or medical acupuncture (in the case of advanced practice nurses) can perform acupuncture. Nurses, however, can provide nursing care for the patient receiving TCM and acupuncture.

CASE STUDY:
REFINING THE ELEMENTS OF CULTURAL SKILL

Mei Fong is an 80-year-old woman with a diagnosis of acute leukemia. Her oncologist tells you that she has had the leukemia for some time and that it is remarkable that she is still alive. Upon assessment, you learn that Mrs. Fong has been taking Chinese herbs and receiving acupuncture for her whole life. For the past 18 years, she received these treatments specifically for her health concerns related to leukemia, a complex pattern of excess and deficiency with symptoms such as fatigue. The TCM treatments are no longer sufficient for managing her symptoms, and the disease has progressed. Mrs. Fong is now seeking biomedical care at the cancer center, where you are her nurse.

Questions
1. Give an example of how you would apply integrative holistic nursing philosophy in the care of Mrs. Fong.
2. How would you demonstrate cultural diplomacy?

Nurse's Answers
1. Using a person-centered, relationship-centered approach, the holistic nurse would demonstrate respect for the 18 years of health and health care that Mrs. Fong received. Although some people in the biomedical culture might hold a bias and suggest to Mrs. Fong that she might have fared better had she sought biomedical treatment 18 years ago, the diplomatic approach would be for the nurse to pace with the patient and demonstrate respect for her choices of care then and now.
2. This response is drawn from an actual case that the author encountered. The physician was very enthusiastic to learn from the patient about what she had done to live so long with leukemia, which the physician thought "should have killed her long ago" according to her medical belief and knowledge. Although the patient might not take the herbs and TCM treatments on the same days as her chemotherapy, the physician determined that the patient was still planning to take her herbs and TCM treatments at some point while accepting her month's-long chemotherapy regimen. The team's scientific and diplomatic question was not if the herbs would interact with the chemotherapy but how

they might interact. The plan was to investigate on behalf of the patient and then use a shared-decision model of care to plan care that met the patient's needs of receiving TCM and chemotherapy.

3. The nurse and the traditional Chinese herbalist (this author) were asked to review the herbal formula (decoction or tea) that Mrs. Fong was receiving and explain it to the physician, the pharmacy, and nurse team members. At that time, it was determined (together with the patient and her family) that the patient would continue her TCM care and herbs but discontinue her herbs for 2 days before and after chemotherapy, which the patient was having every few weeks. Diplomacy is person-centered and relationship-centered, and in this case chemotherapy and TCM were able to be integrated. The rationale was based on the science that most of the chemotherapy drugs would be excreted within 2 to 3 days. Although this case is not typical or considered "standard of care," the purpose of showing it is to exemplify diplomacy in action and what can result from that process.

HOLISTIC TRANSFORMATION

- What is the first step for incorporating what I have learned about integrative holistic nursing practice and cultural skills in my work with patients?

- Using the five Elements of Care® as a reference point, what have I learned from this chapter content about traditional and indigenous healing?

SUMMARY

Traditional healing practices are common to every culture. Traditional and indigenous healing practices and the modalities associated with them are different than complementary therapies. Complementary therapies are healthcare practices and modalities that are not part of a country's tradition system(s) but are not fully integrated into the dominant healthcare system (WHO, 2014). Traditional and indigenous healing systems are part of culture and communities around the globe. The integrative holistic nursing approach prepares nurses to provide diplomatic care to the people who are actively engaged in their culture's healing heritage.

RESOURCES

The Accreditation Commission for Acupuncture and Oriental Medicine (ACAOM)
    http://www.acaom.org

American Academy of Medical Acupuncture
    http://www.medicalacupuncture.org

American Association of Acupuncture and Oriental Medicine
http://www.aaaomonline.org

National Alaska Native American Indian Nurses Association
    https://nanaina.org

National Ayurvedic Medical Association
    http://www.ayurvedanama.org

Transcultural Nursing Society
    http://www.tcns.org

REFERENCES

Alvord, L. A., & Van Pelt, E. C. (1999). *The scalpel and the silver bear: The first Navajo woman surgeon combines Western medicine and traditional healing.* New York, NY: Bantam Books.

American Academy of Medical Acupuncture. (n.d.) Retrieved from American Academy of Medical Acupuncture website: http://www.medicalacupuncture.orFor-Patients/Articles-By-Physicians-About-Acupuncture/An-Overview-Of-Medical-Acupuncture

Anderson, W. (1998). Green man: *The archetype of our oneness with the earth.* Fakenham, England: Compass Books.

Beecher, C. E., & Stowe, H. B. (2002). *The American woman's home.* New Brunswick, NJ: Rutgers University Press. (Original work published 1869)

Benner, P., Sutphen, M., Leonard, V., & Day, L. (2010). *Educating nurses: A call for radical transformation. In The Carnegie Foundation for the Advancement of Teaching: Preparation for the Professions Series.* San Francisco, CA: Jossey-Bass.

Bonomi, P. U. (2003). *Under the cope of heaven: Religion, society, and politics in colonial America* (updated ed.). Oxford, England: Oxford University Press.

Bunson, M. (1992). *Kateri Tekakwitha: Mystic of the wilderness.* Huntington, IN: Our Sunday Visitor Publishing.

Caraka Samhita. (1988). *Caraka Samhita*, Volumes II and III. Varanasi, India: Chowkhamba Sanskrit Series Office.

Clouser, K. D., & Hufford, D. J. (1993). Nonorthodox healing systems and their knowledge claims. *Journal of Medicine and Philosophy, 18*(2), 101-106.

de Smet, P. A. G. M. (1999). *Herbs, health, & healers: Africa as ethnopharmacological treasury.* Berg en Dal, The Netherlands: Afrika Museum.

Du Toit, B. M. (1998). Modern folk medicine in South Africa. *South African Journal of Ethnology, 21*(4), 145-152.

Fett, S. M. (2002). *Working cures: Healing, health, and power on Southern slave plantations.* Chapel Hill, NC: University of North Carolina Press.

Flaws, B. (1994). *Imperial secrets of health and longevity.* Boulder, CO: Blue Poppy Press.

Green, R. R., Santoro, N., Allhouse, A. A., Neal-Perry, G., & Derby, C. (2017). Prevalence of complementary and alternative medicine and herbal remedy use in Hispanic and non-Hispanic white women: Results from the Study of Women's Health Across the Nation. *Journal of Alternative and Complementary Medicine, 23*(10), 805-811.

Greymorning, S. N. (2016). Beyond the IHS: Indigenous knowledge and traditional approaches to health and healing [e-book Chapter 6]. In M. P. Moss (Ed.), *American Indian health and nursing.* New York, NY: Springer.

Grzywacz, J. G., Arcury, T. A., Bell, R. A., Lang, W., Suerken, C. K., Smith, S. L., & Quandt, S. A. (2006). Ethnic differences in elders' home remedy use: Sociocultural explanations. *American Journal of Health Behavior*, 30(1), 39-50.

Hildegard of Bingen. (1994). *Holistic healing* (M. Pawlik, Trans.). Collegeville, MN: The Liturgical Press.

Iwu, M. M. (1993). *Handbook of African medicinal plants*. Boca Raton, FL: CRC Press.

Lad, V. (1984). Ayurveda: *The science of self-healing*. Santa Fe, NM: Lotus Press.

Lao Tsu. (1989). *Tao Te Ching*. New York, NY: Vintage Books.

Leininger, M. M. (Ed.). (1984). *Care: The essence of nursing and health*. Detroit, MI: Wayne State University Press.

Levin, L. S., & Idler, E. (2010). *The hidden health care system: Social resources in health care*. Farmville, NC: Golden Apple Publications.

Libster, M. M. (2004). *Herbal diplomats: The contribution of early American nurses (1830-1860) to 19th century health care reform and the Botanical Medical Movement*. Wauwatosa, WI: Golden Apple Publications.

Libster, M. M. (2015). Cultural diplomacy: Demonstrating person-centered care and coaching. *Perspectives on Cultural Diplomacy* (Vol. I., Nursing). [e-publication series]. Available from www.goldenapplepublications.com

Libster, M. M. (2017). Spiritual formation, secularization, and reform of professional nursing in antebellum America. *Journal of Professional Nursing*. Retrieved from http://dx.doi.or10.1016/j.profnurs.2017.05.002

Libster, M. M., Phillips, S. G., Smith-Taylor, J., Southard, M. E., & Bryant, S. (2015). The Cultural Diplomacy Model™ for demonstrating person-centered care and coaching. *Perspectives on Cultural Diplomacy* (Vol. I., Nursing.) [e-publication series]. Available from www.goldenapplepublications.com.

Libster, M.M. (2022, In press). The Tao of Integrative Nursing Assessment (TINA): An East-West Model for Precision, Complementarity, and Inclusion in Relationship-Centered Care. *Holistic Nursing Practice*.

Lock, S., Last, J. M., Dunea, G., Walton, J., Beeson, P. B., & Barondess, J. A. (2001). *The Oxford illustrated companion to medicine*. New York, NY: Oxford University Press.

Merchant, C. (1980). *The Death of nature: women, ecology, and the scientific revolution*. San Francisco: Harper.

Metzner, R. (1999). *Green psychology: Transforming our relationship to the earth*. Rochester, VT: Park Street Press.

National Center for Complementary and Integrative Health. (2017). *Acupuncture*. Retrieved from https://nccih.nih.gov/health/acupuncture

Orem, D. (2001). *Nursing concepts of practice* (6th ed.). St. Louis, MO: Mosby.

Reid, D. P. (1986). *Chinese herbal medicine*. Boston, MA: Shambhala Publications.

Sandelowski, M. (2000). *Devices and desires: Gender, technology, and American nursing (Studies in social medicine)*. Chapel Hill, NC: University of North Carolina Press.

Sirois, F. M., Riess, H., & Upchurch, D. M. (2017). Implicit reasons for disclosure of the use of complementary health approaches (CHA): A consumer commitment perspective. *Annals of Behavioral Medicine, 51*(5), 764-774.

Starr, P. (1982). *The social transformation of American medicine*. New York, NY: Basic Books.

Sun Bear & Wabun (1980). The Medicine wheel. New York: Simon and Schuster.

Thorne, S. (1993). Health belief systems in perspective. *Journal of Advanced Nursing, 18*(12), 1931-1941.

Wall, S. (2001). *To become a human being: The message of Tadodaho Chief Leon Shenandoah.* Charlottesville, VA: Hampton Roads Publishing.

Wallace, P. A. W. (1946). *The white roots of peace.* Philadelphia, PA: University of Pennsylvania Press.

Walling, A. (2006). Therapeutic modulation of the psychoneuroimmune system by medical acupuncture creates enhance feelings of well-being. *Journal of the American Association of Nurse Practitioners, 18*(4), 135-143.

Wicke, R. W. (1992). *Clinical handbook of herbal medicine* (2nd ed.). Hot Springs, MT: Rocky Mountain Herbal Institute Publications.

Wigmore, A. (1982). *Be your own doctor: A positive guide to natural living.* Wayne, NJ: Avery Publishing Group.

World Health Organization. (2014). *WHO Traditional medicine strategy: 2014-2023*. Geneva, Switzerland:Author.

Retrieved from http://www.who.int/medicines/publications/traditional/trm_strategy14_23/en/

Xiang, A., Cheng, K., Shen, X., Xu, P., & Liu, S. (2017). The immediate analgesic effect of acupuncture for pain: A systemic review and meta-analysis. *Evidence-based Complementary and Alternative Medicine.* Retrieved from https://doi.or10.1155/2017/3837194

PART II
PRECISION NURSING SCIENCE: INTEGRATIVE HOLISTIC NURSING INTERVENTIONS

CHAPTER 4

OVERVIEW OF INTERVENTIONS

LEARNING OUTCOME

After completing this chapter, the learner will be able to explain integrative holistic nursing philosophy and practice.

CHAPTER OBJECTIVES

After completing this chapter, the learner will be able to:
1. Describe integrative holistic nursing philosophy of care.
2. Identify the role of discernment in integrative holistic nursing practice.
3. List safety considerations in integrative holistic nursing.
4. Discuss examples of the 3 T's of integrative care.

INTRODUCTION

"Health is a condition in which all parts and subparts are in harmony with the whole of the client." – Dr. Betty Neuman, Author of *The Systems Model of Nursing*

Integrative holistic nurses demonstrate care when they create the time and space for a healing relationship to occur with a patient – be they a person, a family, or a community. Building healing relationships with patients is a creative process. When an integrative holistic nurse fully engages in this creative process with his or her whole being, all of the Elements of Care® are present: thought (Air – mind element), desire (Water – emotion element), strength (Earth – physical element), and spirit (Ether/Fire Elements – spiritual element). Nurses have their own process for this work, called *the nursing process*. The nursing process, while focusing on the nurse's thoughts, desires, strengths, and spiritual preparation, can provide a patient-centered, relationship-centered framework for finding solutions and demonstrating care. Creating the healing relationship in partnership with the patient and then choosing interventions for a plan of care that is meaningful to them demonstrates precision nursing science that is rooted in respect for the whole person and their healing process. Peplau (1952) wrote:

> Nursing is a process that seeks to facilitate development of personality by aiding individuals to use those compelling forces and experiences that influence personality in ways that ensure maximum productivity. Nurses are assistants and helpers, rather than manipulators of people. (p. 73)

The function of the human personality is to grow and develop. Growth and development promote health. Precision nursing science focuses on the adaptation response of patients to perceived or actual internal and external stressors. Nurses often interact with people who are "stressed," ill, or out of balance. They are seeking adaptation during a critical and often sensitive period for growth and development of the personality when the human experience of change, transition, and transformation is very physical. Integrative holistic nursing that is patient-centered, relationship-centered is not seeking to impose the nurse's own will, healing experience, cultural beliefs, and practices on another but to access knowledge of the science of nursing and the healing arts to offer suggestions for care based on observation and analysis of a patient's unique energetic health patterns.

There are hundreds of complementary therapies, biomedical treatments, and traditional remedies that people can choose to receive from a health practitioner or to try in self-care. How does a person choose what to do? Peplau (1952) is suggesting that choices are made on the basis of need. However, many people do not know what they need because they often do not perceive or understand their own health patterns. People may not even know the anatomy and physiology of their own body, let alone understand the energetic imbalances that may be manifesting as illness. They may have body awareness, or they may not. They may have no insight about their own thoughts and decision-making processes. Patients may or may not have any emotional intelligence, and they may or may not have any spiritual or religious practices that guide them to greater peace and happiness.

Integrative holistic nurses help their patients to choose interventions that will help them to develop and grow physically, emotionally, mentally, and spiritually. Complementary therapies are chosen that match the person's need and their energetic health pattern(s). Although nurses will develop and grow in the process of caring for another in the healing relationship, the interventions that are chosen are not the ones that have or will serve the nurse's needs or fulfill what the nurse believes to be "best" for the patient. The nurse and the patient engage in the creative process of finding and applying those interventions that help the patient. The model for that creative process presented in this text is called the Elements of Care®.

During the nursing process, a nurse has numerous opportunities to make choices. These choices follow a logical problem-solving process that starts with assessment, diagnosis, and planning, moves to implementation or intervention, and then concludes with evaluation. The American Holistic Nurses Association (AHNA) *Scope and Standards* (2018) document cites competencies for each of these phases of the process that are congruent with any scope of practice in nursing. *Integrative nursing* is the activation and demonstration of a holistic philosophy of care. Integrative nursing is defined as "the creation of evolving, healing, relationships" in which the nurse "observes the patient's needs for greater harmony and balance in their life and then addresses those needs by offering care that is a holistic blend of biomedical and caring modalities" (Libster, 2001, p. 26). Part II of this text is about using the nursing process when engaging with the patient to find that unique, creative blend of interventions that will help the patient to grow, develop, and move toward greater healing as balance in body and peace of mind.

PRECISION NURSING SCIENCE AND INTEGRATIVE HOLISTIC NURSING

As stated previously, integrative holistic nursing is a philosophy of care rather than a set of prescribed nursing actions and complementary therapies done to or for a patient. Integrative nursing is the demonstration of that holistic philosophy, to which there is a science and an art. The beliefs and practices of the biomedical culture have great meaning for nurses and patients alike. But ongoing issues of medical waste, unnecessary hospitalizations and diagnostic tests, and over-prescription (particularly of opiates) often compel nurses to seek other paradigms for practice. Integrative nursing is a demonstration of cultural diplomacy in which nurses form a creative blend of biomedical, complementary therapies, self-care, and traditional and indigenous beliefs and practices that best meet the needs of the patient. This process lends itself to "integrative insight" (Libster, 2012), or deep understanding of the approach to the transformation of self of the patient and the nurse who engage in the healing relationship.

Welcoming Integrative Insights

The nursing process begins with assessment, and the first part of that assessment is the engagement, or welcome. During the first contact, be it by phone, the Web, or face-to-face, patients and nurses make impressions on each other. First impressions often last. An integrative holistic nursing approach includes creating a caring space by utilizing holistic philosophy and the Elements of Care®. A nurse's appearance, mannerisms, voice, and use of space tell the patient about the nurse's culture and beliefs. How nurses walk into a room can set the tone for a relationship. Therapeutic use of self, according to theorist Lydia Hall, is the "core" of the nursing process. She wrote of the core of nursing in 1964:

> It is impossible to nurse any more of a person than that person allows us to see. In the process of exploring with a nurse – who he is, where he is, where he wants to go and will he take or refuse help in getting there – the patient will make rapid progress toward recovery and rehabilitation. (p. 152)

Creating a space for the relationship begins at the very beginning of the assessment phase of the nursing process to support patients as they try to "get clear on the meaning of their experience" (Peplau, 1952, p. 20). The holistic integrative healing process supports that which nurses often define as "a lifelong journey into wholeness" (AHNA, 2018). But in that moment of the first encounter together, nurse and patient have an important opportunity to set a pattern for the relationship. Appreciation engages the heart and allows for the possibility of moving beyond the "clinicalization" of care (Cowling, 2000) so that incorporation of solutions from self-care, healing traditions, and complementary therapies domains can emerge. Demonstrating appreciation through communication skills opens nurses' and patients' hearts so that modeling, entering the world of another, can begin.

Accents to the Nursing Process

The five-phase nursing process is taught in prelicensure nursing programs and is a guiding structure for discussion of best practice in state practice acts and scope and standards documents, such as the AHNA *Scope and Standards* (2018). However, professional integrative holistic nurses must still utilize their skill, training, and insight to create their own personal, professional approach to meeting those standards within the five-phase nursing process. The following are some "accents" to the nursing process that are intended to be thought-provoking regarding how to demonstrate a holistic philosophy of care.

Assessment

The accent to integrative holistic nursing assessment is to *begin with the patient's experience.* When a nurse has his or her task as the goal of an encounter with a patient, then that task, such as a list of questions and a perceived time limit, drives the care that is given. As will be shown in the next section in Clinical Vignette #1, that care may or may not be "holistic." It is possible to have a task to do and employ a holistic philosophy of care. The assessment competency in the AHNA *Scope and Standards* (2018) document states, "The holistic registered nurse collects comprehensive data," but how this competency is demonstrated differentiates that care which is holistic from that which is not. The following is an example of two approaches to address the integrative holistic nursing assessment competency using the same scenario.

Clinical Vignette #1

#1. *Michael is an 18-year-old man whose mother died 2 weeks ago. He develops cold/flu symptoms. He believes that his cough and fever are getting worse and decides to go to the urgent care center for help. The nurse says, "I am so sorry that you do not feel well, Michael. Let's take your temperature." The nurse asks him about his symptoms and concerns while completing the questions on the intake assessment. Michael sees the advanced practice registered nurse (APRN) and is then sent home with instructions about home remedies for fever reduction and a handout on elderberry syrup, which can be taken to shorten the length of time that one experiences flu symptoms.*

#2. *Michael is an 18-year-old man whose mother died in a car accident 2 weeks ago. He develops cold/flu symptoms. He believes that his cough and fever are getting worse and decides to go to the urgent care center for help. The nurse says, "I am so sorry that you do not feel well, Michael. Let's take your temperature." While taking his temperature, the nurse says to Michael (modeling), "You know that people often get sick when they are stressed out. How's everything going for you, Michael?" Michael tells the nurse that his mother died 2 weeks ago. The nurse pauses and says, "Oh, my." Michael says, "Yeah, it's been really rough for my dad ... such a shock." The nurse says, "And how about you?" Michael says, "Well, I thought I was okay, and then I got sick and couldn't see what to do for the fever and stuff – always asked my mom." The* nurse says, "I can certainly see how hard that is. I can help you with that, and the APRN is going to help too. Would it be helpful to talk about some suggestions for ways that you and your dad can get help dealing with this sudden shock of losing your mom?" Michael sees the APRN and is then sent home with a list of different people who provide grief counseling in the community, instructions about home remedies for fever reduction, and a handout on elderberry syrup, which can be taken to shorten the length of time that one experiences flu symptoms.

An urgent care visit is expected to be brief, which often compels caregivers to try to control the direction of the visit so as to manage the amount of time that they spend in a room. If the nurse and the APRN approach the competency merely as a list of tasks to be checked off, they would not be able to do their jobs. Holistic philosophy suggests doing an assessment of the patient's spiritual, emotional, mental, and physical self. But meeting the integrative holistic nursing assessment competency by employing holistic philosophy does not have to take hours! In approach #2, the nurse used modeling to enter into Michael's world while she "collected data" on Michael's acute physical symptoms. Modeling does not have to be time-consuming, but it is a skill that requires practice. Modeling during assessment requires relationship-building and communication skills, such as "essence" listening (Libster, 2001). The nurse in the #2 approach asked open-ended questions that invited Michael to tell her what his most important concern was: the sudden death of his mom. He left the urgent care center with some insight about how to deal with his grief and better attend to self-care.

The accent to integrative holistic nursing assessment is to begin with the patient's experience. Some tips for doing this are to use modeling and to hold the question "Why now?" in mind when encountering a patient. As nurses advance their communication skills, techniques such as pacing can be used to more quickly and efficiently assess a patient and their true needs for care. *Pacing* is a specific means of gaining rapport in which the nurse matches the information processes of the patient (Bandler & Grinder, as cited in Walter & Peller, 1992). The nurse paces with the patient by listening for the way that a patient speaks, either in visual, auditory, or kinesthetic terms, and then matches their way of processing information. In Clinical Vignette #2, Michael spoke in visual terms, and the nurse then paced with him by doing the same.

Diagnosis

The accent for the integrative holistic nursing diagnosis is to *focus squarely on the meaning of health patterns* rather than medical diagnoses. Health patterns include words, such as sleep and rest, energy, elimination, and pain relief. A diagnosis is a conclusion drawn from assessment. What can differentiate integrative holistic nursing is how that conclusion is communicated. A diagnosis can be rendered as a judgment or an opinion. Health beliefs and perceptions are underlying factors in any diagnosis. Medical diagnosis has a long history of being problem-focused, whereas health pattern diagnosis so often used in nursing also includes a wellness and prevention solution-orientation in addition to problems.

Problem orientation is often utilized in nursing care as a default strategy when time management is the intention. Person-centered, relationship-centered care offers another view. The key is to ask patients what they think, feel, or have experienced as solutions. An example of this care from Clinical Vignette #1 might be to ask Michael, "What is helping so far?" In that case, he might have explained that he really does not know what to do because his mother always helped him. Solution-focused therapy techniques can be learned and easily applied in patient care by nurses who are not psychotherapists. A solution-focused approach, which focuses on patient strengths, is helpful in time management and has been shown to be highly effective in construction of meaning (Franklin, Zhang, Froerer, & Johnson, 2016).

Many skills can be used to diagnose according to health patterns. One example is to address the person's sense of the meaning of their health concern for which they have sought care. Margaret Newman suggests in her Health as Expanding Consciousness theory, for example, that nurses shift their paradigm and consider that "disease is a manifestation of health" and not a "separate entity that invades our bodies but as a manifestation of the evolving pattern of person-environment interaction" (1994, pp. 5, 17). Therefore, the assessment of what a disease, illness, or health concern means to a patient can lead to a diagnosis that is meaningful to the patient as well. Meaning is pattern. Understanding patients' patterns leads to interventions that are then also meaningful. In Clinical Vignette #1, the meaning of Michael's illness was related to the change, transition, and transformation related to the sudden loss of his mother at a young age when he was still relying on her for care.

Planning and Implementation

The accent for integrative holistic nursing implementation or intervention is to *create plans of care that are unique blends of the Elements of Care®*. Person-centered, relationship-centered care suggests that nurses will partner with patients and create care plans that are unique in that they are specific and meaningful for the patient. The impetus, then, for evolving outcomes identification and the plan of care, according to AHNA Standards 3 and 4 (2018), comes from the patient. However, as nurses in the United Kingdom have discovered after years of implementing a patient/consumer/person-centered, relationship-centered approach to care (PCC), PCC should not be construed as meaning that nurses abdicate their role as caregivers (Nolan, Davies, Brown, Keady, & Nolan, 2004). Also, when caring for the unique patient as an individual, a patient's patterns are still understood as existing within the context of relationships with others, the environment, and the Divine Consciousness or God.

After a patient's health patterns are assessed and summarized in health pattern and nursing diagnoses, the nurse and the patient begin discussion of short- and long-term goals for care. During this process, the integrative holistic nurse receives feedback as to how well he or she has modeled the patient's world. Goal setting is an important step toward pacing with a patient. Patients learn that healing "evolves" and "unfolds" and that outcomes that nurses are held accountable for in practice may not be immediately evident because of the nonlinear nature of the healing process (AHNA, 2018, p. 53). The nurse learns whether his or her thoughts about what the patient's meaningful goals would be are congruent with the patient's. The nurse and the patient then partner to create the best care that will address the change, transition, and transformation process that the patient is experiencing. All five elements can be incorporated within one intervention or can be represented within the total plan of care. The balancing of the elements in a therapeutic herbal bath intervention (Figure 4-1) is demonstrated in Clinical Vignette #2 (Below).

Therapeutic herbal baths have been used throughout history in the care and treatment of the ill. They are a part of the therapeutic modality known as hydrotherapy, or water treatment that is discussed in greater detail in chapter 9. Baths can be taken by submerging the whole body or parts of the body, as in footbaths. Baths have a therapeutic effect on the circulation, the immune and nervous systems, the skin, and the whole person. The therapeutic potential of an herbal bath is determined by the duration and temperature of the bath, the herbs used in the bath, and the person's interest and desire for the modality. A footbath is essentially a water element application.

Clinical Vignette #2

Eloise is a 75-year-old woman whose feet and hands are always cold to the touch. She also "feels cold and achy" most of the time, even though she wears warm clothing and lives in a warm house. Eloise asks her visiting nurse, Ann, what she would recommend. Ann suggests a warm footbath with an herb, such as rosemary (Rosmarinus officinalis), that is energetically warming (Libster, 2012). She also recommends that they add Epsom salt. Eloise loves the taste and smell of rosemary. Eloise and Ann make a infusion, or tea, from the herb together by using rosemary that Eloise finds in the kitchen. After steeping the rosemary for 15 minutes, the nurse strains the infusion into a basin big enough to put Eloise's feet into and covers Eloise's shoulders with a warm blanket.

The elements represented in this intervention are: footbath (Water); rosemary inhalation (Air); Epsom salt (Earth); warm blanket and water (Fire); kindness – making remedy together (Ether).

FIGURE 4-1: HOW TO PREPARE A ROSEMARY FOOTBATH

Heat 2 oz. (50 g) of rosemary leaf in 1 quart (1 L) of water until the water boils, and then remove the pan from the heat. Cover the pan to retain the essential oils in the plant, and let the mixture steep for 15 minutes. Lift the cover and tap the water (which contains essential oil) accumulated on the lid so that it goes into the infusion. Strain the infusion into a container for the footbath, such as a rectangular dishpan. It is best to do this early in the day because rosemary can be very stimulating.

Evaluation

The integrative holistic nurse and the patient evaluate the progress toward the patient's health goals and make revisions as needed. The nurse also evaluates any changes in the patient's health pattern. For example, visiting nurse Ann would evaluate the warmth of Eloise's hands and feet by touching them. Ann would also ask about Eloise's perception of temperature and pain before and after the rosemary footbath. So much information about the patient's growth and development is gleaned by opening the dialogue to evaluate the patient's progress. Course corrections can be made immediately by nurses who are open and responsive to the patient's process.

Evaluation is also a part of the process when boundaries can be evaluated and reset. If the nurse – at some point in the process of developing the healing relationship – has seen to place his or her ideas for care before the patient's current, pressing concerns, then the care can be adjusted. Using interventions with patients that do not address their most important concerns typically do not "work." This principle holds true for biomedical care, such as surgery and drug treatment, as well. This phenomenon is not only a matter of belief or whether or not the patient trusts the caregiver. Trust is built when the nurse or caregiver trusts the patient to express his or her true needs in the moment and create the psychological-emotional-spiritual space for that action to occur.

Clinical Vignette #3

Barbara is a 45-year-old woman who had surgery to repair a hiatal hernia 1 year ago. Parish nurse Julie knew Barbara at church and noticed that she was becoming pale and had an ashen color over the course of a few weeks. They were talking at coffee hour and Julie said, "Barbara, I do not mean to intrude, but I notice that you seem a bit pale. Are you okay?" Barbara was surprised, smiled, and said, "How did you know? Can I talk with you?"

They made an appointment, during which Barbara revealed that she had a surgery a year ago but that the incision, which had removed her belly button, never fully healed and was dripping a few drops of blood every day. Barbara went to her physician, who told her that she had become anemic. The recommendation was to return to her surgeon. Barbara told Julie that she had seen the surgeon, who said that the plan was to open the incision and resuture it. Barbara did not believe that "doing the same thing again would solve the problem."

Julie and Barbara talked about what Barbara wanted to do to heal the wound. Julie provided an imagery session with Barbara in which Barbara had perceived some images of medicinal plants. Julie and Barbara talked about the plants that Barbara described from her imagery. Julie suggested that Barbara read about the use of some of the herbs, which she knew, on the wound. Barbara also had some insights during the imagery session about her belly button and the significance of the removal of it during the surgery. They were directly related to the transitions and transformations she was going through in her life. The wound that had not healed in a year was closed and healed within a week of the session and applying the herbs. Barbara and Julie both experienced the beauty and power of the inner healer in Barbara. Julie was the midwife for the birth of that experience.

There is no requirement in the AHNA *Scope and Standards* for an integrative holistic nurse to employ one or any number of complementary therapies. Provision 2 of the American Nurses Association (ANA) *Code of Ethics for Nurses* states that the nurse's primary commitment is to the patient, whether an individual, family, group or community" (ANA, 2010). As Clinical Vignette #3 demonstrates, complementary therapies that are chosen in congruence with patient's current need can really "work." By modeling the patient's world, the nurse understands the best approach for the patient. The next step after modeling is *role-modeling*. The term is used differently in nursing theory than in common use, where it means "to demonstrate for another." Role-modeling in holistic integrative nursing care is the "facilitation of the individual in attaining, maintaining, or promoting health through purposeful interventions" (Erickson, Tomlin, & Swain, 1983, p. 95). Role-modeling in nursing requires unconditional and nonjudgmental acceptance of the person during the process of nurturing and supporting their growth and development that occurs within the patient's model.

Discernment

How does a nurse choose which remedies, therapies, or treatments to provide or recommend for a patient? Much of the time, those decisions are the patient's. Patients may ask the nurse for advice or support, which then means that the nurse must have an understanding of the patient's worldview and health beliefs as well as their own knowledge of the therapy. The choice of modalities is still very much a creative process. It is also a scientific process. There are five general categories of complementary therapies that nurses have known historically as nursing "fundamentals": touch, environment, nutrition, communication, and energy (Libster, 2001). Examples of modalities from these five areas are included and highlighted in the remaining chapters of this text. Some may be familiar and others not so familiar, but all five areas have been foundational to nursing practice for centuries. New modalities, such as new drugs or biomedical treatments, emerge from time to time. The number of treatment options can be overwhelming. So, how does a person know what to do? Some people, given their beliefs, just eliminate all that does not concur with those beliefs. Some dabble endlessly without discrimination and end up exhausted physically, emotionally, energetically, and financially, when they need their energy for healing a serious concern.

Nurses are often called upon by people in their communities to help them sort out their options and make tough decisions. The integrative holistic nursing process is particularly helpful to nurses who would be those guides in times of great need. In 1633 in France, when the Daughters of Charity were first being sent out into the community to minister to the sick poor, they asked Vincent de Paul, one of their spiritual leaders, how they would know what to do, what treatment to suggest, what care to provide, and whom to treat first. Hundreds of people were in need at the time, and they were overwhelming the city streets. Vincent gave a teaching that actually resonates with some of the instruction given today to nurses. Vincent taught that *discernment* was a three-part process: unrestricted readiness, weighing the evidence, and taking counsel (Libster & McNeil, 2009, p. 38). "Unrestricted readiness" for these early nurses meant that they would pray for understanding of God's will and not impose their own agenda when caring for others. It was in the state of readiness that the nurse would be able to weigh the evidence of a given situation. Seeking wise counsel was also helpful in discerning the best course of action. This Vincentian process of discernment is similar in many respects to evidence-based practice. Through the process of discernment, applying cultural diplomacy and a person-centered, relationship-centered approach, integrative holistic nurses become "ready." They become willing to hear about a patient's self-cares and health beliefs, traditional ways of healing, and complementary therapies that they may be engaged in or wish to explore. They do so without imposing their own religious, spiritual, personal, or professional views in such a way as to manipulate a patient at a moment of change, transition, and transformation.

Clinical Vignette #4

Monica is a 23-year-old newlywed from the Netherlands who is living with her husband, an American, in the United States. She is 2 months pregnant and experiencing extreme hyperemesis. Joan, the home care nurse, visits Monica and starts an intravenous (IV) line to give her some fluids. After she starts the IV and gives Monica some medication, Joan asks Monica a solution-focused question. "Is there one food that you can think of that you could possibly hold down?" Monica says, "Yes, but, ..." She seems shy to answer, but Joan shows authentic interest, so Monica continues. "Well, you might think it is funny, but there is a food that my mother used to make for me back home in Amsterdam when I was child whenever I was sick." That food was mashed potatoes with wilted lettuce. Joan had never had that food, and it really did not sound appetizing to her, but she joyfully made it for Monica. The potatoes and lettuce were in the kitchen. Monica was so fatigued that Joan made her the potatoes to order. Because Monica had already received fluids and the medication, the timing was perfect to try to eat her favorite comfort food, just like her mother used to make. Monica ate a whole bowl and kept it down. She continued to improve after that important moment she said that she really felt the importance of becoming the mom to her own baby.

Safety Considerations

Patients and nurses exercise discernment about which therapies and remedies to use in care. Safety considerations also need to be taken into account as to when, where, and how a modality (remedy or therapy) should be applied at any given time, and the frequency, duration, or amount of the modality. Each and every decision point requires discernment. Some modalities require additional years of study and separate licensure. Some require continuing education or apprenticeships. Other actions associated with the Elements of Care® of integrative holistic nursing are simpler, subtler, and require, for the most part, additional thought. For example, a nurse working in a hospital might provide a warm blanket for someone who is cold after surgery, understanding the importance of vitality and warmth to patient progress and survival. The safe application of therapies is imperative, but the risk of safety to patients is also a matter of degree. Nurses assess the risk of therapeutic interventions, such as in the area of touch, where there may be different risks associated with holding a patient's hand as they walk down a hallway versus offering healing touch session to a patient undergoing chemotherapy.

There is also risk to the process of creative blending of caring modalities with biomedical care that is integrative holistic nursing. Safety and risk assessment includes evaluation of the appropriateness of the modality for the patient, the knowledge and experience of the nurse with the modality, and the context in which it is to be applied. This assessment includes knowledge of the other modalities that a patient is engaged in, and it also involves knowledge of the health beliefs that are associated with that modality so as not to introduce a culture clash when offering choices of modalities or referring to others. Withholding judgment about a modality that a patient is engaged in is important to the development of trust in a healing relationship. It is important to assess patient health patterns and then study the modalities in question from a scientific, traditional, and integrative perspective before rendering an opinion about the match. Think about the 3 T's of timing, type, and tuning (Libster, 2003) guiding the discernment process. *Timing* is the process in which the patient and nurse explore whether or not a therapy should be used at all, used simultaneously, or staggered over time. In Clinical Vignette #4, for example, the risk was very low that the food chosen to address Monica's nutrition concern would be a safety risk to her or her baby. It also was a nutrition intervention (potatoes and lettuce) that had no known risk when given with the antiemetic drug or IV fluids. Integrative holistic nurses need discernment of the *"type"* of therapy or remedy that would be most safe and of less risk to the patient by pacing with the patient, modeling their world and their health beliefs. *Tuning* is similar to dose but applied to all nursing cares and complementary therapies. For example, infant massage instructors teach parents to watch their babies for nonverbal cues of readiness when they are considering massage for them.

Biomedical care is often done to a patient. Complementary therapies can also be done to a patient. Attention to the 3 T's helps the nurse focus on the patient's process of integration and creative blending of cares as well as what the product or outcome of care will be. The energy and impetus for integration come from the heart, rather than the ego. When a patient is in imminent danger, it is the best time and type of care to prescribe interventions and employ them, sometimes without discussion (as in the case of an unresponsive patient). Nurses, in their heart of hearts, know when to act for someone (as in emergency situations). But nurses engaged with patients for most other health decisions that do not involve crisis or emergency response can take the time to do a proper assessment and work through the nursing process mindfully (Chapter 6).

HOLISTIC TRANSFORMATION

- *What new ideas do I have for accenting the nursing process in my caring practice?*
- *What modalities do I currently use in nursing practice from a biomedical view?*
- *What modalities do I currently use in nursing practice from an integrative nursing view?*

SUMMARY

The AHNA *Scope and Standards* has no requirement for an integrative holistic nurse to employ one or any number of complementary therapies. Nurses begin with the patient's understanding of the modality and may become educators, clinicians, and researchers as to how that modality might become an integrated part of the plan of care for that person. Nurses have a responsibility to know the safety of a modality and to learn about it as thoroughly as they would any other treatment in nursing. If and when warranted, nurses modify and adapt that modality to the unique needs of the patient and their health patterns. Integrative holistic nurses use the nursing process when applying the modalities that are described in this text and beyond. Integrative holistic nursing involves discernment at each stage of the nursing process.

REFERENCES

American Holistic Nurses Association. (2018). *Holistic nursing: Scope and standards.* Silver Spring, MD: American Holistic Nurses Association and American Nurses Association.

American Nurses Association. (2010 reissue). In Fowler, M. D. M. (Ed.), *Guide to the code of ethics for nurses: Interpretation and application.* Silver Spring, MD: American Nurses Association. Retrieved from http://www.nursesbooks.org.

Cowling, W. R. (2000). Healing as appreciating wholeness. *Advances in Nursing Science,* 22(3), 16-32.

Erickson, H. C., Tomlin, E. M., & Swain, M. A. P. (1983). *Modeling and role-modeling.* Englewood Cliffs, NJ: Prentice-Hall.

Franklin, C., Zhang, A., Froerer, A., & Johnson, S. (2016). Solution focused brief therapy: A systematic review and meta-summary of process research. *Journal of Marital and Family Therapy*, 43(1), 16-30.

Hall, L. (1964). Nursing: What is it? *The Canadian Nurse*, 60(2), 150-153.

Libster, M. (2001). *Demonstrating care: The art of integrative nursing.* Albany, NY: Delmar Cengage Learning.

Libster, M. (2003). Integrative care – Product and process: Considering the three T's of timing, type, and tuning [Guest Editorial]. *Complementary Therapies in Nursing & Midwifery*, 9(1), 1-4.

Libster, M. (2012). *The nurse herbalist: Integrative insights for holistic practice.* Wauwatosa, WI: Golden Apple Publications.

Libster, M. M., & McNeil, B. A. (2009). *Enlightened charity: The holistic care, education and "Advices Concerning the Sick" of Sister Matilda Coskery (1799-1870).* Wauwatosa, WI: Golden Apple Publications.

Newman, M. (1994). *Health as expanding consciousness.* New York, NY: National League for Nursing Press.

Nolan, M. R., Davies, S., Brown, J., Keady, J., & Nolan, J. (2004). Beyond person-centred care: A new vision for gerontological nursing. *Journal of Clinical Nursing,* 13(3a), 45-53.

Peplau, H. E. (1952). *Interpersonal relations in nursing: A conceptual frame of reference for psychodynamic nursing.* New York, NY: G. P. Putnam's Sons.

Walter, J., & Peller, J. (1992). *Becoming solution-focused in brief therapy.* New York, NY: Brunner/Mazel Publishers.

CHAPTER 5

PAIN RELIEF AND COMFORT: NONPHARMACOLOGICAL INTERVENTIONS

LEARNING OUTCOME

After completing this chapter, the learner will be able to explain the role of integrative care in pain relief and comfort with nonpharmacological interventions.

CHAPTER OBJECTIVES

After completing this chapter, the learner will be able to:
1. Discuss the differences between approaching pain relief in terms of either reductionism or holism.
2. Explain the placebo effect.
3. Summarize the role of stress relief in pain relief and comfort.
4. Identify the nature of pain and at least one nonpharmacological intervention for each of the five Elements of Care®.
5. Describe the Freeze-Frame technique.

INTRODUCTION

Plato once said, "The cause of many diseases is unknown to the physicians of Hellas because they are ignorant of the whole. For the part can never be well unless the whole is well." The knowledge of the whole is nowhere more important than in the care of those in pain. Pain is the most common reason for seeking medical care and the most common reason people use complementary therapies (National Center for Complementary and Integrative Health, 2022). Millions of tax dollars are spent each year funding research into solutions for treating chronic pain in particular (National Center for Complementary and Integrative Health, 2022). To provide integrative holistic nursing support for those seeking pain relief and comfort, nurses begin modeling the whole person and think about role-modeling a plan of care that will address the patient's present concerns with meaningful solutions.

Patients, caregivers, and researchers seek the simplest solutions to alleviating a person's pain. Some drugs, such as opiates and opioids, relieve pain very well, but not without significant risk to the person and communities. This chapter is about solutions that, in general, carry low risk compared with pharmacological methods. To offer integrative holistic nursing with nonpharmacological complementary therapies and self-care suggestions to relieve pain and offer comfort to the whole patient, consider the five Elements of Care®. The five elements position integrative holistic nursing interventions within the professional scope of nursing practice. The reason this is necessary to differentiate is because complementary therapies are practiced by other clinicians who are not nurses. Nurses who practice complementary therapies do so first within their license to practice as a nurse. This chapter and the remaining chapters on modalities will apply the five elements and accents to integrative holistic practice. This chapter, and the remaining chapters in Part II, discuss modalities for health patterns in general, but the responsibility still lies with the discerning nurse caregiver to adapt and apply the information presented to each individual patient, family, or community.

A PATH BEYOND DISEASE AND CURE

The goal and the values of those offering biomedical care, referred to in some nations' health systems as *allopathy*, is the removal of a symptom causing distress, discomfort, or pain. For example, when someone is bleeding profusely, the bleeding must be stopped. The action of stopping bleeding is an example of allopathy. Direct pressure and elevation can stop bleeding, as can some medications. Registered nurses (RNs) know that within the scope of professional practice, they can perform first aid to stop bleeding, and they are legally bound to do so. Prescribing pharmacological medication is not within the RN's scope of practice. The same principles of discernment regarding scope of practice are applied with complementary therapies. The following is some practice background information regarding nursing practice and complementary therapies for pain relief and comfort and any other health pattern:

1. Integrative holistic nursing is a worldview, or philosophy of care. A nurse can practice from an integrative holistic philosophy and not use complementary therapies.
2. Nurses are responsible for being educated in the modalities of their choice for use in practice. If a modality is licensed in a state, a nurse may be required to obtain separate licensure. For example, nurses are licensed to touch and therefore are not typically required to obtain massage licenses to provide massage to patients. However, nurses who promote their massage skills to the public must be educated and skilled in the modality.
3. Nurses who provide complementary therapies to patients may in some states be able to receive training in their chosen complementary therapies for continuing education credit.

4. Prelicensure nursing education typically focuses on specialties that originate with the biomedical model's focus on disease and cure.

Study and practice of integrative holistic nursing provides a path for expansion beyond the biomedical focus on disease and cure. The health belief underlying allopathic biomedical care is the philosophy of "one cause, one cure." This view, often referred to as *reductionism* (in which a person's problems are reduced to a cause and cure of a single body part or system), can be traced back to the colonial period and physicians, such as Benjamin Rush, who trained in European medicine. Rush told his students in 1796, "Be not startled, gentlemen; follow me and I will say there is but one disease in the world. The one disease was a 'morbid excitement induced by capillary tension' and it had but one remedy" (Starr, 1982, p. 42). For this, Rush and his students used "heroic therapies": bloodletting until a person was unconscious and powerful emetics and cathartics, such as calomel (mercurous chloride), until the person was salivating excessively. The belief was that every health problem could be reduced to one primary cause and that there was one cure, heroics, that would help in all cases. This view may be the wish of many who are suffering and in pain.

A desire to remove pain immediately is a natural human response. Numerous studies, a sampling of which are highlighted in this text, demonstrate that using a one cause, one cure approach requires serious reform. A major healthcare reform movement has already begun to address what is being described as a "rapidly evolving public health crisis" (National Institutes of Health, 2022) in that an estimated 25 million people suffer from chronic pain and 2 million Americans are addicted to opioids (National Institutes of Health, 2022). The number of drug overdoses is alarming. Nurses, clinicians, and the public and its representatives are now questioning the use of opiates and opioids and seeking effective and accessible alternatives.

Opiates is a term that has been used traditionally to describe natural drugs derived from poppies *(Papaver somniferum)*. Examples are morphine, oxycodone, and heroin (which is illegal). *Opioids* are synthetic and semisynthetic pain-relieving medications, such as fentanyl. The terms have often been used interchangeably; but the National Institutes of Health uses the term *"opioid"* now in reference to the current public health crisis. *Opioid* is the term that will be used here for ease of reading. The focus of this chapter on integrative holistic nursing is nonpharmacological interventions that provide, directly or indirectly, pain relief and comfort. These interventions may be complementary to biomedical treatments, such as drugs and surgery, or they may be alternatives to biomedical treatments.

The concern and question of most people in the biomedical culture is whether these interventions actually "work." The risk cited with complementary therapies for pain relief and comfort, especially in the case of chronic pain, is that they may not be effective, may be costly, and may delay biomedical treatment (National Center for Complementary and Integrative Health, 2022). The science community is often concerned about a placebo effect from complementary and traditional healing modalities.

The word *placebo* comes from the Latin psalm verse, *'placebo Domino in regione vivorum'* (Psalm 116:6): "I shall please the Lord in the land of the living" (Walach & Jonas, 2004). This psalm was typically sung as part of someone's death rites; however, it gets its meaning from the practice of some people, who would fraudulently pay others to do the singing. Placebo emerged in the 18th and 19th centuries in medicine in such forms as sugar pills or colored water when physicians had no idea what to prescribe (Elliott, 2016). Placebo *treatment* was common by the 20th century. In the 1930s, researchers of the randomized controlled trial began to design studies to compare a drug intervention to placebo – but that was after they realized that the powerful effects of so many effective treatments were inexplicable. By the 1950s, the "placebo effect," viewed as an "unreal" effect or "no effect," had been found to be 32% effective (Elliott, 2016). Placebo was examined within the context of knowledge of self-limited disease. An example of this approach is giving a medication to someone with a common cold on day 7 of the cold when they would be expected to be feeling better already without intervention. If the person has no more cold symptoms on day 8 after receiving medication, was the relief because of the medication or because of the placebo effect (i.e., the nature of self-limited disease)?

Placebos are known to work as a result of people's beliefs. Holistic nurses who model someone's world will know very quickly what beliefs are involved in the effects of complementary therapies and self-care. In the vignette from Chapter 4 about the woman with hyperemesis, the effect of the mashed potatoes with lettuce could be the placebo effect. It did not seem that the woman's emesis was going away, and she did keep the potatoes down. The comfort food also had deep meaning for the patient. The holistic nurse would not judge, critique, or interfere with the process, let alone question the validity of the successful response in front of the patient.

Biological hypotheses for the placebo effect have been studied and clearly explain the human response. The placebo effect is thought to be correlated with increases in neural activity in areas of the brain linked with reward/aversion and anticipation systems before pain reduction, suggesting that pain reduction was instigated by an expectation response that also stimulates dopamine and serotonin release (Elliott, 2016). Medical science acknowledges that placebo provides information that may be critical to our understanding of how the mind and body heal. According to Walach & Jonas (2004):

> This has fueled a debate and obscured the real issue, namely, whether psychologic processes and social contexts that facilitate hope, expectation, positive feelings, relief of anxiety and anticipation of improvement are able to truly affect physiologic processes and contribute to healing over and above pharma-cologically mediated processes. (p. S103)

The newer definition typically ascribed to today is the "effect that is due to the meaning of a therapeutic intervention for a particular patient and context" (Walach & Jonas, 2004, p. S104). Therefore, the context of the healing environment becomes a critical component in health and healing and as a "powerful antidote to illness" that is nonspecific and relieves multiple conditions (Brown, 1998). It is important to remember that biomedical cures, such as therapeutics, medications, and surgeries, are as much a part of the placebo effect and placebo ethics debate as are healing traditions and complementary therapies. There are so many unknowns in medical science that both clinicians and patients alike are willing to overlook when chronic, intractable pain is the issue. Integrative holistic nurses are perfectly positioned to offer the Elements of Care® to make the healing environment with their patients that can be powerful antidotes to illness and potent pain relievers. Although some seek cause and cure, nurses make tremendous impact with healing environments (see Chapters 9-13) that reduce patient stress and allow nature to effect a cure with the Elements of Care®.

STRESS RELIEF

Stress relief plays an important role in pain relief and comfort as well as health and disease. Hungarian endocrinologist Hans Selye wrote *Stress in Health and Disease* in 1976. He defined stress as "the nonspecific response of the body to any demand" (p. 15). There are three phases of the general adaptation syndrome: alarm reaction, stage of resistance, and stage of exhaustion. How a person perceives change within or without, such as alarms or triggers, plays a major role in adaptation and stress response. Nurses realize that minimizing patient "fight-or-flight" response, the term coined by physiologist Walter Cannon, promotes health and well-being. Selye acknowledges that stress is part of our daily experience as human beings, but that it also is associated with surgical trauma, burns, emotional arousal, mental and physical effort, fatigue, fear, frustration, loss of blood, intoxication, environmental pollutants, and pain (1976, p. 14). Stress cannot be avoided, and therefore pain and discomfort cannot be avoided.

Selye and others recognized the homeostatic mechanisms in the body that work to create balance and "normality" as the status quo. Homeostasis is a word that is derived from two Greek words: *homeo* (meaning the same), and *stasis* (meaning standing still). Homeostasis is regulated by the nervous and endocrine systems. The notion that the body-mind-spirit can actually achieve homeostasis and return to its previous state is questionable. The Adaptive Calibration Model, however, a theory of stress based on evolutionary and developmental biology, suggests otherwise. The model "assumes that individual differences in stress response are mainly the result of conditional adaptation ... this model includes the body's ability to use the acquired information from stressful situations for adaptive processing of developmental changes" (Tonhajzerova & Mestanik, 2017).

Allostasis, from the Greek words meaning unstable and mutable, is the process of achieving stability *through* physiological and behavioral adaptation to change. It includes the adaptive effect of learning. Psychological allostasis in which a person exhibits tolerance of stress conditions is termed *resilience*. *Vulnerability* is a tendency toward disruption of adaptive processes. Frequent or continual activation of the allostatic process is referred to as allostatic *load*. In essence, people have the ability to learn and develop, and that is a powerful mechanism for dealing with the stress of change, transition, and transformation in body-mind-spirit. Much of this foundational knowledge for learning from stress comes from research in biological and physiological science. The scholar Rupert Sheldrake (1995), for example, has published extensively on *morphic resonance*, the understanding that past patterns of activity influence the patterns of similar systems in a cumulative fashion. Nursing science and practice also contribute to the understanding that human beings learn and adapt to stress as they create their environment, a symbolic expression of system wholeness (Neuman & Fawcett, 2011; Roy, 2008).

Healing as change involves stress. Holistic nurses can engage patients' perceptions of their stressors and shape, if not reframe, those perceptions through the healing and learning experiences that are nursing care. The *Healing Relationship Model* represents the healing, learning, and growing experience of the patient and their nurse caregiver as a double helix (see Figure 5-1). A helix, as opposed to a line, circle, or spiral, demonstrates learning and growth over time. For example, a patient who walks for the first time after surgery may only walk a short distance, feeling little pain and fatigue. The next day, she increases her distance but goes a bit too far, feeling pain and shortness of breath. In thinking about what happened, the patient spirals back (thinks back) on her experience, what she has learned, and how she has adapted. Much of the process may not even be conscious until the nurse reflects on her behaviors. The next day, the patient does not walk

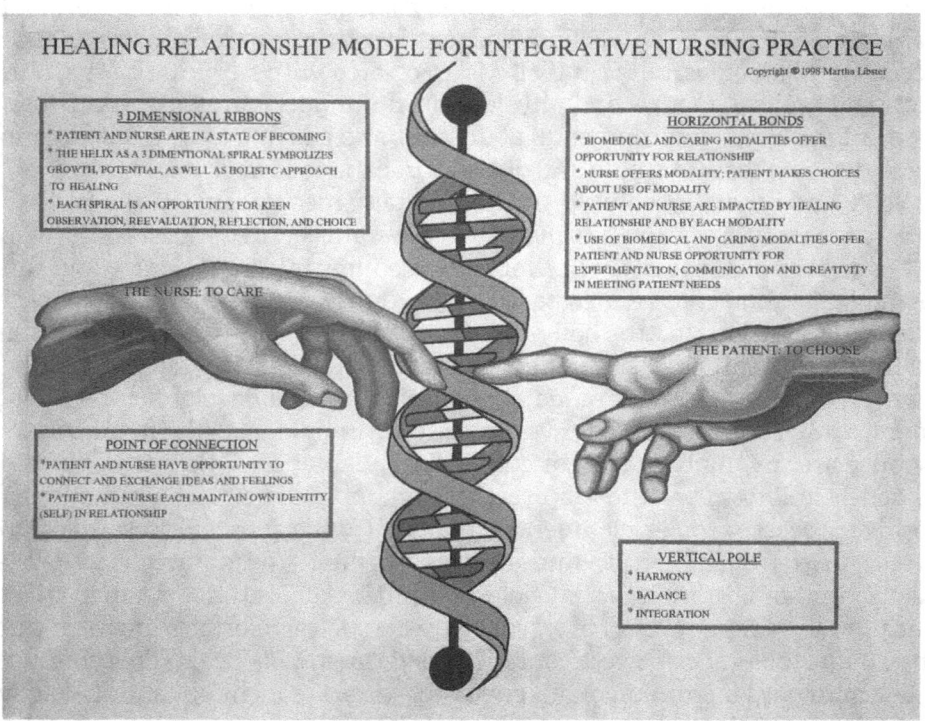

FIGURE 5-1: © 1998 Martha M. Libster

walk quite as far and experiences improvement. The multidimensional, vertically expanded helix is a visual expression of how patients and their caregivers grow and evolve in understanding each person's unique perceptions of stress, change, transition, and transformation that is foundational to the process of healing (Libster, 2001).

Maintaining a "normal steady state by physiologic means" in which the interior environment is passive (1976, p. 31). Drug treatments are so often merciful, especially during crisis. However, while taking medications, people may not develop the insight that they need to grow and develop as a result of what they have learned from their experience of pain and suffering. Alternatively, focusing on the present moment, as will be discussed in further detail in Chapter 6 on mindfulness practice, and learning new coping strategies that address the challenges of the present moment, are effective in supporting physical, mental, emotional, and spiritual adaptation responses and the allostasis associated with change, transition, and transformation.

Complementary therapies support allostasis. The purpose of complementary therapies is to help a person to learn about self and promote adaptation and healing. Stress reduction, although it sounds like a great idea, is only one dimension. Like biomedical reductionism, stress reduction suggests that there is one cause and one cure to stress. The stressor is environmental (outside the patient), and the patient simply has to reduce interaction with that stressor. For example, it is true that if a person is stressed from not sleeping because of construction noise outside their bedroom window, elimination of the noise most likely will reduce the stress response and increase sleep. The complementary therapies nurses provide in holistic practice often focus directly on moving the patient toward solutions for increasing adaptation of internal responses *and* decreasing interactions with external stressors.

Selye used the word *heterostasis* to describe establishment of a "steady state by treatment with agents that stimulate the physiologic adaptive mechanisms" (p. 31). During the process of heterostasis, the body resets the "thermostat of resistance to a heightened defensive capacity by artificial interventions from the outside" (p. 31). Heterostasis strengthens the body's own natural and nonspecific defenses. Sigmund Freud suffered for years from jaw cancer and many operations. When he was asked how he dealt with the physical pain, he is commonly quoted as saying, he worked to surround his pain with *tranquility*.

In seeking tranquility, or whatever they may call their coping with the stress and pain response, people manage not only the physical experience of stress and pain but also manage their perceptions of pain, their feelings about the pain, and their beliefs about the pain experience. Stress is an actual phenomenon, the manifestation of which is largely determined by the person experiencing it. Stress can inspire creativity and good works. But excessive stress as an effect of overactivity of the sympathetic nervous system can produce physical, psychological, emotional, social, economic, political, and spiritual imbalance and distress. The wide-ranging effects of stress make it a foundational concern when seeking to understand how to approach pain relief and comfort holistically.

The following list includes types of stress and what they have been linked to:
- **Physical stress:** Heart attack, angina, physical illnesses, open wounds, peptic ulcers, and motor vehicle and other accidents
- **Psychological stress:** Overthinking, education
- **Emotional stress:** Emotional imbalance, panic attacks, depression, psychosis, and eating disorders
- **Social stress:** Group crises, dysfunctional families, family role crises, sociopathy, and homelessness
- **Economic stress:** Inability to pay bills, loss of job or house, bankruptcy, and budget crises
- **Political stress:** Job politics, elections, management, power, arrogant bosses, ineffective employees, political statements, riots, and wars
- **Spiritual stress:** Love, religious conflict, loneliness, and loss of faith

The American Psychological Association focuses on the length of stress, making generalizations about the differences between acute and chronic stress, such as "Because it is short term, acute stress doesn't have enough time to do the extensive damage associated with long-term stress" (American Psychological Association, 2018). Nurses, who work closely with patients, may find this view wide of the mark. For example, an acute stress, such as acute illness and hospitalization of an infant, can have a long-lasting effect on an infant's growth and development. In some infants, that acute period of stress can, in fact, do extensive damage, not just to the infant but to the family as well. Nursing care should be individualized for those in distress so that care will meet their unique needs for stress, pain relief, and comfort (Tonhajzerova & Mestanik, 2017).

ELEMENTS AND REMEDIES

Numerous complementary therapies and combinations of complementary therapies are nonpharmacological interventions considered by holistic nurses for inclusion in the care of those seeking pain relief and comfort. The remainder of this chapter utilizes the Elements of Care® as a guide for highlighting the nature of five different types of pain and examples of remedies and complementary therapies that might be used for pain relief and comfort for a person experiencing each type. Helping patients to cope with and learn from stress utilizing nonpharmacological complementary therapies and remedies nourishes body, mind, emotions, relationships, and spirit. The complementary therapies included here are just a few examples. Read through these examples using the five elements as a guide for producing a holistic plan of care for pain relief and comfort. Then think about the remedies and complementary therapies that you have used to relieve pain and provide comfort for yourself and others. You will have an opportunity to reflect on your favorite choices of remedies and therapies in the Holistic Transformation section at the end of the chapter.

Earth Element (Physical Pain and Suffering)

The earth element is associated with the physical dimension. The nature of physical pain is suffering. Suffering is a human experience. People suffer in public or private, but when they signal distress through facial cues and sounds, nurses (and others inclined to care) respond. "Suffering is a shared experience and in this light is contagious ... we are moved to assist" (Morse, 2000, p. 5). When suffering is experienced physically, a person is in discomfort. One of the major goals of integrative holistic nursing is to assist the patient in finding pain relief and comfort through self-soothing self-care practices and engagement with those in the healing arts that offer remedies for easing suffering.

Hope for healing as the alleviation of suffering and pain is universal. Remedies for physical suffering exist in all healthcare cultures. Biomedical cures such as surgery and pharmaceutical drugs can ease physical pain and suffering. The healing traditions discussed in Chapter 3 all focus on the relief of human suffering as well. Complementary therapies and self-care offer a patient an opportunity for engagement in choosing and designing care that alleviates suffering and pain. These therapies can be prescribed by a nurse, but this intention of telling people what to do (i.e., prescribing) is the practice of *medicine*. Integrative holistic nurses (including Advanced Practice Integrative Holistic Nurse prescribers) who follow the nursing process utilizing integrative holistic nursing theories – such as modeling and role-modeling – first honor the inherent wisdom of the patient by offering choices of complementary therapies and self-care as they plan care with patients before considering prescribing *for* the patient

The first step is recognizing that the patient is sending a signal of suffering. All patients of every age, infants to elders, experience stress, distress, pain, and suffering. Scientific and ethical debate as to whether infants in the womb feel pain is ongoing (Derbyshire, 2006). The cues and signals of suffering are different for infants than they are for children and adults. Researchers often use videotape of infants to capture their behavioral cues that might signal suffering. For example, Solberg and Morse (as cited in Morse, 2000) found that because the hard cry of infants who are intubated after major chest or abdominal surgery is silent, nurses' comfort actions were absent.

This author worked in a renowned children's hospital in the 1980s and witnessed surgeons who would prescribe no pain medication or Tylenol for infants who had open chest surgeries. When asked for an order for pain medication, the surgeons would ask how the nurses knew that the babies were in pain. The nurses often taught the surgical residents about infant behavior and cues of suffering. One example is the infant who is sleeping fairly soundly with respirations that are even and regular. Then, suddenly, the infant shakes and awakens without any environmental stimulus and begins deep cries. After the infant receives medication, the sudden shake-wake does not occur, and the baby sleeps.

Seminal nursing research on comfort by Morse (1992) has demonstrated the challenges nurses face in providing comfort for patients:

Because of the acute care and curing orientation of the hospital, nursing comfort tasks are devalued and regarded by patients as nontechnical, ordinary, kind, and helpful (but not essential or critical for cure). Thus, the comfort work becomes invisible, despite its therapeutic indications, and when nurses are busy, comfort work receives a lower priority in the work schedule than medical or mechanical tasks. (p. 99)

Pain Measures

Pain scales are effective in helping patients to measure and monitor changes in their behaviors. The experience of pain can be so debilitating for people that they become unable to think well and process things, let alone track their changes and improvements that result from interventions. Therefore, the holistic nurse's presence and feedback act as a guide for evaluation as well as shared decision making about the effectiveness of care.

The simplest scale to use is a Likert or Visual Analog Scale. The nurse asks the patient to rate their experience of pain on a scale of 1 to 5 or 1 to 10, with zero being no pain. The response is recorded so that the pattern can be shown to the patient over time as feedback about the plan of care. If the patient has any pain, a follow-up question is then offered that can move the patient toward constructing creative solutions. That question, based in solution-focused counseling technique (Strong, Pyle, & Sutherland, 2009), invites the patient to identify one thing they can do next in their care that will take them one step, or even a half step, closer to zero pain. For example, if the patient rated pain as 9 on a 10-point scale, the follow-up question would be, "What one thing can you do next that will bring your pain to a 7 or an 8?" The numbers provide a framework, a mutual language, for the nurse and the patient to use to discuss the patient's subjective experience. A patient might say, "I need to get some extra sleep this weekend," or "I need to swim more." The nurse who is modeling the patient then role-models a plan of care that incorporates the particulars of what the patient envisioned. The nurse would clarify what the patient means by "extra" sleep or "more" swimming and then follow up with the patient at the next visit, asking if the goal that they set for themselves to lower their pain scale by a half step was achieved.

Remedy to Alleviate Physical Pain and Suffering

Herbal remedies can be used topically to relieve physical pain very effectively. Numerous over the counter and home herbal remedies, such as capsaicin cream and ginger *(Zingiber officinale),* relieve pain. Some types of pain respond better to warm applications and some to cold applications. Ginger and capsaicin are both warm applications.

Capsaicin is a constituent in cayenne pepper *(Capsicum frutescens)*. Its mechanism of action for pain relief is to reduce the amount of substance P, a neurotransmitter, that is known to deplete serotonin. Substance P also is a mediator of inflammation in the skin (McCarty, Csuka, McCarthy, & Trotter, 1994).

Common ginger root *(Zingiber officinale)* has been relieving pain for centuries. Traditionally, ginger compresses (Figure 5-2) are used to warm the body and therefore would be used for cold pain. Ginger also is a stimulant, anti-inflammatory, and analgesic that, when applied topically as a warm compress to the kidney area on the back, has a deep, penetrating relaxation effect for the whole body (Therkleson, 2010).

FIGURE 5-2: RECIPE FOR GINGER COMPRESS FOR PAIN

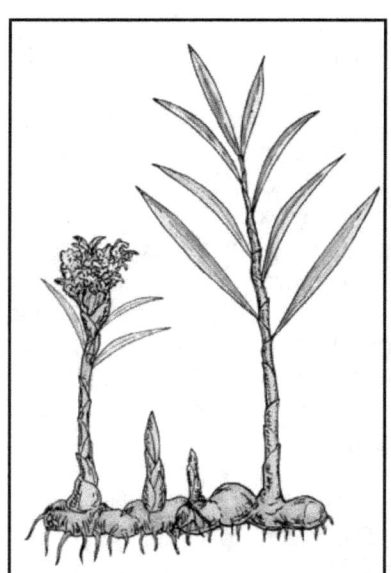

First, prepare the ginger root decoction. Grate 4 to 5 ounces (150 g) of fresh ginger root. Put the ginger into a small cloth bag and add it to 1 gallon (3.8 L) of simmering (not boiling) water. Allow the decoction to steep gently for 5 minutes.

Then prepare and apply the compress. Holding both ends of a cotton hand-size towel (the compress), dip the middle into the ginger water. Wring it out, and place it over the patient's midback where the kidneys are. Touch the skin lightly to make sure that the patient tolerates the level of heat before fully placing the compress. The compress should be applied as hot as is tolerated. Place a dry towel over the compress and then a blanket over that towel, tucking each layer around the patient so that air does not enter the compress and cool it down. Prepare a second compress in the same way as the first. Replace the first compress after 3 to 4 minutes. To replace the compress: Fold the blanket and dry towel away from the kidney area. Place the second hot ginger compress on top of the first and flip the compress over, again making sure that the temperature is tolerated. Remove the first compress from the back to be prepared again in the hot ginger decoction. This technique ensures that the connection between the patient's back and the ginger moist heat compress is maintained. Tuck the dry towel and blanket back in place as the replacement compress is prepared. The compresses should be flipped every 3 to 4 minutes for 20 minutes. The ginger compress will create increased circulation (redness). It decreases pain, inflammation, and stiffness. Ginger compresses are too warming and should not be used when high fever is present, on the head area, on the abdomen during pregnancy, or for infants or the elderly.

Air Element (Psychological Pain and Perception)

The air element is associated with the psychological dimension. The nature of psychological pain is perception. Psychological factors in the perception and response to pain and its treatment include cultural background, previous experience, social environment, attitudes, expectations, gender, personality, and beliefs. Pain as a complex process includes cognitive dimensions that are related to physical effects. Mental stress, for example, involves "exhilarating or aggressive reactions associated with increased norepinephrine excretion" (Selye, 1976, p. 104).

Psychological processes influence the gating mechanisms involved in the pain response discussed in gate control theory. *Gate control theory* suggests that non-painful input closes the "gate" in the nervous system that is open to painful input, thereby preventing pain perception. Activities such as touch, pressure, and vibration excite inhibitory cells, thereby inhibiting transmission cell activity, with the result of feeling or perceiving less pain. Gate control theory suggests that activation of nerves that do not transmit pain signals (called nonnociceptive fibers) interfere with signals from pain fibers, thereby inhibiting pain. Effective remedies for psychological pain address perception of the pain that is experienced physically.

Patients who utilize complementary therapies and remedies can exhibit an increase in their sense of empowerment through the process of choosing those remedies and assigning the timing of remedies in dealing with their pain. Engagement decreases pain and increases the learning experience. Patient-controlled analgesia is a familiar example. Nurses are also adept at helping patients with their coping and communication skills, both important interventions for psychological pain relief and comfort (Field & Adams, 2001).

Biofeedback

One complementary therapy that is highly effective for psychological pain is biofeedback. Biofeedback is a process that "enables a person to learn how to change physiological activity for the purposes of improving health and performance" (Biofeedback Certification International Alliance, 2018). Biofeedback utilizes precise measuring devices that monitor physiological activity, such as heart function, breathing, skin temperature, muscle activity, and brain waves. Holistic nurses may use pulse oximetry and blood pressure and heart rate monitors (such as smart watches and fitness bands) as indicators of physiological changes or responses to stress.

To demonstrate the level of stress that people have, nurses may offer inexpensive biofeedback stress dots at health fairs (Figure 5-3). These dots are made of heat-sensitive material that changes with skin temperature. A tense, stressed state is associated with cold extremities, and warmth is associated with relaxation. When the device demonstrates to the user that the user is tense or stressed, nurses give the users a relaxation strategy or series of exercises that they can do to increase relaxation and thereby improve blood flow. The feedback that the nurse identifies with the user includes places, people, things, and situations that the patient experiences as a stressor. Without the device, the person may not be aware that they have specifically identified stressors. The identification and action cycle lead to empowerment, growth, and development.

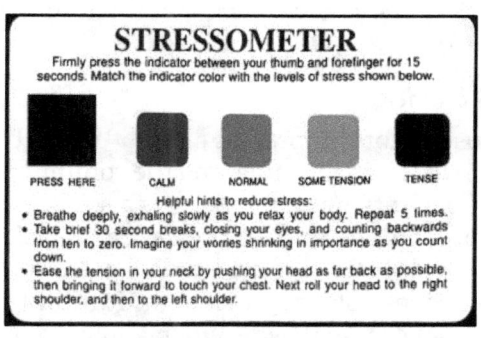

FIGURE 5-3: SIMPLE BIOFEEDBACK DEVICE

Biofeedback is a modality that engages patients as active participants in the use of external equipment that will monitor the effects of any pain relief, stress reduction, or comfort therapies and techniques they employ. In the device, patients have an external barometer of the results of their efforts. Anecdotal evidence of the efficacy of biofeedback in pain relief and comfort is complemented by clinical studies looking at chronic disease and health promotion, such as in reducing early postpartum psychological stress (namely, anxiety and sleeping difficulty; Kudo, Shinohara, & Kodama, 2014). Biofeedback training with stress management, specifically slow deep breathing training, is considered by some to be the most successful therapy for acute stress-related disorders (as cited in Tonhajzerova & Mestanik, 2017).

Nurses, with their specialized knowledge in physiology, psychology, and health promotion, are ideal professionals to provide biofeedback to patients. The Association for Applied Psychobiology and Biofeedback provides certification in biofeedback for nurses who meet professional requirements.

Water Element (Emotional Pain)

The water element is associated with the emotional dimension. The nature of emotional pain is stagnation, and the remedy is movement. E-motion is energy in motion. When emotion as energy gets stuck or stagnates in that its natural tendency to move and flow is blocked in some way, pain results. If it is not addressed, emotional stress characterized as apprehension, anxiety, pain, or general discomfort – accompanied by epinephrine excretion – can transform and deepen into recurrent patterns of pain and discomfort.

Muscle tension is often a result of emotional tension and stagnation. The most common example is the tension-type headache (TTH). TTH are associated with an increase in tension in the muscles of the face, neck, and scalp. They account for 70% of headaches in some populations and can occur at any age (World Health Organization, 2016). A very effective treatment for relieving pain and tightness and comforting the muscles in the neck and head is to use hydrotherapy, or water therapy. A simple and accessible hydrotherapy is a hot-water bottle. For TTH, the holistic nurse can recommend or apply hot-water bottles to the back of the neck and then alternating to the base of the spine, three or four times a day for 15- to

30-minute periods. It is best to try the hot-water bottle at the end of a stressful day before trying to go to sleep.

Hot-Water Bottles to Hug

Nurses have been using hot compresses and hot-water bottles for centuries (Libster & McNeil, 2009). Nurses in hospitals and the community around the globe still use them in care of patients, although there is a science and an art to applying them safely. Hot-water bottles and compresses can physically shut down the normal pain response involved in tension headache, stomachaches, menstrual period pain, or colic. Heat does not just provide comfort, and it is not just a placebo effect. Heat of more than 43 °C or 109 °F, when applied to the skin near where internal pain is felt, switches on heat receptors at the site of pain. These receptor channels, such as transient receptor potential vanilloid 1 (TRPV1), block the body's ability to detect pain in response to heat at around 104 °F (Patwardhan et al., 2010). Receptors called P2X3 detect adenosine triphosphate (ATP), a chemical that leaves cells when they are damaged. The heat response is thought to shut these receptors down. The heat receptor is on one side and the ATP receptor is on the other side that will recognize the pain. Both are present in our cells. When one is activated, it switches off the other.

The science of applying a hot-water bottle includes knowing how to prepare it and where to position it. A hot-water bottle is a thick rubber bag with a stopper. It often comes with a cloth cover. Check the bag to see that it has no signs of damage or potential leakage. Run the tap and fill the bottle to 75% capacity. Do not use water that is hotter than 120 °F, and *do not use boiling water*. After filling the bottle, squeeze the bottle until the water level rises to the top of the neck of the bag to release the remaining air. Screw in the stopper most of the way and burp the bag one more time. Dry the bottle and stopper area carefully and place in the cloth bag. A pillowcase can be used in lieu of a bag cover. The bottle can be held to the abdomen, placed at the feet, and in the case of TTH, placed at the neck as a pillow and then alternating to the base of the spine to release the tension along the spine and neck.

Do not leave hot-water bottles unattended with people who are comatose, young, or elderly. They should also not be used in people with neuropathies or patients who are confused. Sensory perception is an important factor. People need to be able to move away from the bottle should it get too hot and be able to feel that a bottle has gotten too hot. Be sure not to use water that is boiled or over 120 °F. One study identified 85 cases from 2004 to 2013 in the United Kingdom that resulted in serious burns requiring intervention (Jabir, Frew, El-Muttardi, & Dziewulski, 2013). Safety measures when using hot-water bottles begin with careful inspection of the bottle so that it does not leak or break when in contact with a patient. There also is an art to applying a hot-water bottle in integrative holistic nursing practice.

Clinical Vignette: School Nurse – Hug the Bear Therapy

Rose is a licensed school nurse who has noticed a pattern in that several of the younger children in kindergarten and first grade seem to visit her office most often after lunch in the cafeteria. Her assessment reveals that the noise level in the cafeteria is extremely high and the children all complain of abdominal discomfort or headaches after eating lunch. They all bring their lunches, so she does not suspect the food as the trigger for the stomachaches and headaches. Rose considers a nonpharmacological intervention for the children. She offers the children a 5- to 10-minute rest with a teddy bear cloth covering a hot-water bottle. She asks the children if they would like to "hug the bear" as they rest for a few minutes. Each child relaxes in a dark room in the nurse's office and then returns to class refreshed and comfortable. Rose then works with the administration to deal with the noise issues in the cafeteria.

Fire Element (Religious and Spiritual Pain)

The fire element is associated with the spiritual dimension. The nature of spiritual and religious pain is often guilt and shame, and a remedy is heartfelt appreciation and forgiveness. Spiritual and religious pain are parts of the same dimension of a pain experience. Religious pain is a "condition in which a patient is feeling guilty over the violation of moral codes and values of his or her religious tradition" (Satterly, 2001, p. 32). Religious pain is rooted in the guilt of failure and fear related to the imminence of punishment.

Pain is highly subjective. Religious pain is subtle and deeply rooted in belief about God. Integrative holistic nurses model the world of the patient, and they do not have to believe as the patient believes to be able to connect with them spiritually and have an appreciation for their pain. Spirituality, for many, is the search for meaning and life purpose (Wachholtz & Pearce, 2009). His Holiness, the 14th Dalai Lama and 1989 Nobel Peace Prize winner, writes of the difference between spirituality and religiosity:

> Religion I take to be concerned with belief in the claims of one faith tradition or another ... Connected with this are religious teachings of dogma, ritual prayer, and so on. Spirituality I take to be concerned with those qualities of the human spirit – such as love and compassion ... which bring happiness to both self and others. While ritual and prayer, along with the questions of nirvana and salvation, are directly connected to religious faith, these inner qualities need not be. (1999, p. 22)

Another perception of the difference between religion and spirituality is that religion focuses on the moral codes and individual behavior, whereas spirituality focuses on a person's relationship with God (Satterly, 2001). "Patients in spiritual pain are those who have concluded, through their own self-judgments, that there is something wrong with them at their core" (Satterly, 2001, p. 35). A pattern emerging from the research on spiritual pain suggests that hope, meaning, and dignity are common to those experiencing its impact on their ability to cope (Stirling, 2011). People experience spiritual pain when their spiritual needs are not met, when they are fearful, when they are grieving, and when they are dealing with death. Unrelieved physical, mental, and emotional pain can cause spiritual pain (O'Neill & Mako, 2011). Prayer is either the primary or second most frequently used coping strategy to deal with pain, and frequent church attendance is related to decreased pain and related anxiety and depression (Wachholtz & Pearce, 2009). The outcomes of spiritual and religious pain relief are better coping, and a more peaceful resolution in relationship issues, vision and clearer communication. One brief spiritual assessment (Maugans, T., as cited in Wachholtz & Pearce, 2009) that can be used to assess the strengths and resources of people seeking pain relief is the SPIRIT assessment:

>S - Spiritual Belief System
>P - Personal Spirituality
>I - Integration With a Spiritual Community
>R – Ritualized Practices and Restrictions
>I - Implications for Health Care
>T – Terminal Events Planning

Heartfelt Appreciation Experiment

Appreciation as a quality of heart is an extension of gratitude and understanding. It is defined by Doc Childre and researchers at the HeartMath Institute as an "active emotional state in which one has clear perception or recognition of the quality or magnitude of that to be thankful for. Appreciation also leads to improved physiological balance, as measured in cardio-vascular and immune system function" (Childre, 1998, p. 129). They measure heart rate variability (HRV) in persons with different emotional states and in spiritual distress. When a person generates feelings of sincere appreciation within themselves, they create a smooth HRV pattern in which the sympathetic and parasympathetic nervous systems entrain (synchronize) and work together (Childre, 1998, p. 31) rather than oppose each other at biological, emotional, mental, and spiritual levels. An internal peace replaces internal conflict created by disturbing emotional responses to change, transition, and transformation, such as guilt and shame.

The Freeze-Frame technique is easy to learn and to teach to those who are entering the stress and distress of change, transition, and transformation. It is particularly helpful for those whose hearts are heavy with spiritual and religious pain and the burden of the associated feelings of guilt and shame. It includes these steps:

1. Have the patient write down some details about their current stressful situation.
2. Second, have them describe in writing what their current reaction is to that stressful situation.
3. Help them find a comfortable, quiet place, if possible, to close their eyes and take their own pulse in their wrist.
4. Coach them to acknowledge the stressful situation and where they feel

the stress in their body. Then move their attention from the stressful situation to the pulse in their wrist and then to their heart in the center of their chest.
5. Invite them to "Breathe as if you could breathe into your heart" and then exhale through the solar plexus in the center of the belly below the ribs.
6. Next, invite them to activate their own feelings of appreciation for someone or something that they care about.
7. Then, in that moment of appreciation, ask the heart what an efficient, effective attitude or action would be that de-stresses and balances their system (Childre, 1998, p. 22).
8. Invite them to listen carefully to the still small voice of their heart's intuit-intelligence (Childre, 1998) that never guilts or shames them. Have them write down the solution that they witnessed in the experiment.

The Freeze-Frame technique has been used with groups as well as individuals. It is used in solving tough problems of the spirit. In addition to individual work, being willing and able to work on religious and spiritual pain of community, national, and international disputes with large groups and communities is an important and emerging integrative holistic nursing skill. Arnold Mindell, an expert in large-group transformation, writes in his 1995 book, *Sitting in the Fire:*

> Thomas Jefferson said that the price of liberty is vigilance. Vigilance means awareness of the manifold ideas and feelings in yourself and in the world around you. This awareness is part of the price of democracy and peace. ... Many of us shudder at violence. We want to insist on peaceful behavior ... if we don't permit hostilities a legitimate outlet, they are bound to take illegitimate routes ... the fire that burns in the social, psychological and spiritual dimensions of humanity can ruin the world. Or this fire can transform trouble into community. It's up to us." (pp. 12, 18)

Focusing on resolving religious and spiritual pain can have tremendous trickle-down impact on physical, emotional, and mental health and well-being.

Ether Element
(Multidimensional Pain and the Elements)

The ether element is the unity of all dimensions and all elements. The nature of multidimensional pain is isolation, and a remedy is to nurture belonging with conscious breathing and community building. Spiritual pain and distress can threaten an individual with spiritual disintegration, loss of meaning, and isolation. Isolation is remedied by belonging. The need to belong is "among the most fundamental of all personality processes" (DeWall, Deckman, Pond, & Bonser, 2011, p. 979). Isolation is a risk factor for aggression in society, decrease in prosocial behaviors (such as caring), and decreased ability to self-regulate (there is no incentive to control one's behaviors). Research has shown that the nature of many is to "tend and befriend" during stress in addition to "fight or flight." "A working model of affiliation under stress suggests that oxytocin may be a biomarker of social distress that accompanies gaps or problems with social relationships and that may provide an impetus for affiliation" (Taylor, 2006). Patients have been cared for historically in their community and by their community. Today, the pain of isolation for many is intensely real and enduring. Nurses – who have historically worked in spiritual and faith community rather than in isolated private practices (Libster & McNeil, 2009) and innately understand the benefits of community building – are often the trusted professionals the public turns to when they need pain relief and comfort.

Conscious Breathing

Activating a sense of belonging in community is a solution to the experience of multidimensional pain. One way to first address this issue is to focus on one's own sense of self "belonging" to a place and space through the practice of conscious breathing. As will be discussed further in chapter 13, ether is the element that suggests that all of the elements be integrated in interventions for pain. Breath is a product of the engagement of all of the elements. When the vagus nerve is inflamed, breathing becomes shallower. When a person encounters a perceived stressor, their fight-or-flight response engages. People panic, and their respiratory rate goes up. When they are spiritually distressed, breathing can become affected. Engaging all of the elements described here, one could consider saying "Stop that" and then take a time-out for the Freeze-Frame technique and some slow, deep, mindful breaths. The practice does not have to be pranayama. The patient could also lie down with a hot-water bottle under their head or a ginger compress on their back while they use their biofeedback card or instrument to monitor their adaptation to the pain that they are experiencing.

CASE STUDY: REFINING THE ELEMENTS OF COMFORT SKILL

Mark is a 28-year-old stockbroker on Wall Street. He has suffered from severe headaches since graduation from university 6 years ago. Mark visits his advanced practice registered nurse (APRN) because he is not sleeping well and his pain is not fully relieved by over-the-counter pain medications. He tells the nurse and the APRN that he came to the office for a "stronger painkiller." After assessment, the nurse and the APRN agree that Mark has a knowledge deficit about self-care for pain. He also has several high-stress risk factors related to his perception of his job.

Questions

1. How might complementary therapies and self-care remedies be used before advancing Mark's allopathic treatment?
2. Describe one or more interventions you might use that represent all five Elements of Care®.

Nurse's Answers

1. Modeling his world, the APRN acknowledges Mark's severe pain by asking him to tell her more about it and using a pain scale. She asks Mark to rank his headache pain on a scale from 0 to 10, and he says "8." She asks Mark, "If there was any one thing that could lower your pain level to a 7.5, what would it be?" Offering the patient a half step is a therapeutic technique that allows people to consider the possibility of a solution. He says, "Change jobs!" The APRN gives Mark a list of three therapists in the community who counsel people about work-related stress and job change. She explains to Mark that headaches most often result from neck tension, and she asks Mark if he would be willing to learn some remedies and choose some complementary therapies before moving to stronger painkillers. She considers discussing lifestyle and diet choices, which may also be underlying triggers for his headaches. The APRN decides to order education with the nurse to discuss these topics rather than prescribe a drug treatment.

2. In his appointment with the nurse, Mark is taught about diaphragmatic breathing (air, ether) and how to use a hot-water bottle and a ginger compress (water, fire, earth) for his neck while putting his feet up at the end of a long day at the stock exchange. The nurse reviews all of the skills at the office and then gives Mark educational resources (website links and handouts). His pain level after doing the breathing exercise with the nurse is a 4. The plan is to try the breathing exercises and self-care every day for a week and add over-the-counter pain relievers the first day and then as needed after that. Mark will use the pain scale each day, record the results, and be rechecked in a week.

HOLISTIC TRANSFORMATION

1. Create a list of complementary therapies and remedies that you prefer to incorporate in plans of care when working with people seeking pain relief and comfort.

2. Assign each complementary therapy or remedy an element. Does your plan include a representative of all five elements? If not, what might you add to increase the balance of your approach?

SUMMARY

All complementary therapies and self-care remedies have their place in time and space. The premise of holistic care for pain relief and comfort is that all interventions (even placebos) have the potential to heal; that is, they can create change, ease transition, and support transformation that will lead to pain relief, comfort, and healing of the body, mind, emotions, and spirit. Integrative holistic nursing care never guarantees that a person's pain and discomfort is removed or cured. Someone can continue to have pain and yet experience a shift in perception that allows them to integrate that pain experience and continue on the journey of life. Pain and suffering for many is an impetus for isolation or an impetus for self-reflection and discovery. Breathing reconnects oneself with one's inner (heart) intelligence and then compels solutions that allow the pain to lead to meaningful life work and participation in community building. Complementary therapies and self-care remedies provide much-needed nonpharmacological support for the thousands of people seeking pain relief and comfort every day. Holistic nurses engage the five Elements of Care® to role-model balanced and inclusive care plans with their patients.

RESOURCES

Association for Applied Psychophysiology and Biofeedback
https://www.aapb.ori4a/pages/index.cfm?pageid=1&activateFull=false

Chronic Pain: In Depth (fact sheet)
https://nccih.nih.gov/health/pain/chronic.htm

HeartMath Institute
https://www.heartmath.org

REFERENCES

American Psychological Association. (2018). *The different kinds of stress.* Retrieved from http://www.apa.orhelpcenter/stress-kinds.aspx

Biofeedback Certification International Alliance. (2018). Retrieved from http://www.bcia.org.

Brown, W. (1998, January). The Placebo effect. *Scientific American.* 90-95.

Childre, D. (1998). *Freeze frame: A scientifically proven technique for clear decision making and improved health* (2nd ed.). Boulder Creek, CA: Planetary Publications.

Dalai Lama (1999). *Ethics for the new millennium.* New York, NY: Riverhead Books.

Derbyshire, S. W. (2006). Can fetuses feel pain? *BMJ: British Medical Journal*, 332(7546), 909-912.

DeWall, C., Deckman, T., Pond, R., & Bonser, I. (2011). Belongingness as a core personality trait: How social exclusion influences social functioning and personality expression. *Journal of Personality,* 79(6), 1281-1314.

Elliott, D. B. (2016). The placebo effect: Is it unethical to use it or unethical not to? *Ophthalmic & Physiological Optics*, 36, 513-518.

Field, L., & Adams, N. (2001). Pain management 2: The use of psychological approaches to pain. *British Journal of Nursing*, 10(15), 971-974.

Jabir, S., Frew, Q., El-Muttardi, N., & Dziewulski, P. (2013). Burn injuries resulting from hot water bottle use: A retrospective review of cases presenting to a regional burns unit in the United Kingdom. *Plastic Surgery International*, 2013(#736368), 1-8.

Kudo, N., Shinohara, H., & Kodama, H. (2014). Heart rate variability biofeedback intervention for reduction of psychological stress during the early postpartum period. *Applied Psychophysiology and Biofeedback*, 39(3-4), 203-211.

Libster, M. (2001). *Demonstrating care: The art of integrative nursing.* Albany, NY: Delmar Cengage Learning.

Libster, M., & McNeil, B. (2009). *Enlightened charity: The holistic nursing care, education, and "Advices Concerning the Sick" of Sister Matilda Coskery (1799-1870).* Wauwatosa, WI: Golden Apple Publications.

McCarty, D., Csuka, M., McCarthy, G., & Trotter, D. (1994). Treatment of pain due to fibromyalgia with topical capsaicin: A pilot study. *Seminars in Arthritis & Rheumatism,* 23(6, S3), 41-47.

Mindell, A. (1995). *Sitting in the fire: Large group transformation using conflict and diversity.* Portland, OR: Lao Tse Press.

Morse, J. (1992). Comfort: The refocusing of nursing care. *Clinical Nursing Research*, 1(1), 91-106.

Morse, J. (2000). Responding to the cues of suffering. *Health Care for Women International*, 21, 1-9.

National Center for Complementary and Integrative Health. (2022). *Chronic pain: in depth.* Retrieved from https://www.nccih.nih.gov/health/chronic-pain-in-depth

National Institutes of Health. (2022). *NIH HEAL initiative.* Retrieved from https://heal.nih.gov.

Neuman, B. & Fawcett, J. (2011). *The Neuman systems model.* New York, NY: Pearson.

O'Neill, M. & Mako, C. (2011). Addressing spiritual pain. *Health Progress* (January-February), 42-45.

Patwardhan, A. M., Akopian, A. N., Ruparel, N. B., Diogenes, A., Weintraub, S. T., Uhlson, C., ... Hargreaves, K. M. (2010). Heat generates oxidized linoleic acid metabolites that activate TRPV1 and produce pain in rodents. *Journal of Clinical Investigation*, 120(5), 1617-1626.

Roy, C. (2008). *The Roy adaptation model* (3rd ed.). New York, NY: Pearson.

Satterly, L. (2001). Guilt, shame, and religious and spiritual pain. *Holistic Nursing Practice*, 15(2), 30-39.

Selye, H. (1976). *Stress in health and disease.* Boston, MA: Butterworth-Heinemann.

Sheldrake, R. (1995). *Morphic resonance and the presence of the past: The habits of nature.* Rochester, VT: Park Street Press.

Starr, P. (1982). *The social transformation of American medicine.* New York, NY: Basic Books.

Stirling, I. (2011). Spiritual pain. *Scottish Journal of Healthcare Chaplaincy*, 14(2), 22-29.

Strong, T., Pyle, N. R., & Sutherland, O. (2009). Scaling questions: Asking and answering them in counselling 1. *Counselling Psychology Quarterly*, 22(2), 171-185.

Taylor, S. E. (2006). Tend and befriend: Biobehavioral bases of affiliation under stress. *Current Directions in Psychological Science*, 15(6), 273-277.

Therkleson, T. (2010). Ginger compress therapy for adults with osteoporosis. *Journal of Advanced Nursing*, 66(10), 2225-2233.

Tonhajzerova, I., & Mestanik, M. (2017). New perspectives in the model of stress response. *Physiological Research*, 66(Suppl 2), S173-S185.

Wachholtz, A. B., & Pearce, M. J. (2009). Does spirituality as a coping mechanism help or hinder coping with chronic pain? *Current Pain and Headache Reports*, 13, 127-132.

Walach, H., & Jonas, W. B. (2004). Placebo research: The evidence base for harnessing self-healing capacities. *Journal of Alternative and Complementary Medicine*, 10(1), S103-S112.

World Health Organization. (2016). *Headache disorders.* WHO Fact Sheets. Retrieved from http://www.who.int/mediacentre/factsheets/fs277/en/

CHAPTER 6

MINDFULNESS PRACTICE INTERVENTIONS

LEARNING OUTCOME

After completing this chapter, the learner will be able to explain the mechanism of mindfulness and mindfulness practice interventions in integrative holistic nursing care.

CHAPTER OBJECTIVES

After completing this chapter, the learner will be able to:

1. Define mindfulness.
2. Explain Thich Naht Hanh's *Five Mindfulness Trainings* to cultivate loving kindness.
3. Discuss the mechanism of mindfulness.
4. Cite one intervention for use in mindfulness practice.
5. List examples of health concerns and diseases with a clinical research base related to mindfulness.

INTRODUCTION

Mindfulness, historically a Buddhist practice to cultivate compassion, also refers to a mind-body intervention and intentional practice of cultivating moment-to-moment access to awareness. This trait already exists within us, according to Dr. Jon Kabat-Zinn (Shonin, 2016), one of three seminal scholars in the field. This chapter highlights the views and practice interventions of Kabat-Zinn and two others: Thich Nhat Hanh, a Buddhist monk, and Dr. Ellen Langer, about mindfulness, mindlessness, awareness, and consciousness, and present moment meditation.

BACKGROUND

Mindfulness practice has become a media sensation in the last few years, with coverage by Oprah Winfrey, Anderson Cooper of *60 Minutes*, and *Time* magazine, to name a few. Dr. Jon Kabat-Zinn, founder of mindfulness-based stress reduction (MBSR) practice, has had much to say about the emergent trends since he established the Stress Reduction Clinic at the University of Massachusetts Medical Center in the 1990s. Kabat-Zinn originally appeared in the Bill Moyers special called Healing and the Mind on the Public Broadcasting System in 1993. Kabat-Zinn has written and taught for decades that mindfulness, which is rooted in ancient Buddhist practice, is "waking up and living in harmony with oneself and with the world" and can be practiced by anyone (Kabat-Zinn, 1994, p. 3). MBSR focuses on awareness of the present moment, from moment to moment, to suspend judgment of what is happening in life and replace it with discernment. Kabat-Zinn teaches that discernment is the "kind of operation of wisdom where you can see the subtleties ... the thousand shades of gray between black and white, which is absolutely essential to and part and parcel of the cultivation of mindfulness" (Shonin, 2016, p. 124).

The ordinary waking state of consciousness resembles a dream, according to Buddhist tradition. The remedy is to meditate. "Meditation helps us wake up from the sleep of automaticity and unconsciousness, thereby making it possible for us to live our lives with access to the full spectrum of our conscious and unconscious possibilities" (Kabat-Zinn, 1994, p. 3). Mindfulness practice centers on focusing one's consciousness on the present moment, intentionally and without judgment.

Mindfulness Versus Mindlessness

Mindfulness refers to a "meditation practice that cultivates present moment awareness" (Ludwig & Kabat-Zinn, 2008) that will transform mind and body. The focus of mindfulness practice is kindness toward oneself and openness to what might be possible. The foundational belief is that change is not affected in the past or the future, but we affect the past and the future in what we do in the present moment.

Thich Nhat Hanh was a Vietnamese monk, dharmacharya (teacher), and Zen master who was nominated for the Nobel Peace Prize in 1967. He died in January 2022 at the age of 95. His teachings on the *Five Mindfulness Trainings* are carried on by peoples of all faiths as practices of compassion. These five precepts were developed for the lay community during the time of the Buddha as a foundation for all spiritual practice. The Thich Nhat Hanh mindfulness trainings cultivate loving kindness by:

1. Protecting life and decreasing violence in oneself, family and society.
2. Practicing social justice, generosity, not stealing or exploiting other living beings.
3. Practicing responsible sexual behavior in order to protect individuals, couples, families, and children.
4. Deep listening and loving speech to restore communication and reconcile.
5. Mindful consumption, so as to not bring toxins and poisons into our body or mind. (Thich Nhat Hanh, n.d.).

Transforming Mindless Habits

Harvard psychology professor Ellen Langer's definition of mindfulness is based on principles of learning and achieved *without meditation*. Mindfulness is "simply the process of noticing new things. It is seeing the similarities in things thought different and the differences in things taken to be similar" (Langer, 2005, p. 16). Langer writes that when we are learning mindfully rather than just acting on beliefs about learning that have been mindlessly accepted, we avoid forming mind-sets that unnecessarily limit us and keep us from learning (Langer, 2000).

Langer defines mindlessness as "automatic behavior" and "acting from a single perspective" (1989, p. 10). Mindfulness is an antidote to acting from a place of habit or what Langer refers to as "premature cognitive commitments." Langer differentiates the Eastern concept of mindfulness meditation from her work. She writes that in Eastern mindfulness meditation, a person is encouraged to quiet the mind, whereas in this mindfulness work, the mind is actively engaged. It is human nature to seek familiarity and be cautious, if not fearful, of uncertainty. Yet, there are benefits to embracing uncertainty in that our choices may increase as we see possibilities that are not readily apparent. Langer's view is that "certainty breeds mindlessness. Uncertainty, then, is a friend rather than something to be avoided or feared (Langer, 2005, p. 22).

The way we learn sets the pattern for mindfulness or mindlessness. Repetition and single exposure (without question) nurture mindlessness rather than mindfulness. When educational content is delivered as packaged fact without attention to context or different perspective, mindlessness – rather than mindful learning – is cultivated. Life is full of uncertainty but often is presented as fact. Langer uses the example of a scientific statement, such as that "most of the time, under the stated circumstances, horses are herbivorous." When these kinds of findings are reported by teachers or in textbooks, they are translated from statements of probability into absolutes, such as "horses are herbivorous." People automatically translate the uncertainty into false certainty as a process of mindlessness. Probability leads us to wonder about the universe. It drives creativity and invention and a search for truth. The mind is nurtured to consider possibilities and opposites, such as, "When might a horse eat meat?" With the habitual mental process of rooting out uncertainty comes judgment. Mindfulness practice cultivates the suspension of the mindless habit of judgment.

Mindfulness reinforces a mind-set of being receptive, accepting, and compassionate while noticing one's natural tendency to judge (Cameron, 2018). Mindfulness cultivates a healthier mind-set. A *mind-set*, according to Dweck (2016), is a self-perception or self-theory that people hold about themselves. One example of a mind-set is believing that you are either intelligent or unintelligent. Mindfulness trains the mind to be in the present moment, a state that cultivates flexibility of thought and belief and an ability to move through any preoccupation with unproductive judgmental habits.

Consciousness and the Mechanism of Mindfulness

Despite the exponential growth of interest in mindfulness practice and use of the term, there is still a limited understanding of the mechanism of mindfulness, of how it "works." One cognitive model suggested by Holas and Jankowski (2013) is based on Schooler's model of consciousness that discusses the relationship between conscious, unconscious, and meta-conscious cognitive processes. Holas and Jankowski refer to the meta-conscious processes as "meta-awareness" when discussing the relationship between the explanatory model and mindfulness. This model proposes that mindfulness is a cognitive state in which links are forged between consciousness, meta-awareness, and the unconscious. There is a reduction in self-focused attention and an increase in self-regulation that allow for "behaviors of a more natural and spontaneous nature to be evoked, thus increasing the likelihood of achieving the goal... making the ego quiet and lessening the intrapersonal and interpersonal costs of excessive self-identification" (Holas & Jankowski, 2013, p. 241).

A behavioral model suggests that mindfulness involves "re-perceiving," or a shift in perception that is significant for the person. This shift is not to be confused with detachment or distancing oneself from one's experience. Re-perceiving supports the deepening of intimacy and knowing about self and others (i.e., *relationship with* whatever arises in the present moment without judgment). Re-perceiving allows for the psychological and emotional distance that enables clarity of mind. But those who engage in mindfulness practice are clear that they are not disconnecting or dissociating with life, a common misunderstanding of those who begin mindfulness work. "Rather than being immersed in the drama of our personal narrative or life story, we are able to stand back and simply witness it" (Shapiro, Carlson, Astin, & Freedman, 2006, p. 377). Mindfulness practice and meditation, MBSR, and all mindfulness practice-based interventions promote wholeness and peace through association (also called "intimate detachment"), rather than dissociation (Shapiro et al., 2006).

The ego attempts to judge experiences as good and bad. The skill of nonjudgment (i.e., suspending judgment), is one of the mechanisms of how mindfulness works. The mind is constantly evaluating life experiences and comparing them to memories, held beliefs, and expectations. This process of judgment is often stimulated by fear, such as fear of not being good enough or fear of being hurt. When people start to meditate or still the mind and body long enough to tune in to their own thoughts, they often realize how bowed down they are by the constant, unrelenting judgment. They can even become judgmental of attempts at the practice of mindfulness itself. Suspending judgment skill involves stopping the labeling of each thought and each moment as good or bad.

Mindfulness meditation practice encourages one to "witness whatever comes up in the mind or the body and to recognize it without condemning it or pursuing it, knowing that our judgments are unavoidable and necessarily limiting thoughts *about* experience" (Kabat-Zinn, 1994, p. 56) rather than direct contact with experience itself. The mechanism of mindfulness meditation practice is being in the present moment to experience possibility rather than being consumed by prejudice. Mindlessness as "states of liking and disliking ... unconsciously feed addictive behaviors in all domains of life ... they have a chronic viral-like toxicity that prevents us from seeing things as they actually are and mobilizing our true potential" (Kabat-Zinn, 1994, p. 57).

On the biological level, how mindfulness practice and mindfulness meditation practice work, what the mechanism of action is, is basically unknown. However, studies are being conducted on applications for specific diseases and conditions from which inferences may be able to be made. We can also draw upon the biological literature on the mind, some of which is presented here, as well as knowledge of the development of human consciousness documented by people of different traditions, a sample of which is presented in the following sections.

The science behind mindfulness has much to do with understanding of the conscious and subcons-cious minds as well as consciousness. Bruce Lipton, a biologist and author and teacher of the new biology, discusses the power of the beliefs programmed in the subconscious mind during childhood to thwart the ability of the conscious mind that is self-reflective and able to create our future (Lipton, 2008, p. 138). The subconscious mind runs on habitual patterns, whereas the conscious mind can create new responses. However, the place to make any change is in the present moment. Therefore, we need the subconscious mind anchoring our awareness in the present moment – and the conscious mind realizing new beliefs and dreams and responding to environmental stimuli – to work together. In this way, they can help us to replace habitual thoughts and practices as we carve out a new reality for ourselves.

Mindfulness begins with being conscious, or aware of self and surrounding. One ancient way of teaching consciousness is by telling stories. In the Zen tradition, stories support the "self-searching through meditation to realize one's true nature, with disregard of formalism, with insistence on self-discipline, and simplicity of living" (Reps & Senzaki, [1939] 1998). The first story is about a cup of tea. Nan-in, a 19th-century Japanese master, served tea to a university professor who was inquiring about Zen. Nan-in poured the professor's cup of tea in front of him until it was quite full and then kept pouring. He said nothing as he poured, and eventually the professor, who could no longer contain himself, said, "The cup is overfull! No more will go in!" Nan-in said to the professor, "Like this cup, you are full of your own opinions and speculations. How can I show you Zen unless you first empty your cup?" (Reps & Senzaki, [1939] 1998, p. 5).

Sri Aurobindo (1872 – 1950), Indian philosopher of human evolution in consciousness, is known for his maxim that "Man is a transitional being" (Satprem, 1993). He teaches that "consciousness is not a commodity" but "something to kindle like a fire" (Satprem, 1993, p. 52). It is a force or fire *(agni)* that warms and animates everything (Satprem, 1993, pp. 54-55). Sri Aurobindo suggests that there is a flow between that which is outside ourselves and that which is inside ourselves. There is no inner versus outer life. The "adventure" in consciousness shows that what is outside of us is also inside of us. Some may think that to access that inner life they must actually sit in meditation. However, the ancient wisdom underpinning mindfulness practice and meditation is that *"action is meditation* whether a person is taking a shower, or going about his business, the Force flows and flows in him" (Satprem, 1993, p. 42). The stillness in the mental being leads to action that is more mindful, effective, and powerful. The key to mastery is always silence, at every level, because silence enables us to discern the vibrations, and to discern them is to be able to act upon them (Satprem, 1993, p. 62). Energy is consciousness, Matter is consciousness and by acting on consciousness one can act upon Energy and Matter (Satprem, 1993, p. 276). This action begins with the simple process of cultivating mindful learning, of actively drawing distinctions and noticing new things. "Seeing the familiar in the novel and the novel in the familiar is a way to ensure that our minds are active, that we are involved, and that we are situated in the present" (Langer, 2000, p. 222).

The connections between mindfulness and consciousness are also apparent in Western as well as Eastern philosophies of healing. In his treatise *Heal Thyself: An Explanation of the Real Cause and Cure of Disease*, British physician Edward Bach writes, "The Creator of all things is Love, and everything of which we are conscious is in all its infinite number of forms a manifestation of that Love" ([1931] 1996, p. 8). He suggests experiencing this Love by meditating on the image of the Creator as a "great blazing sun of beneficence and love" and that each of us is a particle at the end of each of the sun's rays whose ultimate purpose is to return to the "great centre" (Bach [1931] 1996, p. 8).

Bach encouraged this image as a reinforcement of the consciousness of unity. Mindfulness meditations promote a sense of connection and unity with all life. It is dissociation between our "souls and our personalities," writes Bach, and "cruelty or wrong to others that brings the conflict that leads to disease" ([1931] 1996, p. 9). It is our thoughts and beliefs that are foundations for and expressions of our relationship with the Creator and therefore each other. Those very same thoughts and beliefs can be a wedge that unifies all Creation or foments the division of the sun's rays and particles, as if that were possible. We are all on that path of the return to a sense of unity and wholeness within ourselves and with all of that which is Created. Suffering, in the realm of mindfulness, then is in itself beneficent. Bach suggests the cultivation of unity and alleviation of suffering through calm thought and meditation "brings ourselves to such an atmosphere of peace that our Souls are able to speak to us through our conscience and intuition" (p. 42).

MINDFULNESS IN PRACTICE

Breath and Present Moment

Thich Nhat Hanh's breathing exercises are used by people around the world for cultivating mindfulness as being in the present moment. "In using conscious breathing, we can transform the present moment into a moment full of wonder and beauty (Thich Nhat Hanh, 1993, p. 16). The exercises link a mantra or affirmations with the cycles of respiration. For example, the Joy of Meditation as Nourishment exercise 3 is designed to "bring the body and mind back into oneness and at the same time to help bring us back to the present moment" where we can effect change.

- Breathing in, I know I am breathing in. (Breathe In)
- Breathing out, I know I am breathing out. (Breathe Out)
- Breathing in, my breath grows deep. (Deep Breath)
- Breathing out, my breath goes slowly. (Slow exhale)
- Breathing in, I feel calm.
- Breathing out, I feel ease.
- Breathing in, I smile. (Smile!)
- Breathing out, I release.
- Dwelling in the present moment.
- I know it is a wonderful moment. (Thich Nhat Hanh, 1993, p. 21)

Mindfulness Experiments

The Orange

Many are surprised at the increased awareness that they have after using their senses to focus on eating fruit mindfully. Somatic (body) experiments reveal much about a person's present state of mindfulness. The following experiment can be done with different foods; oranges or tangerines are often best used for reasons that stem from healing traditions. Oranges and tangerines, particularly the peels, are classified in traditional Chinese medicine as an herb that "regulates the qi." This means that oranges or tangerines move qi, or energy, in the abdomen and aid digestion. This experiment can slow down emotional force and open communication channels for improved internal and external dialog.

- Choose a piece of orange.
- Spend some time in quiet reflection.
- Take 5 minutes to "eat" the orange in a way that utilizes all of your senses.
- Discuss the experience:
  - Smell
  - Sight
  - Sound
  - Touch
  - Taste

Ringing the Bell

Ringing the Bell is a mindfulness practice intervention observed at Thich Nhat Hanh's Plum Village community in France, where many people go for training in mindfulness meditation. The bell rings, and everyone stops to observe a period of mindfulness, paying attention to breathing and thoughts. Thich Nhat Hanh said of the ringing of the bell exercise, "Listen, listen. This wonderful sound brings me back to my true home" (Thich Nhat Hanh, n.d.).

Research

A search of the term "mindfulness" in the EBSCO health databases produces over 10,000 results. Pain, stress, coping, and quality of life were the original foci of mindfulness research. Now there are studies on specific diseases as well, such as depression, psoriasis, diabetes type 2, sleep disturbance, and eating disorders, to name a few. Each study has to be reviewed carefully, however, because articles on studies about the effects of yoga and meditation, for example, are indexed under mindfulness and MBSR when they may not have any mindfulness intervention. Examples are provided here of research on mindfulness and MBSR studies for two diseases: obesity and low back pain.

According to Langer, experimental research conducted over 25 years reveals mindfulness results in an "increase in competence; a decrease in accidents; an increase in memory, creativity, and positive affect; a decrease in stress; and an increase in health and longevity, to name a few of the benefits" (2000, p. 220). Langer conducted several studies involving children and young adults that showed that mindfulness practice can increase recall and positive affect toward tasks, objects, and people (Levy, Jennings, & Langer, 2001). In a study with older adults, findings suggested that contrary to popular belief, one of the best ways to improve attention and recall is to let attention wander and embrace distraction (Levy et al., 2001). The study included 80 participants (39 males and 41 females), aged 60 to 89 years, who were living independently. Participants were randomly assigned to one of four attention interventions involving pictures of such things as motorcycles and surfboard riders and were asked to recall the details in those pictures. In the mindfulness groups, participants were told to notice either three or five distinctions. In the control groups, participants were either told to pay attention or were not given any directions related to attention before they were given the set of pictures. The results indicated that those who looked for distinctions in the pictures were able to remember significantly more pictures than those in the control groups did (Levy et al., 2001).

Some people hypothesize that mindfulness influences susceptibility to, or ability to recover from, discomfort and disease. Mindfulness may decrease a person's perception of pain severity as well as effect physical changes in the immune system. In a small study of 27 participants using functional magnetic resonance imaging, Creswell and colleagues (2007) found that a person's disposition toward mindfulness was associated with widespread prefrontal cortical activation and reduced bilateral amygdala activity (as cited in Ludwig & Kabat-Zinn, 2008). Another study by Davidson and colleagues (2003) randomly assigned participants to either an MBSR group or a wait-list control group. They reported an increased left-sided anterior activation by electroencephalogram (EEG; patterns associated with positive emotional experience) in the MBSR group and a greater increase in antibody titers to influenza vaccine. The magnitude of the EEG change predicted the magnitude of antibody response (as cited in Ludwig & Kabat-Zinn, 2008).

Obesity

A review of mindfulness practice for eating disorders (Wanden-Berghe, Sanz-Valero, & Wanden-Berge, 2011) demonstrates that mindfulness-based practice interventions are effective for bulimia nervosa, anorexia nervosa, and binge eating. After initial review of 60 articles, 30 were retained that met inclusion criteria. The results of the study's systemic review indicate that mindfulness-based therapies may be effective in the treatment of eating disorders. A major contributor to obesity is psychological stress. Mindfulness practice has been shown to abate emotional eating in a study of 157 participants using the Mindful Awareness Attention Scale (MAAS) and depression and anxiety instruments (Pidgeon, Lacota, & Champion, 2013. MAAS measures trait mindfulness skills of attention to the present moment. Higher mindfulness skill was associated with lower levels of depression, anxiety, and stress and lowering the propensity for emotional eating (Pidgeon, Lacota, & Champion, 2013). Other studies have been conducted on the mindfulness-based eating awareness training curriculum in adults and children. Mindful eating practice has been shown to decrease impulsive food decisions and increase the ability to notice hunger and fullness cues (Pierson et al., 2016).

Low Back Pain

Twelve percent to 30% of the population suffers from low back pain annually. MBSR programs are typically 8-week programs with 2.5-hour group sessions each week and one all-day silent retreat. Key components of the program are sitting and walking meditation, body scan, and hatha yoga so that the participant develops a practice that can be incorporated into daily life. A systematic review of the literature following Cochrane Collaboration recommendations was conducted on randomized, controlled trials for MBSR in the care of those with low back pain. MBSR was associated with a statistically significant improvement in pain intensity at short-term follow-up, but the clinical benefit was uncertain. No statistically significant or clinically important group differences were found in pain intensity at long-term follow-up. The findings of this systematic review suggest that MBSR practice interventions may be associated with "short-term improvement in pain intensity and physical functioning compared with usual care, but the difference is neither clinically meaningful nor sustained in the long term" (Anheyer et al., 2017, p. 806).

Many people with chronic low back pain use opioids. One study by Zgierska et al. (2016) sought to determine whether mindfulness meditation might help patients who had been treated with 30 mg of morphine or more per day for at least 3 months. The intervention was 8 weekly 2-hour mindfulness meditation sessions and 30 minutes per day of meditation practice at home (at least 6 days per week). The patients continued their "usual" opioid treatment during the study. The participant group consisted of 35 adult patients, mostly women, aged 42 to

62 years. The study found that mindfulness meditation was "feasible, acceptable and safe," and it was helpful for patients as an "early-on technique" for pain flares. Self-report was the method used for tracking meditation practice. The study demonstrates the challenges, as discussed in Chapter 3, of attempting to engage in clinical trials that, by their very nature, seek to control for those influences or variables that are the human experience inherent in centuries-old traditions, such as mindfulness practice. The limitation of the studies of mindfulness practice begins with the attempt to study and generalize findings from that which is so unique to the one person.

CASE STUDY:
REFINING THE ELEMENTS OF OBSERVATION SKILL

Sam has been a nurse for 6 months in the surgical intensive care unit and is starting to feel the stress of the job. He has headaches when he gets home from work every day. His fear is that his headaches might interfere with his ability to do his job. He is exhausted after his 12-hour shifts and says that he cannot do anything else but work and sleep. He comes to the urgent care center, and you are his nurse.

Questions
1. How can mindfulness practice improve your observation and assessment skill?
2. Would you apply mindfulness practice with Sam?

Nurse's Answers
1. Nurses who work in urgent care centers and clinics have brief interactions with patients. Mindfulness practice can be practiced by anyone to promote awareness and cultivate nonjudgment and compassion. Mindfulness practice also focuses the practitioner on the present moment which, in urgent care work, can help in decreasing stress, thereby increasing job satisfaction.
2. Yes, the senior nurse is in a great position to mentor the junior nurse in self-care with MBSR techniques. The nurse is practicing while teaching the junior nurse the steps of Thich Nhat Hanh's loving kindness training. Demonstrating a short breathing technique and discussing a daily practice with Sam can illustrate mindfulness practice. The senior nurse would also encourage Sam to keep a pain log to monitor his stress or pain level.

HOLISTIC TRANSFORMATION

1. Practice sitting and observing your breath. Notice your thoughts. Journal the judgmental thoughts that you experience about yourself.

2. Pick periods throughout the day to practice walking meditation. How does mindfulness change your perception of yourself and the work that you do?

SUMMARY

As Bach has written, "Knowledge of the Soul's purpose and acquiescence in that knowledge means the relief of earthly suffering and distress and leaves us free to develop our evolution in joy and happiness" ([1931] 1996, p. 9). Mindfulness practice interventions hold the potential to relieve suffering and promote peace, happiness, and awareness at a deep level, the level of consciousness. Although the mechanisms for how mindfulness works in health and healing are hypothesized but not conclusive, there are decades of study and practice that suggest it is worthy of consideration. It is a feasible, safe, and noninvasive complementary therapy that can be learned and shared with patients by integrative holistic nurses.

RESOURCES

Center for Mindfulness in Medicine, Health Care, and Society (Started by Jon Kabat-Zinn). https://www.umassmed.edu/cfm/

Kabat-Zinn, J. (2013). Full catastrophe living: Using the wisdom of your body and mind to face stress, pain, and illness. New York, NY: Bantam.

Plum Village (Founded by Thich Nhat Hanh). https://plumvillage.org

REFERENCES

Anheyer, D., Haller, H., Barth, J., Lauche, R., Dobos, G., & Cramer, H. (2017). Mindfulness-based stress reduction for treating low back pain: A systematic review and meta-analysis. *Annals of Internal Medicine, 166*(11), 799-807.

Bach, E. (1996. *Heal thyself: An explanation of the real cause and cure of disease.* Suffolk, England: C.W. Daniels Co. (Original work published 1931)

Cameron, L. (2018). The power of mindfulness and compassion. *Journal of Medical Practice Management, 33*(4), 251-253.

Dweck, C. S. (2016). *Mindset: The new psychology of success.* New York, NY: Random House.

Holas, P., & Jankowski, T. (2013). A cognitive perspective on mindfulness. *International Journal of Psychology, 48*(3), 232-243.

Kabat-Zinn, J. (1994). *Wherever you go, there you are: Mindfulness meditation in everyday life.* New York, NY: Hyperion.

Langer, E. J. (1989). *Mindfulness.* Cambridge, MA: Perseus Books.

Langer, E. (2000). Mindful learning. *Current Directions in Psychological Science, 9*(6), 220-223.

Langer, E. J. (2005). *On becoming an artist: Reinventing yourself through mindful creativity.* New York, NY: Ballantine Books.

Langer, E., & Moldoveanu, M. (2000). The construct of mindfulness. *Journal of Social Issues, 56*(1), 1-9.

Levy, B. R., Jennings, P., & Langer, E. J. (2001). Improving attention in old age. *Journal of Adult Development, 8*(3), 189-192.

Lipton, B. (2008). *The biology of belief: Unleashing the power of consciousness, matter & miracles.* New York, NY: Hay House.

Ludwig, D. S., & Kabat-Zinn, J. (2008). Mindfulness in medicine. *Journal of the American Medical Association, 300*(11), 1350-1352.

Pidgeon, A., Lacota, K., & Champion, J. (2013). The moderating effects of mindfulness on psychological distress and emotional eating behaviour. *Australian Psychologist, 48*(4), 262-269.

Pierson, S., Goto, K., Giampaoli, J., Wylie, A., Seipel, B., & Buffardi, K. (2016). The development of a mindful-eating intervention program among third through fifth grade elementary school children and their parents. *Californian Journal of Health Promotion, 14*(3), 70-76.

Reps, P., & Senzaki, N. (Compilers). (1998). *Zen flesh, Zen bones: A collection of Zen and Pre-Zen writings.* New York, NY: Doubleday. (Original work published 1939)

Satprem. (1993). *Sri Aurobindo or the adventure of consciousness.* Mount Vernon, WA: Institute for Evolutionary Research.

Shapiro, S. L., Carlson, L. E., Astin, J. A., & Freedman, B. (2006). Mechanisms of mindfulness. *Journal of Clinical Psychology, 62*(3), 373-386.

Shonin, E. (2016). This is not McMindfulness. *The Psychologist*, 29(2), 124-125.

Thich Nhat Hanh. (n.d.). *Plum Village* [website]. Retrieved from https://plumvillage.org

Thich Nhat Hanh (1993). *The Blooming of a lotus*. Boston: Beacon Press.

Wanden-Berghe, R., Sanz-Valero, J., & Wanden-Berghe, C. (2011). The application of mindfulness to eating disorders treatment: A systematic review. *Eating Disorders*, 19(1), 34-48.

Zgierska, A. E., Burzinski, C. A., Cox, J., Kloke, J., Singles, J., Mirgain, S., ... Backonja, M. (2016). Mindfulness meditation-based intervention is feasible, acceptable, and safe for chronic low back pain requiring long-term daily opioid therapy. *Journal of Alternative and Complementary Medicine*, 22(8), 610-620.

CHAPTER 7

TOUCH THERAPIES AND BODYWORK INTERVENTIONS

LEARNING OUTCOME

After completing this chapter, the learner will be able to describe one way to integrate touch therapies and bodywork interventions into their nursing practice.

CHAPTER OBJECTIVES

After completing this chapter, the learner will be able to:
1. Describe a technique used in Swedish massage.
2. Explain the physiological benefits of massage therapy.
3. Identify a research-based study on benefits of massage.
4. Describe infant massage education.
5. Explain one theory for how foot reflexology works.

INTRODUCTION

The first sense that is developed as a baby in utero moves against its mother's uterus is the sense of touch. In his book, *Touching: The Human Significance of the Skin*, world-renowned anthropologist and touch researcher Ashley Montagu writes of the importance of touch that, "The impersonality of life in the Western world has become such that we have produced a race of untouchables. We have become strangers to each other, not only avoiding but even warding off all forms of 'unnecessary' physical contact" (1986, p. xiv). Increased use of social media and personal technologies, such as mobile devices, has served to further distance us from the physical space and, therefore, the physical touch of each other. Social isolation and loneliness, despite the growth in human populations, remain cause for concern in the nursing care of people of all ages. Touch therapies and all forms of bodywork that involve direct human touch are not just luxury amenities. They have proved to be life-saving and health-promoting agencies of care.

The purpose of this chapter is to introduce the use of touch therapies and bodywork interventions that can be considered for use in integrative holistic nursing practice. Three forms of touch therapies and bodywork will be discussed in detail: massage therapy, infant massage education, and foot reflexology.

BACKGROUND

Hippocrates, the father of modern medicine, is commonly quoted as saying that the "way to health is to have an aromatic bath and scented massage every day." Touch therapies and bodywork (TTB), like massage, are often easily accessible. They also have centuries of safe use. TTB includes modalities such as Swedish massage, Japanese shiatsu, Chinese tui na, sports massage, rehabilitative massage, and foot reflexology.

Nursing care has historically included TTB – from simple back and foot rubs to highly researched interventions such as kangaroo care (mother to newborn skin-to-skin contact) and infant massage. Basic touch that is employed in day-to-day care of patients is distinguished from TTB, which is purposefully focused on the therapeutic effect of touch. Estabrooks's (1987) historical findings suggest that nurses touch for three basic reasons: to comfort, to perform a procedure, or both, and that much of nursing care in contemporary times is procedural. Examples of nurses' touch include bathing, giving walking assistance, holding patients' hands, and feeding patients. The meaning of touch for patients and their perception of their nurses' use of touch in caregiving has been the subject of research for some time.

One instrument used in research is the Patient Touch Questionnaire, which cites four kinds of nurses' touch: traditional and instrumental (e.g., bathing, back rubs, and teaching), optional (e.g., giving a comforting touch, such as patting a hand), and essential (e.g., turning or exercising the patient). The patient instrument, developed from the Nurses' Touch Questionnaire, found that the 98 adult patients sampled believed that nurses' touch "demonstrated care" and was important but also "conveyed control" and should be used occasionally (as compared with the touch they preferred from family and friends; Mulaik et al., 1991). Whereas the study from Mulaik and colleagues focused generally on patient perception of nurses' touch, research since the 1990s on patient perceptions of touch has been focused on procedural touch. TTB is the mindful application of touch in care for which there is a supporting body of scientific evidence for its application and centuries of art of expression in a way that models a patient's needs for touch.

The movement analyst Irmgard Bartenieff suggests in her work that touch varies in *shape* and *effort*, from such actions as a sudden poke to a constricting grip to an enveloping hug. Touch that is to be therapeutic, she writes, "should be a form of three-dimensional shaping, which is supportive rather than a form of more linear impositions, such as poking" (Bartenieff & Lewis, 2002, p. 150). Touching another person can be a scientifically based and creative, intimate therapeutic act that nurses can learn. TTB skills can enable nurses, through shape and effort, to convey the exact therapeutic experience that a patient requires for health and healing. Those skills begin with mindfulness practices, such as mindful breathing and being in the present moment, as discussed in Chapter 6.

It also is important in TTB that the nurse models an individual patient's culture because physical touch is perceived differently from culture to culture. Some people use direct touch freely and embrace physical contact, where others value indirect touch. For example, in some religious communities, there is a practice known as "laying on of the hands," in which practitioners do not touch the body directly.

TOUCH THERAPIES AND BODYWORK IN PRACTICE

The term *touch therapies* refers to a broad range of modalities used by practitioners that involve putting the hands on or near the body. The three modalities chosen for this text are massage and bodywork techniques, infant massage education, and foot reflexology. Each represents a different dimension of touch therapies and bodywork interventions.

Massage and Bodywork Techniques

A *massage* involves the use of one's hands in the application of pressure and repetitive motion to the skin and underlying muscles for the beneficial purposes of physical and psychological relaxation, relief of tension and sore muscles, stimulation of nerves, and improvement of blood, lymph, and energy (or qi) circulation. According to traditional Chinese medicine (TCM) theory, a possible explanation for how massage works is that it "promotes circulation of qi, blood and fluid throughout the body, dredges meridians and collaterals to relieve pain, and regulate yin and yang" (Xiong, Li, & Zhang, 2015, p. 143). TCM makes an important distinction in the need for touch. When a person has stagnation of energy or qi in a particular area of the body and someone presses on that area (as occurs during therapeutic massage), the patient will experience the pressure as helpful (in that tension is relieved). The patient may experience some discomfort as a muscle, for example, is being worked, but the overall sense that the patient has is that tension and stress are relieved.

Alternatively, when a person has *blood* stagnation in an area of the body, there may be discomfort during massage, especially deeper massage. The skin may even bruise from being lightly touched. It is best to address the underlying blood stagnation first with hydrotherapies, dietary changes, and topical herbal remedies (which are discussed in the following chapters) before proceeding with deep massage. Hematoma is a known risk factor related to deep tissue massage in those with chronic low back pain, particularly those who are advanced in age and demonstrate blood vessel brittleness (Sun, Yuan, & Zhang, 2015). Deep tissue bodywork can be avoided in those patients.

The general techniques used in massage therapy include stroking, kneading, tapping, compression, vibration, rocking, holding, pressing, and friction. In general, long strokes that move from the heart and the center of the body toward the extremities are relaxing. Strokes toward the heart from the extremities are stimulating and energizing. Massage therapy, by increasing blood flow throughout the body, in turn increases the oxygen-carrying potential of the body and the flow of lymph, thereby increasing the removal of metabolic waste.

Skeletal muscles make up about 40% of the human body. When a muscle group is tensed, its oxygen-carrying capacity is reduced. Lymph fluid is moved throughout the body by muscle movement. When people are not able to move as well as they might (e.g., after they have had surgery or experienced an injury), massage helps to keep lymph fluid moving in the lymph channels. Swedish massage, a common massage technique, incorporates basic strokes such as the following:

- **Effleurage:** Light stroking or touching that is focused horizontally
- **Petrissage:** Kneading with a vertical lift technique
- **Friction (rubbing):** Quick, short movements of the hand and fingertips over superficial tissues transversely
- **Percussion (tapotement):** The application of downward vertical pressure with abrupt release, including tapping, slapping, cupping, and beating
- **Vibration or shaking:** Pressing down and then back and forth in a particular place

Research

In healthy adults, massage therapy has been shown to promote relaxation, increase alertness, improve cognitive performance and mood, and reduce stress hormone levels (cortisol) and symptoms of anxiety. In adolescents suffering from touch deficit, neglect, poor attachment, and abuse in childhood, massage therapy has been shown to significantly decrease aggression and violence and increase empathetic behaviors (Field, 2002). Some researchers suggest that the early physical abuse serves to heighten sensory thresholds (such as pain). This effect slows the response to a stimulus and generates arousal-seeking behavior leading to aggression (as cited in Field, 2002).

Field conducted another study comparing American and French adolescents in terms of their aggression. Even 12-year-olds, who were observed during play and when sitting closely together with their best friends, only touched each other 2% of the time. American children touched *themselves* more often, in behaviors such as wringing their hands, twirling their hair, and wrapping their arms around themselves (Field, 1999). A systematic review of studies on sensory-based interventions, such as massage therapy on children with behavioral disorders related to autism spectrum disorder, attention-deficit disorder, and Down syndrome, found massage to be "highly effective" in reducing troublesome behaviors. Out of 132 studies examined, seven sensory-based intervention studies met the criteria for inclusion in the review (Yunus, Liu, Bissett, & Penkala, 2015).

Some of the leading research done on the effect of touch in general and massage in particular over the past two decades has been conducted by the Touch Research Institute of the University of Miami School of Medicine, led by Tiffany Field. One review of studies of the effect of massage therapy on biochemistry in those with depression, HIV, breast cancer, aging, and pregnancy showed that massage is related to a decreased level of cortisol (a stress hormone) and increased levels of serotonin and dopamine (Field, Hernandez-Reif, Diego, Schanberg, & Kuhn, 2005). Massage therapy effects positive change on biochemistry right after a single treatment and also over the entire treatment period. Cortisol is a by-product of the sympathetic nervous system, the hypothalamic-pituitary-adrenal-cortical axis, and is known to kill the body's natural killer cells. It can be measured with a simple saliva test. Serotonin enhances dopamine production and impedes cortisol. Dopamine and serotonin are involved in reducing depression. Thus, positive changes have been noted in biochemistry after massage therapy, including reduced cortisol and increased serotonin and dopamine levels. Many conditions are positively affected by massage therapy, including depression, pain syndromes, autoimmune and immune chronic illnesses, and stress conditions (Field et al., 2005).

Another study investigated the effects of Swedish massage versus a light touch intervention (with the back of the hand) over 5 weeks on neuroendocrine and immune parameters. The data suggest that massage therapy has cumulative and sustained biological effects and that the "dosage" of massage may result in profoundly different biological actions. This observation may explain why there are problems replicating biological and psychological findings in the massage literature: Studies vary greatly in intervention frequency, length, and type. An additional finding of this study funded by a grant from the National Center for Complementary and Alternative Medicine of the National Institutes of Health is that the light-touch condition, involving gentle, systematic, and comprehensive stroking of an individual for 45 minutes, has biological activity (Rapaport, Schettler, & Bresee, 2012, p. 795). Nurses can use light touch just as effectively as deep touch in creating change, transformation, and healing.

Some studies on massage try to better understand its effect on disease processes. One example is a systematic review for essential hypertension (Xiong et al., 2015) in which massage was tested as a complementary therapy to use in conjunction with antihypertensive drugs. The review included randomized controlled trials comparing massage with any type of control intervention as well as studies comparing the effects of massage with antihypertensive drugs to drugs alone. Meta-analysis of 24 articles involving 1,962 patients with essential hypertension were used. The findings showed that massage combined with antihypertensive drugs may be more effective than antihypertensive drugs alone in lowering systolic blood pressure (Xiong et al., 2015). However, the investigators had "numerous concerns" with the methodologies used in most of the studies. The review did not state what type of massage was used in the studies. The investigators also stated that, "Frequency is one of the most important factors contributing to the positive effects of massage." Massage was practiced 30 to 60 minutes per week in the studies. According to TCM theory, massage should be given every day for relieving uncomfortable symptoms (Xiong et al., 2015).

Some massage therapists specialize in providing massage care to those who received a diagnosis of cancer and are undergoing biomedical cancer treatment. To patients with cancer, massage offers general quality-of-life benefits as well as alleviation of cancer-related symptoms or cancer-treatment-related symptoms, including pain, anxiety, and fatigue (Liu et al., 2015). A review cited studies that demonstrated that massage therapy (modalities unknown) decreased nausea during chemotherapy, increased the number of natural killer cells, showed promise in resolving cancer-related fatigue, and contributed to the lessening of symptoms of depression, anxiety, and pain in those receiving palliative oncology care (Liu et al., 2015).

Massage therapy is also well known for its benefit to those with neck pain, a major health problem worldwide. A large randomized controlled trial of over 600 participants with neck pain is currently underway in Sweden (Skillgate et al., 2015).

A meta-analysis of 14 studies included 1,299 patients. Compared with control groups, the children with asthma who received massage therapy demonstrated improvement in pulmonary function parameters and a reduction of plasma concentrations of platelet aggregating factor and prostaglandins (Wu, Yang, & Zhang, 2017).

Professional Notes

According to the Commission on Massage Therapy Accreditation (COMTA), massage therapy students must choose a licensed and accredited school for their education. (See the Resources section for the website.) They undergo hundreds of hours of class and practice to become certified and are required to follow COMTA standards of practice. Although nurses who are licensed to touch can perform back and foot rubs as part of nursing care, in order to advertise oneself to the public as a "massage therapist," states typically expect that the nurse has completed a hands-on massage therapy program.

Regulation varies from state to state. In the United States, 44 states and the District of Columbia regulate massage therapists (National Center for Complementary and Integrative Health, 2022). Most states that regulate massage therapists require that they have completed 500 hours of training from an accredited program. The National Certification Board for Therapeutic Massage and Bodywork (NCBTMB; see the Resources section) certifies practitioners who pass a national examination and fulfill other requirements.

Massage therapy is either contraindicated or requires modification in patients with acute illness or injury, fever, recent surgery, cardiovascular or respiratory insufficiency, psychosis, or those who may be or are pregnant. Massage should not be performed over varicose veins, suspected or known phlebitis, deep vein thrombosis, skin lesions, or fractures and should not be performed in the presence of an open wound (National Center for Complementary and Integrative Health, 2022).

Infant Massage: An Educational Approach

Infants aged 0 to 5 years experience stress, anxiety, depression, and difficulty adapting to the environment, as do adults. However, the experience of nonverbal and preverbal infants is different from those who are verbal, thus fostering the need for integrative modalities that "role-model" a plan for care that is in a language that they can understand. Touch therapies are that language. Touch is a baby's first communication. They spend 9 months in touch with their mother's uterus. To expect that a baby would instantly disconnect with the mother upon birth is unrealistic, and yet so many adults mindlessly hold this expectation after birth. Nurses, who assist families in labor, often show parents how to practice skin-to-skin (kangaroo) care after birth to assist the baby in transition. This scenario could be said to be the first touch therapy modality that integrative holistic nurses give and a newborn person experiences! Nurses are natural teachers of health touch and healing touch.

Infant massage is a touch therapy modality that is delivered according to an educational model of care rather than direct patient contact. Those who are certified in infant massage are not certified to actually massage babies and therefore do not need to be licensed to touch. Infant massage certification is an educational certification to *teach parents and caregivers* how to communicate and bond with their babies through massage. The International Association of Infant Massage (IAIM) was founded by Vimala Schneider McClure with the purpose of "promote nurturing touch and communication through training, education, and research so that parents, caregivers, and children are loved, valued and respected throughout the world community" (IAIM, n.d.; McClure, 2017). The first step taught to parents and caregivers in an infant massage class is to ask a baby's permission to touch. They then choose an unscented cold-pressed vegetable oil to warm in their hands and use in the massage. Scented oils, including all natural, organic essential oils in small amounts, can be overwhelming for a newborn. The therapeutic purpose of the massage is for the parent to bond with baby. This bonding takes place through all senses, including smell. It is familiar and therefore calming for babies to smell their parents/caregivers.

Infant massage is typically taught in five weekly sessions. Strokes taught during the first session include such techniques as "Indian milking" of the ankle and "toe squeezes." Caregivers are taught to start with the feet and legs rather than the head and face. However, if babies have injuries, such as sore places on their heels from where they were poked for a blood draw in the hospital, caregivers will need to move slowly and invite the baby to tell them, through crying, their story about their body. Infants may cry when their parents put their hands near their heels and ask infants to tell them if their heels are okay.

This touch-focused communication begins the trust-building process between parent and child. The child understands that his or her parent invites their feelings and will listen. The parent sees the immediate result of opening the communication channels with their baby and the positive results that the subsequent massage that heals their baby's heels may have. Subsequent sessions focus on the abdomen, chest and arms, and face and back. The role of the infant massage instructor is more than teaching massage strokes. The effective instructor helps with communication and cue interpretation and conveys unconditional positive regard for parents and babies (McClure, 2017).

Over time, those who have conducted research using the cumulative risk model have demonstrated that the most common risk factors to infant physical, mental, emotional and spiritual health are poverty, parenting skill, maternal depression, and preterm birth (Zeanah, 2009, p. 134). Infant massage is inexpensive, assists parents in developing their infant communication and caregiving skills, and is an effective modality for fathers and depressed mothers to use when seeking to bond with a baby when the mother experiences postpartum depression after birth.

Research

A systematic review of literature on infant massage from 2006 to 2011 was conducted by a Swedish nurse doctoral student using the Cochrane Central Register of Controlled Trials, PubMed, and the Cumulative Index of Nursing and Allied Health Literature (CINAHL). She found no reports of harmful effects from infant massage. It was found to have "positive effects on children's growth, health and behavioral development, and to have beneficial effects on the mothers' psychological well-being when they gave their children massage," and she concluded that "parental education in infant massage is a cost-effective and health promoting measure" (Garmy, 2012). However, one mixed-method study of 39 dyads (mothers and infants) suggests that "high-risk" mothers (i.e., those who had risk factors over and above their demographic risk) may not benefit from an infant massage education program alone and that infant massage programs should be targeted at parents experiencing "moderate" risk problems. The majority of mothers with at-risk interactions did not have access to the teaching about infant cues and signals because they attended programs facilitated by Peter Walker instead of IAIM-trained facilitators. The trainings differ in orientation. The IAIM trainers focus on baby's communication cues, emotional, and behavioral states; the Peter Walker facilitators focus on flexibility and movement and not infant communication and participation (Underdown, Norwood, & Barlow, 2013).

Infants also have a great need for help in neuromotor organization, especially as a result of the birth process. Infant massage is helpful for healthy newborns who are adapting quickly to extrauterine life and developing emotional attachment with their parents and caregivers. Hospitalized premature infants are at particular risk for delays in bonding and maternal attachment. Studies have shown that massage (head-to-toe 15-minute massage three times per day for 5 days) given to premature neonates by their mothers on a daily basis can promote and maintain emotional attachment between the mother and her infant (Shoghi, Sohrabi, & Rasouli 2017).

Massage therapy (specifically, passive limb movements) promotes growth and development in preterm infants as well as improved bone density; yet, as of 2010, it is used in only 38% of neonatal intensive care units (Field, Diego, & Hernandez-Reif, 2010b). Similarly, the use of moderate pressure versus light pressure massage is essential for improving neurobehavioral outcomes in full-term infants (Field, Diego, & Hernandez-Reif, 2010a) and promoting growth in both preterm and full-term infants. In preterm infants, moderate pressure, but not light pressure massage, consistently elicited a parasympathetic nervous system response characterized by an increase in the high-frequency component of heart rate variability (HRV) and an increase in gastric motility (Diego & Field, 2009). These increases in HRV and gastric motility were related to weight gain in the infants, suggesting that the effects of massage therapy may be mediated by increased parasympathetic nervous system activity (Diego & Field, 2009).

Professional Notes

Infant massage practice and research have two different but potentially complementary models. The infant massage practice model is similar to that of adult massage, in which the focus is the therapeutic benefit of massage. The infant massage education model, however, incorporates both the therapeutic benefits of the physical massage and stresses the communication and bonding focus of the interaction between parent/caregiver and infant. The infant still receives the benefits of massage, but the focus is associating that positive effect with a parent or caregiver rather than a massage therapist or nurse. When one is reviewing findings from clinical trial data from infant massage studies, it is important to place findings within their appropriate scientific context.

As discussed previously, infant massage instructors are teachers and infant-parent/caregiver relationship facilitators, and not necessarily massage therapists or health professionals who are licensed to touch.

Foot Reflexology: Adding a Dimension to Touch

Foot reflexology (FR), thought to have possibly originated in Egypt, as depicted on the wall of the tomb of Ankhm'ahor of the Sixth Dynasty, is the practice of using both hands on the feet and stimulating the reflexes in the feet that correspond to body organs, systems, glands, and energy centers with specific hand and finger techniques. This ancient practice is based on the premise that there are zones and reflex areas located on the feet and hands that correspond to all parts of the body. The feet are viewed as maps or mirrors of the body. Each part of a foot represents a certain part of the body. According to this theory, reflexes can communicate with organs, glands, and other parts of the body. In fact, each foot has more than 7,000 nerve endings that facilitate this communication process.

The two feet, together side by side, represent the entire anatomy of the human body with all of its organs, systems, and energy pathways. Each part of the body is referred to as an "area" or "energy field" within a zone on the feet. There are 10 vertical zones, five on each foot, drawn from the toe to the heel. A FR treatment includes touching the whole body, all areas and all 10 zones, in one session. The ability to do this in a short time is what makes FR unique and potentially profound in its impact on balance and integrative holistic health. FR is neither a medical treatment of disease or diseased body organs and systems, nor is it a simple foot rub.

The feet represent a hologram of the entire human anatomy and physiology (processes) scaled down into the feet. Reflexologists work to form a three-dimensional understanding and representation of the hologram. That representation is depicted as a "chart" or map of the hologram of the body scaled down into the feet. The chart is used in teaching and treatment. The position of the organs and how one effects the physiology or flow of movement of energy through the organs is the foundation for foot reflexology practice and skill. Anyone can push points on the feet, but that is not foot reflexology. Foot reflexology has been defined as "moving energy in a way that complements physiology and energy patterns of the unique person" (Libster, 2015, p. 51). Foot reflexologists use a keen knowl-

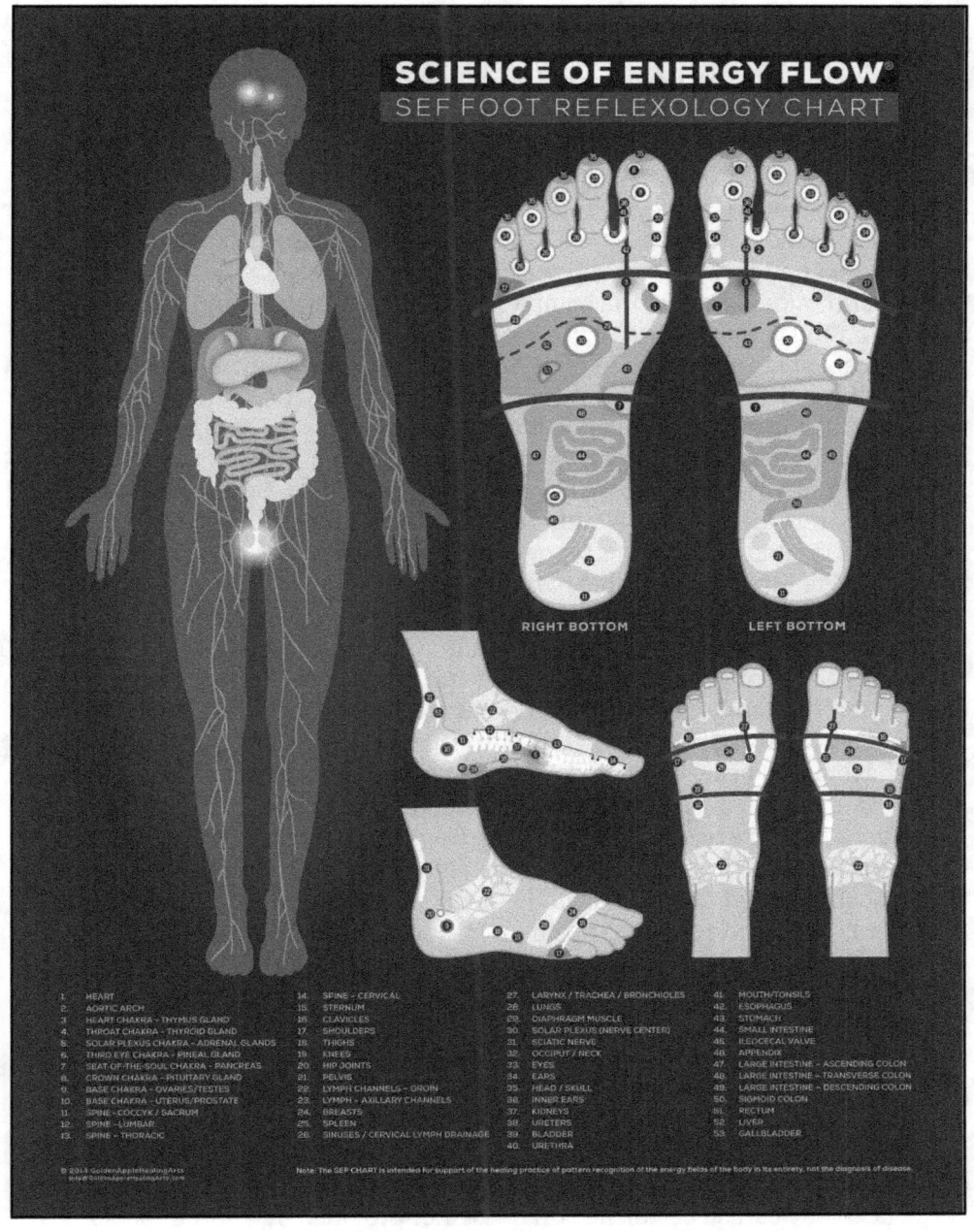

FIGURE 7-1: SCIENCE OF ENERGY FLOW® FOOT REFLEXOLOGY CHART
© 2014 Golden Apple Healing Arts

edge of anatomy and physiology, which they visualize and apply to working the feet. The way the feet are worked depends on the anatomy and physiology of an organ or system. For example, when working the gallbladder, which is anatomically behind the liver on the right side of the body, the reflexologist uses a finger technique to lift the liver area on the right foot and stimulate the gallbladder. The gallbladder has a duct that empties into the small intestine. Therefore, the foot reflexologist's hand and finger techniques should mimic the normal physiological action of the gallbladder and move the energy of the gallbladder area downward into the small intestine area. The same notion of working an organ area according to its physiological function and the flow or movement of energy through it is applied to each organ and system.

The Reflexology Association of America (RAA) defines reflexology as manual techniques "applied to specific reflex areas predominantly on the feet and hands. These techniques stimulate the complex neural pathways linking body systems, supporting the body's efforts to function optimally" (RAA, 2016). Reducing stress and reestablishing the balance of energy are key benefits of reflexology. How this is achieved is still the question driving scientific and clinical research of the modality. Modern reflexology has its roots in the Zone Therapy practice and research of the early 20th-century American physician, William Fitzgerald, who redeveloped the practice in 1913 (Fitzgerald & Bowers, 1917). Dr. Fitzgerald showed that when any part of a zone is stimulated, it affects all of the corresponding parts of the body located in that zone. Many years later, physiotherapist Eunice Ingham (1984) perfected the theory and developed it into a usable therapy. She not only pinpointed which zones affected which parts of the body, but also how.

Reflexology involves the use of the hands and fingers to apply pressure to specific zones, or energy channels, of the feet and hands. These zones correlate with other parts of the body. For example, the toes correspond to the head; the ball of the foot, and the heart and lung areas; and the heel corresponds to the pelvis (see Figure 7-1). Reflexologists believe that poor diet, stress, lack of exercise, illness, and other factors can cause congestion in the feet, resulting in deposits of crystalline-like grains around the nerve endings. By using deep pressure with the fingers, reflexology therapists can break down these crystals so that they can be carried away in the bloodstream and excreted from the body. The crystals can be seen during FR treatments as they are excreted through the pores on the soles of the feet.

Foot reflexology is a commonly used complementary therapy for stress and disease management in Europe (Germany, England, Switzerland), Asia (Korea, Thailand, Taiwan, China), and Russia. Various forms of reflexology exist, some of which have been around for centuries. Examples of techniques include the Ingham Method and Zone Therapy. The Ingham Method is a commonly used technique in the United States. It allows the practitioner to pinpoint the exact zone and location affected by the application of pressure. Different countries have slightly different variations of these techniques.

Reflexology can be performed on oneself or provided by another person. The equipment needed to perform reflexology includes a well-padded table, a chair or stool, and a quiet environment. If reflexology is done in the home or hospital, no padded table is required. A person can be treated in a recliner chair, a bed, or with their feet on a stool or in the lap of the provider. Foot reflexology treatments are complemented by other modalities, such as music, essential oil foot massage and aromatherapy, relaxation and breathing exercises, herbal foot wraps, and hydrotherapy (footbaths).

Science of Energy Flow®

The Science of Energy Flow® Foot Reflexology technique (SEF) (Libster, 2015) was created by a nurse and is used by integrative holistic nurses around the world. The SEF technique is an example of precision nursing science in practice that incorporates the healing traditions of foot reflexology (more than twenty-five hand positions) with herbal applications for stress relief. The treatment begins with a "Five Element" herbal footbath ablution of the feet followed by an anointing of the feet with soothing herbal oils. The treatment concludes with an herbal wrap for the sealing of the feet and protection of the person's healing. All herbal applications are customized to meet the precise energetic needs of the patient for balance in body and peace of mind.

The SEF treatment integrates the ancient understanding of foot reflexology and topical herbal applications with emerging scientific understanding of ways to effect whole person healing through the hologram of the feet. A person's divine blueprint for wholeness is activated through SEF foot reflexology. The SEF chart is intended for guiding pattern recognition of the energy fields of the body in its entirety and the SEF treatment through the feet. The SEF chart is not used in the diagnosis and treatment of biomedical disease.

Research

There are several theories for how reflexology works. Fitzgerald, who referred to foot work as "zone analgesia," and other zone therapists suggest that prolonged massage to a particular tender reflex point causes a counterirritant effect (increased circulation) with its accompanying sympathetic healing reflex in the organ associated with the area being treated (Fitzgerald & Bowers, 1917). Another theory is that the foot work breaks up uric acid crystals that form on the nerve endings in the feet and subsequently block energy flow to the nerve endings of the feet that are connected to body organs and systems. Others posit that reflexology works when "proprioceptive centers in the feet stimulate responses in the autonomic and sensorimotor nervous system (Kunz & Kunz, 1995).

In addition to these physical theories, others teach that reflexology may be explained best by the emerging science of memory, holograms, energy fields, and light. Such works include those by Sheldrake (1995) on morphic resonance and Bohm (1980) on implicate order that suggest that the action of reflexology works through the hologram of the feet providing access to a "blueprint" of wholeness. This action is what differentiates this healing modality (foot reflexology) from others, such as the practice of medicine. "The focus is sending a signal to the blueprint" that dictates the change necessary to manifest healing (Libster, 2015, p. 15).

The pressure techniques of reflexology create change in the feet, which are highly sensitive because of their purpose in mobility and in the fight-or-flight response. Any pressure perceived by the foot is a stimulus to which the entire body responds. The perceived result is most often stress relief and a sense of relief and balance, physically through each foot. This result is followed by physical, emotional, and psychological change stimulated by releasing blockages in the corresponding areas in the feet. Effects other than stress relief have been studied. A few examples of clinical research and meta-analyses are provided in the following sections.

Dysmenorrhea

One correlational study compared the effects of foot reflexology and connective tissue manipulation (a bodywork intervention) in participants with dysmenorrhea. FR was applied to 15 participants 3 days a week. Treatments were performed during one cycle, which started at the third or fourth day of menstruation and continued until the onset of the next menstruation. Both treatments provided significant improvements. The FR used in the study did not include treatment of the whole body in the feet. It included application of olive oil and gentle mobilization of the foot. The solar plexus point was pressured to stimulate the whole body. Afterward, the endocrine glands, small and large intestine, spine, uterus, vagina, ovaries, fallopian tube, and breast fields were stimulated, followed by the solar plexus again (Demirtürk et al., 2016).

Sleep

A systematic review and meta-analysis of 44 studies indicates that foot reflexology is a useful nursing intervention to relieve fatigue and to promote sleep (Lee, Han, Chung, Kim, & Choi, 2011).

Blood Pressure

FR is used to increase vagal modulation and decrease blood pressure in both healthy people and patients with coronary artery disease. In the study, FR was performed on participants lying in a comfortable, supine position. A certified foot reflexologist from the Taiwan Association of Reflexology used the "Father Josef's techniques" using the thumb and the fingers to apply pressure to stimulate all reflex zones in both feet. Grapeseed oil was used to prevent friction and discomfort because it is not sticky, is odorless, and absorbs easily into the skin (Lu, Chen, & Kuo, 2011).

Labor

Reflexology has been shown to reduce labor pain intensity, duration of labor, anxiety, and the frequency distribution of natural delivery and to increase Apgar scores. For this study, the sole of the foot was rubbed with sunflower oil, followed by a mild massage of the whole foot. Then pressure was applied to the pituitary gland, solar plexus, and uterus fields for 40 minutes (20 minutes for each foot; Moghimi-Hanjani, Mehdizadeh-Tourzani, & Shoghi, 2015).

Stress, Fatigue, and Depression

A systematic review of the literature was conducted using databases (MEDLINE, Embase, Cochrane, and CINAHL) and Chinese (CNKI), Japanese (J-STAGE), and Korean databases (KoreaMed, KMbase, KISS, NDSL, KISTI, and OASIS) to examine the state of the science of FR as a self-care practice. The search included MeSH terminology and key words (foot reflexology, foot massage, and self). Analysis of three nonrandomized trials and three before-and-after studies showed that self-administered foot reflexology resulted in significant improvement in subjective outcomes such as perceived stress, fatigue, and depression. However, no significant improvement occurred in objective outcomes such as cortisol levels, blood pressure, and pulse rate. No randomized controlled trials were reviewed (Song et al., 2015).

Professional Notes

National certification is available through the Reflexology Association of America (RAA) but is optional. The RAA has a published Code of Ethics and Standards of Practice for a specific technique and areas of application (RAA, n.d.). The process of obtaining reflexology licensure or certification varies from state to state. However, the RAA has formulated and reported the basic standards for obtaining certification in reflexology, which include the completion of a certain number of hours in practice and testing. In some states, a massage license is required to practice reflexology. For the most part, however, any person licensed in nursing can become a reflexologist with properly documented education. No standard curriculum that is mandated for certification and licensure exists nationally.

CASE STUDY:
REFINING THE ELEMENTS OF TOUCH SKILLS

Michael and Jackie Jones just gave birth to their first child, a premature infant, at the hospital. The baby, who is in the neonatal intensive care unit, has not been gaining weight. Michael and Jackie ask their nurse what they can do to help their baby. They say that their friends suggested that they massage the baby but are afraid to do so because they might "hurt the baby" because "she is a preemie." They ask Nurse Brian to massage the baby.

Questions

1. How might Nurse Brian respond to Mr. and Mrs. Jones?

2. What might he recommend for their plan of care to integrate infant massage?

Nurse's Answers

1. Modeling the world of the first-time parents, Nurse Brian can express understanding about their fears. After discussing their concerns, he might offer to discuss massage with them. He lets them know that infant massage has been used to promote growth and development in premature infants. When the nurse observes their readiness for information and education about massage, he focuses his education on massage specifically for premature infants.

2. For a short-term goal, the nurse recommends that he help the parents to become comfortable holding the baby so that they can learn to do some passive limb movements that are "exercise" for the baby. He explains that the loving touch they give the baby can help them to bond with and communicate with their baby, knowing that touch is baby's first communication. His long-term plan includes signing the new parents up for an IAIM course with a nurse instructor on the unit who works with families transitioning to home.

HOLISTIC TRANSFORMATION

Back massage is a massage modality used historically in nursing. Try the following "recipe" for slow stroke back massage relaxation on a friend or family member. It was published originally by Sims in a 1986 article of *Nursing Times* that focused on massage for patients with cancer and then furthered by Somani, Merchant, and Lalani in 2013.

Use equal and gentle pressure for 10 minutes.

Step 1: Effleurage or long strokes. Start from the spine and cover the whole back and shoulder area.

Step 2: Fanning out. Continue the first step but add circular movements to the upper portion of the spine with both hands on either side of the spine.

Step 3: Feathering or light strokes with fingertips. Close the 10 minutes with cupping – gently pat the back with a cupped hand.

After the massage, answer the following questions:

1. What changes did you notice in your friend or family member's body as a result of your nurses' back massage?

2. How did you feel during the nurses' back massage? What are your thoughts about touch therapies?

SUMMARY

Touch therapies and bodywork encompass a broad range of healing techniques, including massage therapy, infant massage education, and foot reflexology. Touch therapy is accessible, cost-effective, and effective. Nurses with education in touch therapies and bodywork are in a position to offer their service in any clinical setting. One important way to learn touch therapies is to experience them personally and try different techniques and strokes on friends and family members while observing for responses. Touch therapies and bodywork may be complemented by other modalities, such as relaxation, guided imagery, music, and mindfulness meditation. Massage, infant massage education, and foot reflexology are known to promote stress relief and have some clinical research evidence for relieving symptoms associated with chronic and acute illness.

RESOURCES

American Massage Therapy Association   https://www.amtamassage.or

Commission on Massage Therapy Accreditation (CMTA)   https://comta.ormassage-therapy-trainincurriculum/

International Association of Infant Massage   https://iaim.net

National Certification Board for Therapeutic Massage & Bodywork (NCBTMB)
　　　http://www.ncbtmb.com

Reflexology Association of America
　　　http://reflexology-usa.org

REFERENCES

Bartenieff, I., & Lewis, D. (2002). Body movement: *Coping with the environment.* London, England: Routledge.

Bohm, D. (1980). *Wholeness and the implicate order.* London, England: Routledge Classics.

Demirtürk, F., Erkek, Z. Y., Alparslan, O., Demirtürk, F., Demir, O., & Inanir, A. (2016). Comparison of reflexology and connective tissue manipulation in participants with primary dysmenorrhea. *Journal of Alternative and Complementary Medicine*, 22(1), 38-44.

Diego, M. A., & Field, T. (2009). Moderate pressure massage elicits a parasympathetic nervous system response. *International Journal of Neuroscience,* 119(5), 630-638.

Estabrooks, C. A. (1987). Touch in nursing practice: A historical perspective. 1900-1920. *Journal of Nursing History*, 2(2), 33-49.

Field, T. (1999). American adolescents touch each other less and are more aggressive toward their peers as compared with French adolescents. *Adolescence,* 34(136), 753-758.

Field, T. (2002). Violence and touch deprivation in adolescents. *Adolescence,* 37(148), 735-749.

Field, T., Diego, M., & Hernandez-Reif, M. (2010a). Moderate pressure is essential for massage therapy effects. *International Journal of Neuroscience*, 120(5), 381-385.

Field, T., Diego, M., & Hernandez-Reif, M. (2010b). Preterm infant massage therapy research: A review. *Infant Behavior and Development,* 33(2), 115-124.

Field, T., Hernandez-Reif, M., Diego, M., Schanberg, S., & Kuhn, C. (2005). Cortisol decreases and serotonin and dopamine increase following massage therapy. *International Journal of Neuroscience*, 115(10), 1397-1413.

Fitzgerald, W. H., & Bowers, E. F. (1917). *Zone therapy, or relieving pain at home.* Columbus, OH: I. W. Long.

Garmy, P. (2012). Aktuellt kunskapsläge om spädbarnsmassage – systematisk litteraturöversikt, 2006-2011. *Nordic Journal of Nursing Research & Clinical Studies,* 32(4), 29-33.

Ingham, E. (1984). *The Original works of Eunice Ingham.* St. Petersburg, FL: Ingham Publishing, Inc.

International Association of Infant Massage. (n.d.) [website]. Retrieved from http://www.iaim.net

Kunz, K., & Kunz, B. (1995, April/May). Understanding the science and art of reflexology. *Alternative & Complementary Therapies*, 183-186.

Lee, J., Han, M., Chung, Y., Kim, J., & Choi, J. (2011). Effects of foot reflexology on fatigue, sleep and pain: A systematic review and meta-analysis. *Journal of the Korean Academy of Academic Nursing,* 41(6), 821-833.

Libster, M. (2015). *Science of energy flow: Foot reflexology with herbal stress relief.* Wauwatosa, WI: Golden Apple Publications.

Liu, S., Qi, W., Li, H., Wang, Y. F., Yang, X. F., Li, Z. M., ... Cong, D. Y. (2015). Recent advances in massage therapy – A review. *European Review for Medical and Pharmacological Sciences*, 19(20), 3843-3849.

Lu, W. A., Chen, G. Y., & Kuo, C. D. (2011). Foot reflexology can increase vagal modulation, decrease sympathetic modulation, and lower blood pressure in healthy subjects and patients with coronary artery disease. *Alternative Therapies in Health and Medicine*, 17(4), 8-14.

McClure, V. (2017). *Infant massage: A handbook for loving parents* (4th ed.). New York, NY: Random House.

Moghimi-Hanjani, S., Mehdizadeh-Tourzani, Z., & Shoghi, M. (2015). The effect of foot reflexology on anxiety, pain, and outcomes of the labor in primigravida women. *Acta Medica Iranica*, 53(8), 507-511.

Montagu, A. (1986). *Touching: The human significance of the skin* (3rd ed.). New York, NY: Harper & Row.

Mulaik, J. S., Megenity, J. S., Cannon, R. B., Chance, K. S., Cannella, K. S., Garland, L. M., & Gilead, M. P. (1991). Patients' perceptions of nurses' use of touch. *Western Journal of Nursing Research*, 13(3), 306-323.

National Center for Complementary and Integrative Health. (2022). *Massage therapy: What you need to know.* Retrieved from https://www.nccih.nih.gov/health/massage-therapy-what-you-need-to-know

Rapaport, M. H., Schettler, P., & Bresee, C. (2012). A preliminary study of the effects of repeated massage on hypothalamic–pituitary–adrenal and immune function in healthy individuals: A study of mechanisms of action and dosage. *Journal of Alternative and Complementary Medicine*, 18(8), 789-797.

Reflexology Association of America. (n.d.) *Reflexology Association of America code of ethics and standards of practice.* Retrieved from http://reflexology-usa.orinformation/standards-and-ethics/

Reflexology Association of America (2016). http://reflexology-usa.orinformation/raas-definition-of-reflexology/

Sheldrake, R. (1995). *The presence of the past: Morphic resonance and the habits of nature.* Rochester, VT: Park Street Press.

Shoghi, M., Sohrabi, S., & Rasouli, M. (2017). The effects of massage by mothers on mother-infant attachment. *Alternative Therapies in Health and Medicine,* 23(7), e-pub ahead of print.

Skillgate, E., Bill, A.-S., Côté, P., Viklund, P., Peterson, A., & Holm, L. W. (2015). The effect of massage therapy and/or exercise therapy on subacute or long-lasting neck pain – The Stockholm neck trial (STONE): A study protocol for a randomized controlled trial. *Trials, 16, 414*. doi:10.1186/s13063-015-0926-4.

Somani, S., Merchant, S., & Lalani, S. (2013). A literature review about effectiveness of massage therapy for cancer pain. *Journal of the Pakistan Medical Association*, 63(11), 1418-1421.

Song, H. J., Son, H., Seo, H. J., Lee, H., Choi, S. M., & Lee, S. (2015). Effect of self-administered foot reflexology for symptom management in healthy persons: A systematic review and meta-analysis. *Complementary Therapies in Medicine*, 23(1), 79-89.

Sun, F., Yuan, Q.-L., & Zhang, Y.-G. (2015). Large buttocks hematoma caused by deep tissue massage therapy. *Pain Medicine*, 16(7), 1445-1447.

Underdown, A., Norwood, R., & Barlow, J. (2013). A realist evaluation of the processes and outcomes of infant massage programs. *Infant Mental Health Journal*, 34(6), 483-495.

Wu, J., Yang, X., & Zhang, M. (2017). Massage therapy in children with asthma: A systematic review and meta-analysis. *Evidence-Based Complementary and Alternative Medicine*, 2017, article 5620568. Retrieved from https://doi.or10.1155/2017/5620568

Xiong, X. J., Li, S. J., & Zhang, Y. Q. (2015). Massage therapy for essential hypertension: A systematic review. *Journal of Human Hypertension*, 29(3), 143-151.

Yunus, F. W., Liu, K. P. Y., Bissett, M., & Penkala, S. (2015). Sensory-based intervention for children with behavioral problems: A systematic review. *Journal of Autism and Developmental Disorders*, 45, 3565-3579.

Zeanah, C. H., Jr. (Ed.). (2009). *Handbook of infant mental health* (3rd ed.). New York, NY: Guilford Press.

CHAPTER 8

COMMUNICATION INTERVENTIONS

LEARNING OUTCOME

After completing this chapter, the learner will be able to identify examples of integrative holistic communication interventions.

CHAPTER OBJECTIVES

After completing this chapter, the learner will be able to:
1. Explain different communication interventions used in cultivating therapeutic relationships.
2. Describe some counseling techniques used in cultivating therapeutic relationships.
3. List applications for music therapy and music-based integrative holistic interventions.
4. Discuss one of the professional nursing implications associated with the use of communication interventions, such as music and animal-assisted therapies.
5. Define animal-assisted therapy as an integrative holistic intervention.

INTRODUCTION

Touch, as discussed in Chapter 7, is one form of communication that is characteristic of integrative holistic nursing. Touch and the other senses are used when developing relationships with people, animals, plants, and the environment. Communication is also a foundational process in the development of therapeutic relationships, which are the cornerstone of integrative holistic nursing interventions. Communication is a reciprocal process involving a receiver and a sender. These two communication roles are defined and expressed in relationships with the environment and with other people. Communication interventions are the modalities that provide the structure from which people in relationships with one another are able to capture and define understanding, expand their repertoire for expression of thoughts and feelings, and initiate insights that form the healing experience. Communication interventions involve verbal and nonverbal approaches that are demonstrated within the boundaries of a therapeutic relationship.

BACKGROUND

The skill of initiating and maintaining a therapeutic relationship is foundational to professional practice in health care. All nurses are taught and tested on some basic methods for developing rapport with patients and utilizing communication skills; however, an integrative holistic paradigm suggests that communication interventions mindfully address all five Elements of Care®. The interventions attend to a patient's thoughts (Air), feelings (Water), physical space and environment (Earth), spirit (Fire), and meaning (Ether).

Incorporating all five elements within a communication intervention is an integrative holistic nursing skill in the cultivation of therapeutic relationships. This chapter provides a review of some skills for cultivating therapeutic relationships and then gives examples of two communication interventions in practice. Some communication modalities can be learned and immediately integrated with nursing practice; others require further education and professional certification or licensure should a an integrative holistic seek to incorporate them in practice.

Cultivating Therapeutic Relationships

Therapeutic relationships address the healing and educational needs of patients. Hildegard Peplau (1952, p. 69) wrote in her classic text, *Interpersonal Relations in Nursing*, that, "Careful observation and skillful listening always precede the giving of advice." When nurses follow the nursing process, they assess before attempting to diagnose or label the health pattern before them or plan care. The nursing process (see Chapter 4) and modeling the patient's world (see Chapter 2) are the scaffold for a mindful listening approach.

According to the American Holistic Nurses Association/American Nurses Association *Holistic Nursing Scope and Standards of Practice* (2018), one of the major focuses of integrative holistic nursing practice is assisting patients to find meaning in their experience. The nurse – as counselor and coach – helps patients to remember and understand what is happening to them in the present situation so that their experiences can be "integrated with rather than dissociated from other experiences in life" (Peplau, 1952, p. 64). During traumatic injuries, illnesses, and other healing crises, people can experience a disconnect from their previous life experience. These moments of great change and transition often represent the point in a person's life when that person seeks meaning as well as care. These opportunities compel nurses to communicate in ways that assist patients in their own processes of coming to understand the meaning of their experiences, gaining insights from those experiences, making life decisions, and developing greater skill in communicating thoughts and feelings as a result.

The integrative holistic nurse in therapeutic relationships often serves the patient as counselor and coach who facilitates a patient's life learning and decision making. The integrative holistic nurse with a master's degree in Psychiatric

Mental Health Nursing is educated and experienced also to provide psychotherapy services to patients. Such psychotherapy services represent a continuum of care starting with promoting wellness (as does the integrative holistic and coach) and include interventions that address serious psychiatric illness. Although both integrative holistic counselors and coaches and nurse psychotherapists work with patients on behavior change and decision making, the "field of consideration of affect and belief systems goes wider and deeper for psychotherapy than is prudent for health coaching" (Jordan, 2013, p. 31). The direction of the general skills discussed here is toward the integrative holistic nurse as counselor and coach.

Nondirective counseling and coaching is an effective overarching communication approach that can be used in integrative holistic nursing to promote a patient's understanding and insight. A nondirective counseling approach has also been thought to cultivate nonjudgment in the counselor and coach and help in the modeling of the world of another. Some people question the validity of the notion that a counselor, coach, or therapist can fully bracket their own values and judgments and provide a truly nondirective space for patient reflection because people in the helping professions are human beings, just as those they serve. However, nondirection and bracketing (or suspending) one's own values are critical in regard to social and moral issues that emerge during the process of cultivating therapeutic relationships so as not to exploit the power that counselors and coaches may have in that relationship (Gaylin, 2000).

Communication modalities, either those geared toward counseling and coaching or those meant to be psychotherapeutic, compel nurses to work on their own instrument, that is, their own self. Self-awareness in the nurse is the instrument used in cultivation of therapeutic relationships. Those nurses who have grappled with their own personality development and interpersonal problems through educa-tion and experience are, according to Peplau (1952, p. xii), better prepared to demonstrate care to patients who are experiencing major life challenges. In self-awareness work, nurses reflect on their own personal and professional rituals or repeating solutions. Some rituals are familiar and therefore can be energizing. Some rituals that are mindless habits repeated for purposes of promoting the nurse's comfort related to familiarity do not support the patient (Hess et al., 2012). The nurse can affirm the rituals and beliefs in a person's cultural background that offer meaning and support for decision making, behavior change, and healing. Capturing context and culture requires relevant ways of knowing from both the nurse and the client. These are unique skills that assist nurses in cultivating deeper self-knowledge while honoring diverse perspectives.

Empathy

The ability to provide care that authentically models the patient's world is the practice of *empathy*. This communication skill, according to participants involved in qualitative research led by Geist-Martin and Bell (2009), suggests that integrative holistic care providers have an "obligation to open their hearts to patients first of all" through looking at and listening closely to patients so as to build therapeutic relationships. The research of the HeartMath Institute supports this premise. The heart's electrical signals permeate every cell of the human body. HeartMath techniques for stress reduction and self-awareness help to improve the quality of the heart's signals to the cells through the two-way communication system between the heart and the brain (Childre, 1998). Heart rate variability (HRV) research at the HeartMath Institute demonstrates that "feelings of sincere appreciation" *create* smooth, even rhythms (HRV) that exemplify cardiovascular efficiency (Childre, 1998, p. 31) in which the two branches of the autonomic nervous system are working together. People who cultivate their own sincere appreciation for another person are able to express empathy and sympathy in their relationships with others.

Empathy and sympathy have been identified as distinct psychological processes since the early 20th century. Whereas sympathy was the term used to describe the shared feelings and the "bond that holds society together" since the 1700s, the term *empathy* (derived from the German *Einfühlung*), meant to project oneself emotionally as "inner imitation" (Jahoda, 2005).

Peplau (1952, p. 173) defines the empathic experience as the ability to feel what is going on in a situation "without specifically being able to discuss and to identify elements of it in awareness." She differentiated the use of the term *empathy* in nursing from "sympathy" in the 1950s. Sympathy had been cultivated as an "essential quality" in nursing in the early 20th century (Harmer & Henderson, 1939). Empathy, as an essential quality of relatedness, stems from the nurse's skill in cultivation of a nonjudgmental attitude and accepting people as they are.

Empathy, respect, and responsibility are the three values aligned with the art of nursing that are the basis for authentic nurse-patient relationships, considered the "hallmark of high quality nursing care" (Alligood & Fawcett, 2017, p. 7). Authenticity in therapeutic relationships is fostered through the development of relatability, a quality achieved through the "genuine expression of knowledge, concern, and empathy for individuals' needs" (Prestia, 2016) and through personal work that cultivates self-awareness.

Nonverbal expressions of empathy varied across cultural groups and had an impact on the quality of communication and care. Lorié, Reinero, Phillips, Zhang, & Riess (2017) conducted a systematic review of studies examining how culture mediates nonverbal expressions of empathy with the aim to improve clinician cross-cultural competency. The authors concluded that mindful and skilled nonverbal communication plays a significant role in fostering trusting provider-patient relationships and is critical to high-quality care.

Self-Awareness

Self-awareness can be cultivated through observation of self-talk, boundaries and use of personal space and through managing feelings of uncertainty. Communication includes verbal and nonverbal expression. The words that are used in communication reflect thought processes. For example, when a patient asks for something and the nurse replies, "I am sorry, but I can't get that for you right now," the patient may hear the words "I can't" rather than the nurse's heartfelt apology for not being able to help "right now." Mindfully reframing a response according to what *can* be done often results in energizing communication between the nurse and the patient. One example of a reframe might be: "Yes, I can certainly get that for you in 10 minutes."

Boundaries mark the limits of a professional relationship and define a safe relational space where the patient and the nurse can explore the patient's issues. Boundaries are also the limits of the fiduciary relationship in which a person, the nurse, with "particular knowledge and abilities accepts the trust and confidence of another to act in that person's best interest" (Peternelj-Taylor & Yonge, 2003, p. 57). The complexities of establishing the limits of professional boundaries of the nurse-patient relationship can cause a lot of confusion and concern. Patients expect a nurse to act in their best interest and to respect their dignity. "This means that a nurse abstains from obtaining personal gain at the patient's expense and refrains from inappropriate involvement with a patient or the patient's family members" (National Council of State Boards of Nursing, n.d.).

Even with much training in therapeutic relationships, nurses can still experience new levels of uncertainty when they learn new caring interventions, such as touch therapies and counseling techniques. The nurse has a responsibility to focus the therapeutic relationship on the needs of the patient and to not engage in behavior that exploits the patient's vulnerability when the patient is seeking help. Nurses who engage in complementary therapies, such as touch and communication therapies and interventions, learn additional skills and techniques to manage the uncertainties of the new relationship.

Listening to one's own self-talk or inner dialogue is one way to manage uncertainty. It has been a well-known psychological concept for centuries in which a person adopts two or more different viewpoints and has a dialogue within oneself (Puchalska-Wasyl, 2015). Two Polish studies using the psychological instruments *Dialogical Activity Form and Figure's Emotional Climate Inventory* studied more than 200 participants' "emotional types" of internal viewpoints, called "imaginary interlocutors." Five potential types were identified in the two studies: Faithful Friend (self-reinforcement), Ambivalent Parent (strong, loving, but ambivalent), Proud Rival (pride and self-confidence), Helpless Child (negative affect predominates), and Calm Optimist (relaxed and distant to external pressures). The studies identify seven major functions for self-talk: Support, Substitution, Exploration, Bond, Self-Improvement, Insight, and Self-Guiding (Puchalska-Wasyl, 2015, p. 457).

Some popular psychology strategies that can be helpful in doing one's own self-talk evaluation and personal work include "inner child work." The classic by W. Hugh Missildine (1963), *Your Inner Child of the Past*, teaches self-awareness work that focuses on three major concepts: the inner child of the past, being a parent to oneself, and mutual respect so as to illuminate solutions to personal problems that are the "real causes of loneliness, anxiety, and exhausting conflicts" (Missildine, 1963, p. 8) so that a person can live with themselves and others more "fully, more freely, and more comfortably." Another popular psychology teacher, a woman named Byron Katie, teaches a method of self-inquiry known as *The Work*, which challenges and lessens the harmful effects of long-held beliefs. Katie's experience, as described in her book with husband Stephen Mitchell, *Lov-*

ing What Is: How Four Questions Can Change Your Life (2008), is that all suffering is caused by believing our own stressful thoughts.

Nurses can choose numerous self-help methods to explore their beliefs, habits, self-talk, and life experiences, which can potentially lead to greater self-awareness and more meaningful relationships with patients. The Self-care Institute at Golden Apple Healing Arts that teaches precision self-care to nurses specializes in applying the Elements of Care® program with plants as partners (see Resources) in the creation of a sustainable self-care plan.

Counseling and Coaching Techniques

One of the outcomes of self-awareness personal work is the ability to allow for silence in the healing relationship. Silence cultivates the healing relationship in that it demonstrates the nurse's commitment to supporting the patient's work. This person-centered, relationship-centered approach is often challenging at first to those who work in health care, where doing work *for* (rather than with) a patient is often mandatory. Silence, or the pause in verbal communication, is a time-honored technique in counseling and coaching (Tindall & Robinson, 1947). Silence technique initiated by the nurse allows for organization of thoughts, clarification, and shifting the opportunity for contribution to the conversation to the patient (Tindall & Robinson, 1947).

One of the major purposes of counseling and coaching is the support of behavior change. Change creates feelings of ambivalence and uncertainty. *Motivational interviewing* (MI) is a counseling and coaching method derived from client-centered therapy, which is specifically focused on helping people to resolve ambivalence and uncertainty related to change by finding the internal motivation that they need to make the changes in behavior that they have identified. MI is nondirective in content and directive in process in that the counselor and coach guide the patient into the change process with a "clear sense of what is more adaptive behavior or direction" (Constantino, DeGeorge, Dadlani, & Overtree, 2009, p. 1250). The principles of MI include collaboration, support for autonomy, and empathy, which provide an environment for healing past wounds and promote self-awareness. Two of the most common areas in which MI is used are in counseling those suffering from substance misuse and other chronic illnesses, such as asthma and diabetes. The MI technique is most effective in those who are unmotivated to change and in those who are bound by anger and hostility that impedes their ability to change (Hettema, Steele, & Miller, 2005).

When employing MI techniques, the nurse accepts the patient's ambivalence and resistance to change as normal rather than pathological. The nurse listens carefully as patients talk about their change process and supports references to positive changes that have been made, including the baby steps. To negotiate behavior change successfully, nurses must build on basic communication skills and establish a therapeutic environment. Integrative holistic nurses understand that sacred presence is invaluable in setting the stage for exploring the change process. Practitioner time constraints and the perception by the patient of a hurried approach can be a challenge and a barrier to empathic active listening. This situation can lead to unintended results and patient dissatisfaction (Southard, Bark, & Hess, 2016).

To further the process of nondirective counseling and coaching, nurses prompt further discussion with open-ended questions beginning with the words "how" or "what." Questions that begin with "why" stop the flow of dialogue because people rarely know why they do what they do, at least consciously. Asking "how" or "what" questions is a simple technique that provides answers that can serve the nurse counselor and coach as guideposts to further nondirectional counseling and MI. "Why" questions suggest that the nurse is seeking understanding of causation for problems. "What" and "how" questions flow from an awareness that solutions emerge regardless of whether or not there is understanding of the cause for problems.

Walter & Peller (1992, p. 6) state that solution-focused counseling techniques "shift the focus from the past, where we usually look for causes, to the present, where we map patterns of problem maintenance." Solution-focused counseling and coaching communication support collaboration and shared decision making in the quest for solutions to tough problems. The integrative holistic nurse's reflections about health and wellness patterns can be a time for reframing any of the nurse's own tendencies to respond automatically in a prescriptive and directive way. Focusing on wellness patterns facilitates the development of rapport and trust between the nurse and the patient. The patient learns very quickly that the focus of the relationship is solutions rather than blaming, shaming, and placing guilt upon a person for their health behaviors and habits.

One example of solution-focused communication techniques is the focus on exceptions. Most people enter a healing relationship with a problem in mind. One way of accessing the patient's thoughts about potential solutions is to ask about exceptions, such as, "Has there ever been a time when you have felt or been ___?" The nurse fills in the blank with the goal or opposite of the problem. For example, if a patient says that she seems to have pain "all the time," the nurse might ask the patient to describe a time and place when she has noticed that she is the most comfortable, even for a short time. The nurse takes that response, uses the one exception, and encourages the patient to repeat what has worked in the past, if only for a short time. Solution-focused brief therapy (SFBT) can be learned and utilized as a counseling and coaching technique by nurses.

It is considered more collegial and collaborative in approach because it does not involve confrontation or interpretation, nor does it even require the acceptance of the underlying tenets, as do most other models of psychotherapy" (Institute for Solution-Focused Therapy, n.d.). Empirical studies (77 studies) and two meta-analyses on the effectiveness of SFBT show that the overall success rate is 60% in three to five visits (Institute for Solution-Focused Therapy, n.d.). Margaret McAllister has written extensively on the solution-focused nursing model for those who are working in a public health paradigm, which is based on the application of solution-focused principles spawned by the brief therapy movement in mental health care. She writes that the principles of solution-focused nursing include that the nurse's role is "beyond illness-care" to that of adaptations and recovery, that "working with what's going right can enhance the person's hope, optimism and self-belief" (McAllister, 2010, p. 152), and that care is focused on the individual within their societal and cultural context. Patients are encouraged by strategies that focus on their strengths that come from being active, involved, and committed (McAllister, 2010).

COMMUNICATION INTERVENTIONS IN PRACTICE

The National Center for Complementary and Integrative Health (NCCIH, 2022) website, in its definition of integrative holistic care as "practices and products of non-mainstream origin," categorizes interventions as either natural products or mind and body practices. Communication interventions, such as those discussed previously and in the following sections, are mind and body practices; however, many are not listed or categorized as such by the NCCIH. Integrative holistic communication is demonstrated through verbal and nonverbal acts that begin with the patient's experience, assist in the focus on health patterns and the movement toward meaningful goals, and demonstrate the nurse's incorporation of all of the Elements of Care®: fire, air, water, earth, and ether – whether through a single intervention or through a combination of interventions.

Many examples of integrative holistic communication therapies and interventions incorporate the five elements. Elements of Care® communication involves mindful attention to thought (Air); feeling (Water); nonverbal body movement (Earth); spirituality, belief, and laws (Fire); and meaning or essence (Ether). Two examples of communication interventions that exemplify attention to all five elements have been chosen for this chapter. They are music therapy, one of the "expressive arts therapies" that also includes dance and art therapy, and animal-assisted therapy. In their fullest therapeutic sense, expressive arts and animal-assisted therapies are integrative holistic interventions that required education and mental health experience beyond foundational education in nursing. However, some of the communication principles of these therapies can be applied in integrative holistic nursing practice, just as the solution-focused nursing model utilized communication techniques adapted from brief psychotherapy to general nursing practice.

Expressive Arts Therapies: Music Therapy

Music can be employed for therapeutic as well as aesthetic purposes. It has the power to evoke emotions, memories, and healing. The same can be said for sound. Music therapy is an actual therapeutic intervention that is differentiated from simple sounds and from what are referred to as "music-based interventions," "music listening," and "music medicine interventions." *Music therapy* is defined by the American Music Therapy Association (AMTA, n.d.) as the "clinical and evidence-based use of music interventions to accomplish individualized goals within a therapeutic relationship by a credentialed professional who has completed an approved music therapy program." Music therapists provide therapy using music as their preferred avenue for communication. Clinical music therapy is *not* listening to a musician or a nurse playing music for a patient in a hospital, nor is it being offered when a nurse helps a patient choose music on an iPod. *Music medicine* is defined in one study as "passive listening to prerecorded music provided by medical personnel other than a music therapist" (Yinger & Gooding, 2015). One of the most common and promising uses of music is in the treatment of anxiety and pain during medical procedures (Yinger & Gooding, 2015).

Music therapy is an established health service similar to occupational and physical therapy. Therapists address physical, psychological, cognitive, and social functioning for patients of all ages and cultures. Music therapists treat diseases and mental illnesses and promote health and well-being. The evolution of music as a therapy follows the healing practices of many cultures. Evidence of equating the use of music with healing can be found in biblical, literary, and historical writings. The Greek god Apollo is referred to not only as the god of medicine but also as the god of music. In addition, Plato claimed that various musical scales or "moods" could be successfully prescribed for relaxation.

Research

Psychiatrist and musician Rudolph Dreikurs, a founding member of the National Association of Music Therapy in the early 1950s, promotes the social integration benefits of music therapy, recognizing music's ability to help unite people in community and build communication in relationships without provoking defense mechanisms (Eriksson, 2017). Music therapy is known for its effects in treatment of those who have survived traumatic events, experienced grief and loss, for all ages from children to seniors with a wide range of medical and psychological diagnoses. Some of the patients most commonly referred to a music therapist are those diagnosed with developmental disabilities, autism spectrum disorders, mental health issues, Alzheimer's disease and dementia, and behavioral disorders such as attention-deficit/hyperactivity disorder (Eriksson, 2017). One clinical trial in 42 patients with dementia in which 6 weeks of music therapy was combined with standard treatment in the experimental group showed that dementia reduces agitation and disruptiveness and prevents increases in medication (Ridder, Stige, Qvale, & Gold, 2013). Available evidence suggests that music medicine and music therapy can have a positive impact on pain, anxiety, mood disturbance, and quality of life in patients with cancer (Archie, Bruera, & Cohen, 2013).

In music therapy experience, patients can have four types of musical experiences: "receptive or listening, composition, improvisation, and re-creative or performance," such as a sing-along or music lesson (Eriksson, 2017, p. 248). Music therapists choose or arrange compatible music experiences that challenge the patient and provide an opportunity for their growth and development. There is support for the effectiveness of music therapy's positive effect on the neuroplasticity of the brain in studies using brain scans to measure transformation and change (Doidge, 2007 as cited in Eriksson, 2017). Music therapy is also thought to promote people's creativity as well as their mental health through the harmony and beauty of the music. Music therapy is guided by six principles:

- **Intent:** Informing the patient about what to expect in therapy
- **Authentic presence:** Nonjudgmental acceptance of the patient and nurse
- **Wholeness:** Music promoting feeling one with environment
- **Preference:** Patient selection of music promotes mindful participation
- **Entrainment:** Patient heart rate regulates to match the tone and rhythm of the music
- **Situating the client:** The therapist creates a dedicated and quiet space for therapy (McCaffrey & Locsin, 2002)

Various types of music are used in therapy. Examples include prerecorded background music, improvisational music and songwriting created by the patient and the therapist, and live and recorded music. Each provides the patient with a different mode for expressing emotions and telling their story to the therapist without words while affording the person an experience of being heard. Different types of music can elicit different mood responses. Music can stimulate both positive and negative emotional responses and memories and can elevate or lower one's spirit. Certain music can help reduce stress and feelings of isolation. The trained therapist selects music with the patient that fits the individual's need and mood.

Some of the known physiological benefits of music include improved respiration, decreased blood pressure, improved cardiac output, reduced heart rate, and muscle relaxation. Music therapy is a communication intervention that evokes mostly covert, unobservable responses in people that include mental and emotional associations and memories and may also include pain relief and relaxation (Eriksson, 2017). Music therapy reduces the side effects of chemotherapy, reduces anxiety in patients who have experienced myocardial infarction, and improves mood postoperatively in patients who have been on bypass machines (Larkin, 2001). Current research by psychologists such as Daniel Levitin, a Canadian who studies the neuroscience of music at McGill University in Montreal, is focused on the physiological benefits of music on the function of the immune system and on stress reduction (American Psychological Association, 2013). Music therapy is cost-effective, noninvasive, and easy to administer. It is an effective nonpharmacological therapeutic modality that can be used with people of all ages, cultures, abilities, races, and religions.

Professional Notes

Caution is recommended when considering the use of music with patients who have hearing difficulties and in people while they are experiencing extreme emotional states, such as a child who is crying or upset. Certain music, rhythms, and tones can accentuate and aggravate – rather than allay – certain emotions. Nurses who incorporate music in the care of patients are practicing music-based interventions. No additional education is required. To practice music therapy, however, nurses must be board certified in order to practice. According to the AMTA, the standard curriculum for becoming a music therapist includes courses in research analysis, physiology, acoustics, psychology, and music. To become a certified music therapist, one must hold a bachelor's or higher degree in music therapy from one of the schools listed on the AMTA website and complete an internship at a clinical site approved by the AMTA. Once the internship is completed, the candidate is eligible to take the national certification examination that is offered by the AMTA's Certification Board of Music Therapists. Successful candidates obtain the credentials Music Therapist-Board Certified (MT-BC; AMTA, n.d.). A person who has earned a baccalaureate degree in an area other than music therapy can also become a music therapist by completing the courses required for music therapy. In such cases, the person need not earn another baccalaureate degree but can sit for the certification examination once those courses have been completed.

Additional licensures and certifications awarded in music therapy are Registered Music Therapist (RMT), Certified Music Therapist (CMT), and Advanced Certified Music Therapist (ACMT). All music therapists are listed on the National Music Therapy Registry. A certified music therapist must be reexamined every 5 years or show documentation of 100 contact hours of continuing education to continue to practice. These standards and criteria are set by the AMTA, which has official publications on the subject, including journals, monographs, bibliographies, and brochures. The AMTA has also implemented a code of ethics, standards of practice, a system of peer review, a judicial review board, and an ethics board. Music therapists follow the legal and ethical standards set forth by this professional association.

Animal-Assisted Therapies

Animal-assisted therapy (AAT), also referred to as pet therapy and animal-facilitated therapy, improves the physiological, mental, emotional, and spiritual health of a person with the therapeutic aid of animals in direct contact with patients. The animals discussed here that contribute to human therapy are dogs (canines) and horses (equines). A child psychologist named Dr. Boris Levinson and his dog, Jingles, are credited with pioneering AAT, which Levinson called "pet therapy." Levinson first observed that one of his patients who would not speak in therapy would talk to Jingles before the sessions. Jingles's contribution was considered to be that of a facilitator of rapport and as a "transitional object" for the child (Goddard & Gilmer, 2015). Sigmund Freud recognized that his dog, a Chow Chow named Jo-Fi, had a "special sense" for relationships with humans. Freud found that the presence of his dog was especially calming to children and would include him in therapy sessions (Goddard & Gilmer, 2015).

Each session of AAT includes stated goals and an individualized plan of care for the human patient. Animals assist in goals that address all five elements: physiological, mental, emotional, spiritual, and etheric needs of the patient. As a communication intervention, AAT is effective in increasing verbal interactions in groups, improving patients' willingness to be involved in group activities, reducing loneliness, and increasing self-esteem and confidence in interpersonal interactions (Goddard & Gilmer, 2015).

Proponents of equine AAT or equine facilitated therapy (EFT) suggest that horses' unique characteristics "enhance a number of therapeutic processes, providing patients with interactive and multisensory experiences not otherwise available in traditional mental health treatment settings" (Schroeder & Stroud, 2015). Therapists who work with horses generally blend therapeutic techniques, such as mindfulness and gestalt therapy work, with a variety of horsemanship exercises to support the therapeutic process. Activities include observation of horse behavior, grooming, handling and, in some cases, horseback riding. Therapeutic horseback riding is a treatment modality that seeks to improve the physical and psychosocial skills of the rider but does not involve a licensed therapist. *Hippotherapy* is a "physical, occupational, or speech therapy treatment modality that is conducted by licensed therapists and uses equine movement" (Rigby & Grandjean, 2016, p. 10). In addition to the physical effects of horseback riding on posture, balance, and gait, a calm horse can calm a patient very effectively.

Therapists provide structure, observe processes, and assist patients with making meaning of their experience with the horse as it relates to their treatment goals (Professional Association of Therapeutic Horsemanship, n.d.). Horses are particularly suited to group therapy because they are herd animals with a high level of sociability. They are also prey animals and are therefore highly attuned to their environment. They exhibit a keen sensitivity to human behavior and attitudinal change (Schroeder & Stroud, 2015). One specific psychotherapeutic observation of the effects of EFT is that transference reactions can be addressed without some of the confounding interpersonal factors present in traditional therapy because they occur with a horse. One therapist suggests that, "It is much more difficult to attribute a transference reaction to the shortcomings, inappropriate behaviors, or premeditated offenses of a horse" (as cited in Schroeder & Stroud, 2015, p. 370).

Research

Research has shown that animals facilitate and break barriers in human-to-human communication (Goddard & Gilmer, 2015). A systematic review of the literature on dog-assisted therapy screening more than 400 articles demonstrates that children with autism spectrum disorders have positive outcomes related to a combination of recreational therapy and dog AAT, whether the dog was trained as a service, companion, or therapy dog (Hallyburton & Hinton, 2017). Dog AAT is known to reduce anxiety, pain, and loneliness (Goddard & Gilmer, 2015). A systematic review of 10 research studies demonstrates that institutionalized adults with dementia receive positive quality-of-life experiences and benefits from dog AAT (Wood, Fields, Rose, & McLure, 2017). Dogs have also been shown to help women hospitalized during high-risk pregnancy. Fifteen to 30 minutes of dog AAT each day was shown to reduce anxiety and depression symptoms in the women in a pre- and post- "pet therapy" comparative study using Beck's Depression Inventory and the State-Trait Anxiety Inventory as measurement (Lynch et al., 2014).

EFT research includes several populations, including at-risk youth, people with eating disorders, people experiencing grief, and survivors of severe trauma, such as family violence. Twenty-four studies conducted between 2005 and 2013 were included in a study of the state of the science of EFT. The qualitative research demonstrated the value of EFT for enhancing adolescents' communication and relationship skills. The experimental and quasi-experimental research reviewed provided evidence for the value of EFT for enhancing children's and adolescents' emotional, social, and behavioral function (Lee, Dakin, & McClure, 2016).

Professional Notes

Patients who have allergies and asthma related to animal dander or who have extreme fear of animals may not be able to participate in AAT. Research has addressed the potential concern about dogs introducing infection in elderly populations during therapy sessions. One study on the effects of canine-assisted therapy in an elderly population residing in a long-term care facility ($N = 1,690$) reported that there were no infections reported when the dogs visited over a 5-year period (Banks & Banks, as cited in Goddard & Gilmer, 2015).

Nursing is a recognized primary position for someone who would incorporate AAT in care of patients and groups. Certification programs are available for distance and on-campus learning. Some programs require that students hold undergraduate degrees.

CASE STUDY:
REFINING THE ELEMENTS OF COMMUNICATION SKILLS

Camille, a 15-year-old who is pregnant, has a history of physical abuse by her parents. She has been living in a foster home and is admitted to the obstetrics unit for preeclampsia during the final trimester of her pregnancy. The nurses observe that she seems depressed.

Questions
1. What communication approach can be used to develop a healing relationship with Camille?
2. The team is considering AAT for Camille. How would you approach the integration of this modality in her care plan?

Nurse's Answers
1. Using a nondirective approach facilitates communication and assists nurses in bracketing any judgments they may have about teen pregnancy. The nurses use solution-focused training to focus their efforts in helping Camille focus on her strengths as a new mother-to-be and MI coaching techniques to help Camille deal with goals of the hospitalization and bed rest related to her pregnancy.
2. Although studies have shown that 15 to 30 minutes of dog AAT each day can reduce depression symptoms in pregnant women with high-risk pregnancies (Lynch et al., 2014), it is important to first assess Camille. The

nurse includes a "pet assessment" during the health assessment, and Camille smiles for the first time since admission when she talks about her foster family's dog, Sunny, a collie. The nurse can have Camille fill out a modified depression assessment and then work with the AAT team at the hospital to bring in a dog, preferably a collie.

HOLISTIC TRANSFORMATION

- How would you describe your preferred communication pattern in terms of the Elements of Care®?

- What is your favorite type of music? How do you feel when you hear someone else playing music that you do not like? What do you do?

SUMMARY

Communication interventions are foundational to all integrative holistic nursing care. All registered nurses incorporate excellent communication skills that begin with modeling the world of a person, family, or group. Integrative holistic nursing communication mindfully incorporates all five Elements of Care®, regardless of the modality. Numerous modalities can be used to facilitate communication with and by patients. Nurses can seek continuing education, certification, and advanced-degree work in communication interventions and therapeutic techniques. Music and AAT are two evidence-based interventions that nurses can consider in development of the healing relationship with persons and families and in building caring communities.

RESOURCES

American Music Therapy Association   http://www.musictherapy.org

HeartMath Institute   https://www.heartmath.org

Institute for Music and Neurologic Function   http://www.imnf.org

Institute for Solution-focused Therapy   https://solutionfocused.net/research/

Professional Association of Therapeutic Horsemanship International   https://www.pathintl.org

Self-care Institute at Golden Apple Healing Arts   www.GoldenAppleHealingArts.com

World Federation of Music Therapy   http://www.wfmt.info

REFERENCES

Alligood, M. R., & Fawcett, J. (2017). The theory of the art of nursing and the practice of human care quality. *Visions: The Journal of the Rogerian Nursing Science*, 23(1), 4-12.

American Holistic Nurses Association. (2018). *Holistic nursing: Scope and standards of practice* (3rd ed.). Silver Spring, MD: American Nurses Association Press.

American Music Therapy Association. (n.d.). *What is music therapy?* Retrieved from https://www.musictherapy.org

American Psychological Association. (2013). *Science watch: Music as medicine.* Retrieved from http://www.apa.ormonitor/2013/11/music.aspx

Archie, P., Bruera, E., & Cohen, L. (2013). Music-based interventions in palliative cancer care: A review of quantitative studies and neurobiological literature. *Supportive Care in Cancer*, 21(9), 2609-2624.

Childre, D. (1998). *Freeze frame: A scientifically proven technique for clear decision making and improved health* (2nd ed.) Boulder Creek, CA: Planetary Publications.

Constantino, M. J., DeGeorge, J., Dadlani, M. B., & Overtree, C. E. (2009). Motivational interviewing: A bellwether for context-responsive psychotherapy integration. *Journal of Clinical Psychology*, 65(11), 1246-1253.

Eriksson, C. (2017). Adlerian psychology and music therapy: The harmony of sound and matter and community feeling. *The Journal of Individual Psychology*, 73(3), 243-264.

Gaylin, W. (2000). Nondirective counseling or advice? Psychotherapy as value laden. *Hastings Center Report*, 30(3), 31-33.

Geist-Martin, P., & Bell, K. K. (2009). "Open your heart first of all": Perspectives of holistic providers in Costa Rica about communication in the provision of health care. *Health Communication*, 24(7), 631-646.

Goddard, A. T., & Gilmer, M. J. (2015). The role and impact of animals with pediatric patients. *Pediatric Nursing*, 41(2), 65-71.

Hallyburton, A., & Hinton, J. (2017). Canine-assisted therapies in autism: A systematic review of published studies relevant to recreational therapy. *Therapeutic Recreation Journal*, 51(2), 127-142.

Harmer, B., & Henderson, V. (1939). *Textbook of the principles and practice of nursing* (4th ed.). New York, NY: Macmillan.

Hess, D. R., Dossey, B. M., Southard, M. E., Luck, S., Schaub, B. G., & Bark, L. (2012). *The art and science of nurse coaching: The provider's guide to coaching scope and competencies.* Silver Spring, MD: American Nurses Association.

Hettema, J., Steele, J., & Miller, W. R. (2005). Motivational interviewing. *Annual Review of Clinical Psychology*, 1, 91-111.

Institute for Solution-Focused Therapy. (n.d.). *What does the research say about solution-focused brief therapy?* Retrieved from https://solutionfocused.net/research/

Jahoda, G. (2005). Theodor Lipps and the shift from "sympathy" to "empathy." *Journal of the History of the Behavioral Sciences*, 41(2), 151-163.

Jordan, M. (2013). *How to be a health coach: An integrated wellness approach*. San Rafael, CA: Global Medicine Enterprises.

Katie, B., & Mitchell, S. (2008). *Loving what is: How four questions can change your life*. New York, NY: Random House.

Larkin, M. (2001). Music tunes up memory in dementia patients. *Lancet*, 357(9249), 47-49.

Lee, P. T., Dakin, E., & McClure, M. (2016). Narrative synthesis of equine-assisted psychotherapy literature: Current knowledge and future research directions. *Health and Social Care in the Community*, 24(3), 225-246.

Lorié, Á., Reinero, D. A., Phillips, M., Zhang, L., & Riess, H. (2017). Culture and nonverbal expressions of empathy in clinical settings: A systematic review. *Patient Education and Counseling*, 100(3), 411-424.

Lynch, C. E., Magann, E. F., Barringer, S. N., Ounpraseuth, S. T., Eastham, D. G., Lewis, S. D., & Stowe, Z. N. (2014). Pet therapy program for antepartum high-risk pregnancies: A pilot study. *Journal of Perinatology*, 34(11), 816-818.

McAllister, M. (2010). Solution focused nursing: A fitting model for mental health nurses working in a public health paradigm. *Contemporary Nurse*, 34(2), 149-157.

McCaffrey, R., & Locsin, R. (2002). Music listening as a nursing intervention: A symphony of practice. *Holistic Nursing Practice*, 16(3), 70-77.

Missildine, W. H. (1963). *Your inner child of the past*. New York: Pocket Books.

National Center for Complementary and Integrative Health. (2022). *Complementary, alternative, or integrative health: What's in a name?* Retrieved from https://nccih.nih.gov/health/integrative-health#types

National Council of State Boards of Nursing. (n.d.). *Professional boundaries*. Retrieved from https://www.ncsbn.orprofessional-boundaries.htm

Peplau, H. E. (1952). *Interpersonal relations in nursing*. New York, NY: G. P. Putnam's Sons.

Peternelj-Taylor, C. A., & Yonge, O. (2003). Exploring boundaries in the nurse-client relationship: Professional roles and responsibilities. *Perspectives in Psychiatric Care*, 39(2), 55-66.

Prestia, A. S. (2016). Existential authenticity: Caring strategies for living leadership presence. *International Journal for Human Caring*, 20(1), 8-11.

Professional Association of Therapeutic Horsemanship International. (n.d.). *PATH International*. Retrieved from https://www.pathintl.org

Puchalska-Wasyl, M. (2015). Self-talk: Conversation with oneself? On the types of internal interlocutors. *The Journal of Psychology*, 149(5), 443-460.

Ridder, H. M., Stige, B., Qvale, L., & Gold, C. (2013). Individual music therapy for agitation in dementia: An exploratory randomized controlled trial. *Aging & Mental Health*, 17(6), 667-678.

Rigby, B. R., & Grandjean, P. W. (2016). The efficacy of equine-assisted activities and therapies on improving physical function. *Journal of Alternative and Complementary Medicine*, 22(1), 9-24.

Schroeder, K. & Stroud, D. (2015). Equine-facilitated group work for women survivors of interpersonal violence. *The Journal for Specialists in Group Work*. 40(4): 365-386.

Southard, M. E., Bark, L., & Hess, D. (2016). Facilitating change: Motivational interviewing and appreciative inquiry. In B. M. Dossey, L. Keegan, C. C. Barrere, M. A. Blaszko Helming, D. A. Shields, & K. M. Avino (Eds.), *Holistic nursing: A handbook for practice* (7th ed., pp. 541-556). Burlington, MA: Jones & Bartlett Learning.

Tindall, R. H., & Robinson, F. P. (1947). The use of silence as a technique in counseling. *Journal of Clinical Psychology*, 3(2), 136-141.

Walter, J. L., & Peller, J. E. (1992). *Becoming solution-focused in brief therapy*. New York, NY: Brunner Mazel Publishers.

Wood, W., Fields, B., Rose, M., & McLure, M. (2017). Animal-assisted therapies and dementia: A systematic mapping review using the Lived Environment Life Quality (LELQ) model. *American Journal of Occupational Therapy*, 71(5).

Yinger, O. S., & Gooding, L. F. (2015). A systematic review of music-based interventions for procedural support. *Journal of Music Therapy*, 52(1), 1-77.

CHAPTER 9

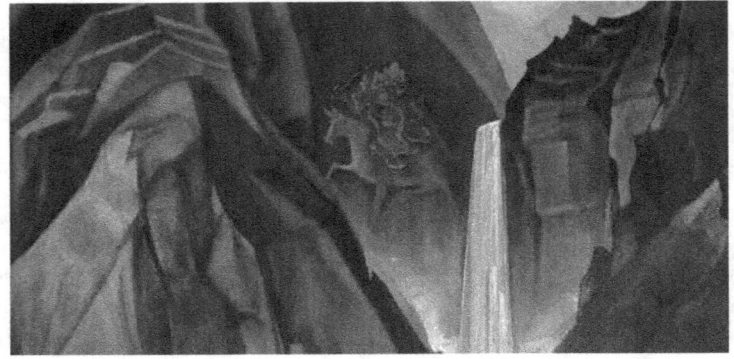

Palden Llamo, Nicholas Roerich, 1931
Courtesy, Nicholas Roerich Museum, New York, NY

WATER ELEMENT: HYDROTHERAPY

LEARNING OUTCOME

After completing this chapter, the learner will be able to discuss hydrotherapy interventions in integrative holistic nursing practice.

CHAPTER OBJECTIVES

After completing this chapter, the learner will be able to:
1. Discuss the history of hydrotherapy.
2. Describe some of the scientific properties of water thought to be responsible for its healing effects.
3. Identify two hydrotherapies used in patient care.
4. Discuss the professional nursing issues associated with hydrotherapy.

INTRODUCTION

Water therapy has been an integral part of the healing arts dated at least to the time of Aesculapius, Hippocrates, Galen, and Celsus (Bender et al., 2005). Two primary categories of water therapy are used for treatment of disease, cleansing, exercise, and relaxation: hydrotherapy and balneotherapy. *Hydrotherapy* is the use of water, and *balneotherapy* is the use of natural thermal mineral spring water. Water has been the central focus of the nature-cure system for centuries, which began as the *water-cure method* (Czaranko, 2013). Whole institutions were, and in some countries still are, dedicated to the application of water cure. Hydrotherapy, in the general sense, typically refers to the *external* application of water.

Hydrotherapy methods have been used for centuries in many religious and cultural purification rites and healing practices. Water is, for many people, the symbol of the means for the purification of the soul and the body. Water *ablution* is the term used in the traditions of Islam, Judaism, Shinto (Misogi), and Christianity, for example, to denote a ritual of purification. Water is also used for the treatment of disease and injury as well as for promoting relaxation and relief of stress, anxiety, and acute and chronic pain. Over centuries, healing shrines and spas have been erected where healing mineral springs bubble up out of the ground or pour through the cracks in caves. These special places are where people "take to the waters" for health, healing, and cure. Various forms of water – from ice to liquid to vapor – are used internally or externally (or both) to promote healing.

The focus of this chapter is the external hydrotherapeutic topical and environmental applications that can be readily applied in integrative holistic nursing practice. Such methods include hot and cold immersion baths, packs and wraps, sauna, thermal spring mineral baths, irrigations, enemas, and footbaths.

BACKGROUND

The nature cure, water-cure movement in the United States was popular in the early and mid-19th century. The theory of water cure was that *psora*, or irritated skin, induced disease (Silver-Isenstadt, 2002). Water cure doctors, such as the renowned Mary Gove Nichols, believed that the body's nervous system was only aroused by the use of medications, which it recognized as poison. The body then spent vital energy ridding itself of the perceived poison rather than healing. Nichols and her patients knew that water cure took time and often demanded a change in lifestyle. One example of a very "active" water cure treatment for croup was detailed by Nichols. She placed a 10-year-old boy in a tub and poured two pails of cold water over his throat and chest. She then rubbed the areas until they were bright red. He was then laid down and wrapped in a wet sheet and covered with blankets. He then started to perspire and with that, his breathing became easier. Upon perspiration, the sheet was removed. The boy was doused with cold water again and then rubbed with coarse towels. He went to bed without croup symptoms (Silver-Isenstadt, 2002).

Hydrotherapy was also foundational to early nursing care, particularly in the care of the mentally ill (Harmon, 2009). Nurses, particularly those who practiced in the 19th century, when water cure was very popular, used hydrotherapies in patient care. Historical research describes retired nurses' experiences in administering "the water cure," which included the application of hot or cold wet sheet packs and continuous tub baths. The nurses, who worked in state mental hospitals during the mid-20th century before the invention of neuroleptic drugs, used hydrotherapies to effectively calm agitated or manic patients (Harmon, 2009).

Harmer and Henderson (1939) included the use of hydrotherapies in their textbook for nurses. They taught the different uses for full baths, half baths, hot baths, sedative baths, cold baths, continuous baths, hot packs, cold packs, sedative packs, and full-body sheet packs. They also learned about adding certain substances to a bath, such as sea salt and mustard powder, to affect body and bath temperature. Their instructions included the proper use of water temperature for affecting certain conditions. Hot baths and packs were used to increase circulation and to relieve inflammation and congestion of internal organs. Hot baths increase perspiration and subsequent elimination through the skin, thereby resting inflamed, congested kidneys (Harmer & Henderson, 1939). Baths at 92 °F / 33 °C were used for sedation and comfort. Baths at body temperature and cold packs were used as sedatives:

> A bath at body temperature produces no marked changes in the body, either thermic or circulatory, but surrounds it with a medium that shields it from all external stimuli, or irritation of nerve endings from air, clothing, pressure, changes in temperature, and the like. As a result, the nerve centers and whole nervous system are protected and allowed to rest. The bath is therefore soothing and quieting in its effects and gives a chance for repair and the storage of vital energy (Harmer & Henderson, 1939, p. 475).

Today, hydrotherapies are used in boutique services, such as spas and salons, as well as in rehabilitation, sports medicine, chiropractic, naturopathy, and physical therapy clinics. They are used by nurses in hospitals, home care, clinics, and skilled nursing facilities. However, they are so much a part of the basic skills of nursing care that they may be easily overlooked for research funding and practice guideline development as nursing science evolves. The science and art of hydrotherapy includes water temperature regulation, timing patterns of external applications incorporating the use of water, and pro-moting comfort with water. Hydrotherapies effect healing of the whole person.

Water has many properties that account for the proposed mechanisms of action for its healing effects. These properties include density and specific gravity, buoyancy factor, hydrostatic pressure, refraction and reflection factor, viscosity, stream flow, and turbulence. Knowledge of water's properties can be used to construct care.

Density is defined as mass per unit volume.

Specific gravity is the relative density, or the ratio of the density of a body to the density of water. The specific gravity of water is 1. The specific gravity for a female is 0.75 and for a male is 0.95. Lungs deflate at a specific gravity of 1.05 to 1.08. This concept explains why people can float in water and can swim longer with their heads above water.

Buoyancy factor is the force of gravity that results in a feeling of weightlessness when one is immersed in water. Buoyancy factor decreases weight-bearing and joint compression forces, decreases the effort required with slow movements against gravity, and increases functional ability (Prins & Cutner, 1999).

Hydrostatic pressure is the pressure exerted by molecules upon an immersed body. The fluid pressure is equal at a given depth. Because of this property, swelling decreases with increased pressure, offsetting the tendency of blood to pool in extremities and helping to build the muscles of inspiration and exhalation. This factor also has a diuretic effect by increasing the amount of residual urine output.

Viscosity refers to the amount of cohesion molecules have to other matter. This property provides **resistance** with increased speed, which improves strength (Prins & Cutner, 1999).

Turbulence refers to uneven patterns of water movement that can establish patterns of low-pressure areas following in the wake of an object moving through a fluid.

The human body is 75% water. Water is, for many people, quite valuable and rare, such as in South Africa and some tribal nations in the American Southwest. For others, it may be taken for granted given its abundance. The Austrian naturalist and inventor Viktor Schauberger (1885 to 1958), who referred to water as "the earth's blood," stated that for water to be healthy and life-supporting, it needs to flow along a natural course with winding curves. He predicted that "methods of water control, power stations, and forestry are ruining water" (Alexandersson, 1997, p. 18). His alternative was to employ the movement found in all of nature to promote creativity and growth, the "hyperbolic spiral which externally is centripetal and internally moves towards the centre" (Alexandersson, 1997, p. 77). When water moves through a water course employing this movement pattern (as in Figure 9-1), it becomes productive living water.

Although the hyperbolic spiral, in its centripetal movement, is symptomatic of contraction, concentration, and cooling temperatures, the opposite holds true for centrifugal movement: It is expansive and even explosive. The two exist simultaneously in nature. For growth to occur, the centripetal must predominate. Nurses can simulate the movement of a natural water course when they stir water, such as a bath, in a figure 8 pattern.

FIGURE 9-1: WATER COURSE

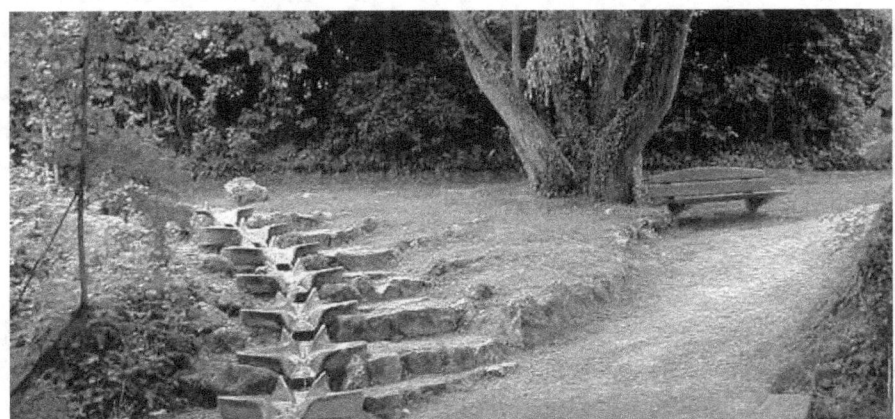

Watercourse at Anthroposophical Society Headquarters, Dornach, Switzerland. ©Martha Libster

The skin is the largest organ of the body, and it provides protection and a physical and psychological boundary distinguishing the self from others and the environment. Physically, hydrotherapy is the use of water to engage the skin in regulation of body warmth, qi, and blood circulation. Water stimulates the immune system, helps increase the body's white blood cell count, aids the body in purging itself of accumulated metabolites and environmental toxins, and produces a state of general relaxation that promotes the healing process. Movement of water is fundamental to hygiene practices such as handwashing.

Hydrotherapy, as a vital part of the nature cure system, can be used by all professionals and the public in self-care. Nature cure is a relatively simple system that does not depend on knowledge of disease, although a working knowledge of anatomy and physiology is helpful.

> The nature-cure system is the same for all diseases, and all cases, even as the origin of all diseases has but one cause, an unnatural mode of life, and there exists a unity in all the laws of nature and in all her manifestations. (Czeranko, 2013, p. 88)

Hydrotherapy was greatly developed by Father Sebastian Kneipp (1821 – 1897), a German priest, considered an early founder of the naturopathic medicine movement and the Kneipp-cure hydrotherapies. He cured himself of tuberculosis with hydrotherapies and herbs. According to the Kneipp tradition, the fundamental rules of hydrotherapy are:

- The shorter the application, the better its effect.
- The colder the water, the shorter is the time of its employment; and the greater will the reaction be. Weak patients must, nevertheless, begin with water at a moderate temperature; at first 66 ° 18 °C, cooler after a time, down to 59 ° 15 °C and 55 ° 13 °C, and at last quite cold. The body must be as warm as possible before the application of cold water. If there is a lack of natural warmth, the first applications must be warm.
- There should be no drying of the body by artificial means, after the use of water; the clothes should be put on quickly, and, in order to help a reaction, exercise should be taken, rapidly at first and slower by degrees. If there is no reaction, or if the patient is very weak, the warmth of a bed should be sought.
- Hardening the body is the best means of preserving the general health, and the protection against attacks of disease. (Czeranko, 2013, p. 72)

Hydrotherapy is an approach to healing that can be used as an alternative or complement to pharmacological treatment. Hydrotherapy has been shown to be effective in invigorating skin, toning muscles, and promoting blood flow. It can also be used in health promotion, such as for prevention of the common cold. In addition, it has been used to treat and manage these conditions:

- Problems with circulation
- Respiratory infections
- Pain caused by pulled back muscles, sciatica, chronic rheumatoid arthritis, bronchial asthma, unstable hypertension, and severely disturbed peripheral blood circulation
- Varicose veins
- Edema
- Headaches
- Low blood pressure
- Circulatory problems
- Sleeplessness

Hydrotherapy enhances mood and promotes self-determination and self-motivation. Hydrotherapy can also help alleviate tension, nervousness, and other symptoms that accompany anxiety attacks.

The healing properties of hydrotherapy are based on water's mechanical and thermal effects. Hydrotherapy and balneotherapy exploit the body's reactions to hot and cold stimuli, the protracted application of heat, water pressure, and the sensa-tions water gives. Nerves carry impulses felt at the skin deeper into the body, where they are instrumental in stimulating the immune system, influencing the production of stress hormones, invigorating circulation and digestion, encouraging blood flow, and lessening pain sensitivity. Generally, heat opens pores, expands blood vessels, and relaxes muscle tissue, allowing for blood flow away from internal organs, which the mind then registers as a calming and soothing effect on the body. In contrast, cold stimulates and invigorates the skin, closes the pores, and forces blood toward internal organs. Hydrotherapy uses this basic knowledge of the body's natural thermal responses in the art and science of hot and cold water applications that produce a desired effect on the body and mind. For example, if a person is feeling tired and stressed, a warm shower or bath followed by a short, invigorating cold shower can help to stimulate the body and the mind. Water also has a hydrostatic effect and massage-like feeling as it gently kneads the body. Cold or warm water in motion stimulates touch receptors on the skin, boosting blood circulation and releasing tight muscles.

HYDROTHERAPY IN PRACTICE

Numerous forms of hydrotherapies are used and recommended by nurses for their patients, such as baths and showers, sitz baths, footbaths, friction rubs, steam inhalation, hot and cold compresses, enemas, irrigations, body wraps, wet sheet packs, and sauna and whirlpool baths. Perhaps the best known and most widely practiced hydrotherapy intervention is the bed bath. Nurses are trained in specific techniques for providing a bed bath that not only promotes hygiene but also increases relaxation and healing when applied mindfully and knowledgably. Bed baths are not without risk to patients, however. Adult patients, in particular, who are used to performing their own hygiene activities may experience feelings of anxiety and vulnerability associated with being dependent on nursing care. One study suggests that when nurses first provide instruction and guidance to patients who are going to receive bed baths do so with the goal of relieving the anxiety, patients do experience decreased anxiety (Lopes, Barbosa, Nogueira-Martins, & de Barros, 2015). Despite its significant history of positive effect and widespread use in patient care, the bed bath has been challenged more recently by the practice of bathing *without* water.

Washing without water practice evolved from the bag bath concept in 1994, which consisted of several nondisposable washcloths put in a bag together with an amount of no-rinse cleansing fluid diluted in water. Washing without water differs from the bag bath concept because it is an all-in-one method (i.e., it has no separate water or cleansing fluid required) and uses a completely disposable solution. Washing without water is claimed to offer several advantages compared to the traditional bed bath with water and soap. Washing without water is believed to decrease physical and emotional strain and increase satisfaction among both patients and caregivers, have a positive influence on skin condition, and be less costly and less time-consuming than the traditional bed bath (Groven et al., 2017).

Although bathing without water is a "worthy alternative" to the traditional bed bath and preserves water resources, there is little to no substantiating evidence as to its hygienic or other health-related benefits when compared with the use of water. In the right hands, the bed bath is a simple but time-honored effective integrative holistic hydrotherapeutic intervention. The following data on other hydrotherapies can be translated to immediate application in nursing practice in some cases for use in structuring activities of daily living with patients and providing basic nursing care, such as the bed bath.

Research

Several different forms of hydrotherapy are discussed here that nurses can consider integrating in plans of care. Hydrotherapies may be applied by the nurse, or they may be recommended for self-care or provided by a therapist to whom the nurse has provided the patient a referral. Hydrotherapy, specifically warm water applications, is most often used in patients with pain resulting from neurological or musculoskeletal conditions. The heat and buoyancy of the water "block nociceptors by acting on thermal receptors and mechanoreceptors and exert a positive effect on spinal segmental mechanisms" (Castro-Sánchez et al., 2012, p. 2). Warm water increases blood flow and promotes muscle relaxation. The hydrostatic effect of water also alleviates pain by reducing peripheral edema and sympathetic nervous system activity. Different hydrotherapy applications are employed to achieve pain relief and promote comfort.

Immersion Baths

Immersion baths are types of baths in which the entire body or parts of the body are submerged in water. Cold or warm water or a combination of both cold and warm water may be selected for their therapeutic effects. Studies have been conducted on the effects of immersion baths. For example, one study (N = 36) compared cold water immersion with ice packs and ice massage. All were applied for 15 minutes, and all were able to reduce skin temperature and exert a hypoalgesic effect; that is, decreased sensitivity to painful stimuli. The results of the study suggest that of the three modalities, cold water immersion generated the least reduction in skin temperature but was the most effective modality in changing motor nerve conduction (Herrera, Sandoval, Camargo, & Salvini, 2010).

Various substances (such as Epsom salt, sea salt, and vinegar) are often added to warm water immersion baths. Herbs are commonly used and will be discussed in Chapter 13 Immersion baths can be applied to different parts of the body, such as the hip, arm, thigh, and feet. Two examples of partial immersion baths are the footbath and the sitz bath.

Footbaths

Footbaths are a healing tradition in nursing dating back nearly 400 years (Libster & McNeil, 2009). The soles of the feet have a high concentration of pores. Therapeutic footbaths are an easy and accessible way to clear waste from the body, such as uric acid, which pools in the feet because of gravitational pull. Warm, sedative footbaths are 92 °F (33 °C). When beginning a footbath for patients, put the basin in front of them the long way so that the feet fit more comfortably in the basin. Footbaths are essentially a water element application; however, herbs (see Chapter 13 and other substances can be added to the footbath to represent the other four Elements of Care®: aromatic bath oils (Air), bath salts (Earth), flowers and leaves (Ether), and a helpful approach and prayers for healing (Fire; Libster, 2014). Therefore, footbaths alone can represent a full five-elements integrative holistic nursing practice.

Research has shown that footbaths are very effective in helping people, especially older adults, to sleep more soundly. One crossover study reports that administering 20-minute warm footbaths at 104° F (40 °C) before sleep in older adults had no effect on sleep outcome (Liao, Wang, Kuo, Chiu, & Ting, 2013). Another study of 60 women post-cesarean section involving hand and foot bathing demonstrated a positive effect on decreasing their anxiety and stress (Cal, Cakiroglu, Kurt, & Dane, 2016). The intervention of the pre-test and post-test design was warm water at a temperature of 96.8°F to 98.6°F (36°C to 37°C) with immersion for 10 minutes in the morning (Cal et al., 2016). Another study of 20 healthy women found that warm footbaths may induce sympathetic/parasympathetic nervous system balance and prevent cardiac arrhythmias (Aydin et al., 2016). Warm footbaths for 15 minutes at a temperature of 104°F to 113°F (40°C to 45°C), given at 8 p.m. for 5 days, were effective in helping 87% of participants who are patients with stage 4 cancer to relax and sleep (Cherian, 2012). Warm footbaths (105.8°F to 109.4°F, or 41°C to 43°C) for 30 minutes also result in improvement of systemic arterial stiffness in both healthy young and older women (Hu et al., 2011).

Cold footbaths are a healing tradition used to promote respiratory and immune health. The third president of the United States, Thomas Jefferson (1743 – 1826), ascribed his freedom from common "catarrhs" (inflammation of the mucous membranes, cough, and phlegm) for 10 years "partly to the habit of bathing my feet in cold water every morning, for sixty years past" (Jefferson, 1944, p. 691). He lived to the age of 83 years. For a cold footbath, the feet are placed into a footbath container filled to calf depth with cool to cold water. Patients are encouraged to take their feet out when they feel very cold or when the water is no longer perceived as being cold. Another hydrotherapy technique for stimulating circulation is to immerse the feet first in a bucket of warm water and then into a cold-water bucket, alternating back and forth. This kind of hydrotherapy is often best tolerated when involving the feet alone rather than the whole body, as may be done at thermal springs.

Ionic footbaths are offered as a highly popular adjunctive treatment at many holistic health centers and spas. They are said to aid in detoxification of heavy metals in the body. The presence of heavy metals in the body is measurable, but these beliefs and claims, while supported by anecdotal evidence, have yet to be supported with clinical trial evidence. Some of the major questions to be answered are whether or not introducing electromagnetic current to the feet has any deleterious effect on negative cell growth patterns, such as in the case of cancer cells. Robert O. Becker, an expert in electromagnetics, writes in his book *Cross Currents* (1990, p. 138), that "extremely small electrical currents have a variety of major biological effects. Most people who employ or promote electrical currents for treatments are either unaware of these effects or choose to ignore them."

Ionic footbaths employ a process called *electrolysis*, during which the water in the ionic footbath with added sea salt is separated into positive and negative ions by using direct electric current. Electrol-ysis, based on the 19th-century science of Michael Faraday, is used in manufacturing and metal purification and in cleaning and preserving historical artifacts, such as coins. Electrolysis of water produces hydrogen.

Inside Edition (2011), an ABC syndicated nighttime news program, worked with an electrical engineer named Steven Fowler, who tested the ionic footbath device in his lab in South Carolina. He reported that the change in water to a brownish orange color had to do with rust, which occurred whether or not feet were in the ionic tub. Fowler said that inside the "array" that is placed in the water are "just two metal electrodes with a positive and negative current. When introduced to salt water, a chemical process called electrolysis takes place and causes the electrodes to rust at an extremely rapid rate." Manufacturers of the ionic footbath state that the device generates positive and negatively charged ions (H^+, OH^-) through electrolysis in water, and that causes the removal of particles or toxins from the body via osmosis and diffusion through the skin when in contact with the ion gradient created in the water. One study on the subject found no evidence that the ionic footbath device removes heavy metals from the body; however, the sample size for phase 1 of the study was 10 and for phase 2, it was 24 (Kennedy, Cooley, Einarson, & Seely, 2012). The study is a Canadian-based naturopathic medicine study that examined the use of the IonCleanse SOLO footbath device in removing heavy metal toxicity as measured by urine and hair analysis. The study compared distilled water and tap water baths. It also investigated the possibility that the metals in the bath device were actually corroding in the process. But that, too, is a measurable process that was only preliminarily investigated (Kennedy et al., 2012).

The practice of using saltwater footbaths alone to purify and detoxify a person is part of traditional healing practices, such as Ayurveda. It is the effect of the addition of the electromagnetic current that is still in question. Ionic footbath products have been approved for use by the Federal Communications Commission and its European counterpart.

Sitz Baths

A *sitz bath* is another type of partial bath in which the hip, rectal, or perineal areas are immersed in water to decrease swelling, inflammation, and pain. A sitz bath can be administered as a cold or warm bath. Parts of the body not immersed in water are covered with a blanket to preserve body heat. Cold or warm sitz baths are effective for improving circulation, reducing swelling, and therefore improving oxygenation and healing of tissues, such as hemorrhoids. They are also complementary therapies for infection or inflammation of the anus, bladder, prostate, and preparation for pregnancy or pain relief after vaginal delivery.

Packs and Wraps

A wrap is primarily used as a supportive measure for treating fever and local inflammation. The person receiving treatment adopts a relaxed position. Next, a cotton flannel or wool cloth is soaked in cold or hot water, wrung out, and wrapped around the patient's specific body parts. A body part when hot will warm the cold pack and the pack will need to be changed to continuously draw off the heat. If the purpose of the pack is to warm an area, such as the feet, the goal of the pack is to keep it warm. To keep the moist heat, the wrap is covered by plastic and then a small towel. The small towel is then secured with a larger towel. Each layer is pressed with the hands to press any air out from the pack to best retain the warmth. A hot-water bottle can be sandwiched between towel layers to retain the heat as well.

Moist heat packs are useful for treating pain and stimulating circulation of qi and blood in an area of the body. Wraps are useful for sore throat (neck wrap); bronchitis and lung disease (chest wrap); pelvic infection, hemorrhoids, or prostate problems (hip wrap); arthritis (joint wrap); phlebitis from intravenous fluid infection, and edema (calf and arm wrap). Cold packs include ice bags and cold wrapping cloths that are placed on the affected part of the body. Ice bags are applied for 1 minute, removed for 4 minutes, and then reapplied. Cold packs are useful for various joint inflammations, sprains and strains, pleurisy, neck pain, and headaches.

Water Irrigations

Nasal irrigation, such as a neti pot, is a hydrotherapy that is in common self-care practice. It is thought to originate with the Ayurvedic Indian tradition and is widely prescribed in pediatric patients, particularly for the treatment of allergic rhinitis, chronic sinusitis, and the prevention of respiratory tract infection. A paper reviewing numerous clinical trials that have been conducted to study the effect of traditional nasal irrigation practice found that many studies had small sample sizes and other "methodological problems," leaving gaps in knowledge about the best devices, solutions, and durations of nasal irrigation treatment to be recommended (Principi & Esposito, 2017). However, a recent study conducted in adults (N = 45) in Shanghai, China, showed that participants who were treated with nasal irrigation (using 100 mL of warm saline) for allergic rhinitis related to house-dust mites had better relief after 30 days than from nasal corticosteroid spray (Lin, Chen, Cao, & Sun, 2017).

Transanal irrigation (TAI) is used when patients are unable to evacuate their bowels as a result of such conditions as multiple sclerosis, neurogenic bowel dysfunction, and spina bifida, and when less invasive interventions have proven ineffective (Wilson, 2017). Tepid water (96.8° 36°C to 100.4° 38°C) is used as irrigating fluid via rectal catheter. Patients who have the dexterity and cognitive ability can be taught to do their own TAI. Patients cannot use TAI if they have bowel problems such as stenosis, active bowel disease, or diverticulitis (Wilson, 2017).

Aquatic Exercise, Aqua or Water Therapy

When the body is submerged in a bath, a pool, or a whirlpool, a person experiences weightlessness as the body is relieved from the constant pull of gravity. During floatation in the water, the combination of weightlessness and the absence of external stimuli causes the body to relax. The brain relaxes in aqua or water therapy during floatation when it and the body are shielded from external stimuli.

Patients with chronic back pain have been found to benefit from aqua therapy combined with other nonpharmacological treatment such as therapeutic education, muscle strengthening exercises, aerobic training, and stretching (Dupeyron et al., 2013). Ai-Chi, a type of aquatic exercise, is also helpful for people in chronic pain, such as those with multiple sclerosis. It is a combination of movements from tai chi, Qi Gong, Shiatsu, and Watsu (see the next paragraph) accompanied by music and conducted in a water environment, such as a pool. It is a combination of deep breathing and slow, broad movements with the arms, legs, and torso that is performed in shoulder-depth water. The 16 movements characteristic of Ai-Chi include floating, folding, gathering, and relaxing postures. The principles of the therapy are as found in tai chi: *Yuan* (circular movements seeking internal and external harmony), *Sung* (promote blood circulation), *Ching* (absence of tension), *Yun* (movement at a given speed directed by the mind), *Cheng* (balance and posture), *Shu* (relaxed movement of the body), and *Tsing* (concentration; Castro-Sánchez et al., 2012). A meta-analysis comparing land and aquatic exercises for people with arthritic joints found that they are equally effective but that people with arthritic hips and knees may find aquatic exercise easier to tolerate (Battterham, Heywood, & Keating, 2011).

One well-known form of aqua therapy is aquatic Shiatsu, or "Watsu." It includes passive stretches and massage techniques administered in warm water

(95 ° 35 °C). Watsu, which means "freeing the body in water," is used in rehabilitation centers and birthing suites. It began in 1980 at the Harbin Hot Springs in Northern California, where Harold Dull brought his knowledge of Zen Shiatsu into a warm pool. Dull discovered that the effects of Zen Shiatsu could be amplified by stretching someone while he or she floated in warm water. Shiatsu, meaning "finger pressure," was developed in Japan, where Zen Shiatsu is the most common technique. Watsu, however, combines the elements of massage, Shiatsu, and movement therapy in warm water.

During Watsu, the patient floats in warm water, lessening resistance in the limbs. Watsu movements include rocking and stretching the whole body while supporting the joints. It helps to decrease muscle tension, increase range of motion, facilitate deep breathing, decrease pain and stress, and improve body awareness. It is also often used in rehabilitation centers to treat traumatic injuries, such as brain and spinal cord injuries; orthopedic disorders; congenital birth defects, including spina bifida and autism; and other neurological disorders in children and adults.

Balneotherapy

Balneotherapy, also known as *spa bathing* or *thermal therapy*, is defined as the use of natural mineral waters, natural peloids and mud, and natural sources of different gases (CO_2, H_2S, and Rn) for medical purposes such as prevention, treatment, and rehabilitation (Latorre-Román, Rentero-Blanco, Laredo-Aguilera, & Garcia-Pinillos, 2015). Balneotherapy, also known as "taking the waters," is a healing tradition in Europe and around the world that involves soaking in natural mineral springs and pools. It has beneficial properties with little or no risk or side effects, particularly in patients with rheumatologic and musculoskeletal disorders, low back pain, dermatological conditions, chronic obstructive pulmonary disease, peripheral vascular disease, hypertension, diabetes, and obesity (Karagülle & Karagülle, 2015; Latorre-Román et al., 2015; Passali et al., 2013).

One study of 52 men and women measured the effect of a 12-day balneotherapy program conducted at Balneario San Andrés, Spain, where the water is a hypothermic (≥68° 20°C) hard water of medium mineralization, with bicarbonate, sulfate, sodium, and magnesium as the dominant ions. The program had significant positive effects on participants' pain, mood, sleep quality, and depression (Latorre-Román et al., 2015).

Saunas and Steam Baths

Saunas and steam baths produce similar effects. Sauna is the use of a hot, dry, wood-lined room for relaxing while sitting or lying down, and it encourages detoxification by opening the pores of the skin and eliminating through perspiration any fat-soluble substances, metabolites from medications, and heavy metals that have been stored in adipose tissue. *Steam baths*, the wet version of a sauna, also promote perspiration and remove body toxins. Saunas and steam baths are relaxing and promote blood and qi circulation. The decision to take one rather than the other is guided by personal preference. In a sauna, the heat acts more quickly to eliminate toxins through the skin, although some consider the moist air of a steam bath more satisfying to the respiratory system. Saunas are deeply relaxing and are a great way to melt away stress. Sauna baths stimulate blood flow, increase heart rate, have an immune-modulating effect, promote hormone production, encourage mucus secretion in the respiratory system, open the airways, reduce resistance to respiration, promote relaxation, and can improve mental outlook. A 2016 study from Finland found that frequently using saunas could reduce the risk of developing dementia (Laukkanen, Kunutsor, Kauhanen, & Laukkanen, 2016).

Saunas and steam baths should be used with caution. Rehydration with water after the therapy is imperative. Saunas should not be used by people with acute rheumatoid arthritis, acute infection, active tuberculosis, sexually transmitted diseases, acute mental disorders, inflammation of an inner organ or blood vessels, significant vascular changes in the brain or heart, circulatory problems, or acute cancer.

Water Immersion During Labor and Water Birth

Pregnant women and their care providers around the world seek natural and noninvasive approaches for easing pain in childbirth. Approximately one third of women in the United States surveyed use complementary therapies during pregnancy and postpartum (as reported in Sullivan & McGuiness, 2015). For some time, the World Health Organization (1996) has recognized the contribution that nonpharmacological traditional methods of pain relief, such as hydrotherapy, make to safe and less invasive childbirth practices. Hydrotherapies can be very effective in reducing pain in childbirth and increasing a women's ability to cope with labor pain when compared with using opiates (Sprawson, 2017).

Water birth, used since the 1800s, is a birthing practice in which the baby is actually born underwater. There is controversy and little research as to the safety of delivering a baby in water. However, water immersion is more widely practiced by women before and during labor as a nonpharmacological method to manage labor pain (Benfield, 2002; Benfield, Herman, Katz, Wilson, & Davis, 2001). Water immersion is a pain management strategy in which a woman's abdomen is completely submerged in warm water before the birth of the baby. According to Prins and Cutner (1999), hydrotherapy is a safe and effective intervention that can be used to help low-risk women cope with labor. The therapeutic benefits of hydrotherapies include increased relaxation, increased satisfaction, increased cervical dilation, lower blood pressure, and increased diuresis with no increased risk of infection (Benfield, 2002). According to a study by Benfield (2002), the use of water immersion during delivery, which is sometimes called "maternal bathing," can also rapidly relieve pain and anxiety. The buoyancy that the woman experiences during the immersion promotes ease in movement, progression of the labor, and reduction in perineal tears (Sullivan & McGuiness, 2015). Women are more inclined to explore water immersion and water birth options when trying for a vaginal birth after having had a cesarean section (McKenna & Symon, 2014).

A review of eight randomized control trials employing water immersion during the first phase of labor found a significant reduction of epidural analgesia use and a reduction in duration of the first stage of labor, with no studies finding adverse effects to the woman or neonate (Cluett & Burns, 2009). One study found pain to be significantly reduced in those receiving a nonpharmacological intervention of a warm water aspersion bath (98.6° 37 °C) while sitting or standing. The water was directed at the lumbosacral area for 30 minutes. A Visual Analog Scale used for measuring pain intensity before and after the intervention (Barbieri, Henrique, Chors, Maia, & Gabrielloni, 2013) showed the hydrotherapy to be effective in managing pain in labor without opiates.

Hydrotherapy, such as swimming, can also be helpful during pregnancy as a woman prepares her body for labor. One clinical study of 17 women, for example, found that Watsu significantly lowered participants' levels of stress and pain and improved their mental health-related quality of life and mood in the third trimester (Schitter, Nedekjkovic, Baur, Fleckenstein, & Raio, 2015).

Professional Notes

Hydrotherapy is used by doctors, nurses, physical therapists (PTs), PT assistants, nursing assistants, and patients for physical fitness and for healing purposes. Hydrotherapy is widely used in sports medicine and in rehabilitation centers by PTs and trained or certified nonlicensed providers, such as PT assistants. Nurses are licensed to touch and therefore, with education, can utilize hydrotherapies such as footbaths, compresses, and nasal irrigations in the care and comfort of patients. Hydrotherapies are hands-on clinical practices that are best learned from knowledgeable practitioners who can impart the nuances of applying various interventions. Nurses involved in the recreational and stress-reduction uses of hydrotherapy for maintaining physical fitness, such as aquatic aerobics, can recommend the use of hydrotherapy for self-care.

The Harbin School of Healing Arts in California, a private institution, originally owned by Harold Dull, the founder of Watsu, has a certification program for the public. Several stages and many hours are involved in Watsu training, with each stage teaching presence, flow, form, adaption, and creativity, which are learned continuously throughout life. Rather than just being a step, each stage becomes a platform that supports and sustains the next (Harbin School of Healing Arts, n.d.). To obtain licensure, certification, or registration, it is important to first check with state, city, and county ordinances for licensing and bodywork training requirements to set up an aquatic therapy practice.

When using hydrotherapy, nurses use their public health knowledge, education, and experience to maintain the hygienic quality of the water and the environment to avoid potential problems such as waterborne infections. Water safety precautions include prevention of drowning, a common cause of unintentional injury and death in the United States. In 2007, the Virginia Graeme Baker Pool and Spa Safety Act was enacted by Congress and signed into law. It was designed "to prevent the tragic and hidden hazard of drain entrapments and eviscerations in pools and spas" (U.S. Consumer Product Safety Commission, n.d.).

It is critical to check the temperature of water before performing any hydrotherapy. People with impaired temperature sensation run the risk of scalding or frostbite at temperature extremes. Caution should also be taken when using hydrotherapy with older adult and very young children. Older adults should avoid long full-body warm immersion baths. Patients with heart disease bathe with the water line below the heart level and should consult their practitioners before participating in any hydrotherapy that involves changes in temperature. Nurses should use caution when considering hydrotherapy with patients who have the following health or medical conditions:

- Raynaud's disease
- High or low blood pressure
- Diabetes mellitus
- Multiple sclerosis
- Pregnancy
- Contagious infections

HOLISTIC TRANSFORMATION

- *Reflect on your personal experience with the water element. How do you feel in water?*

- *What hydrotherapies do you currently use in patient care and what would you like to add to your repertoire?*

SUMMARY

Hydrotherapy, or water therapy, can be performed independently, in a group setting, or one-on-one with a nurse, health practitioner, or therapist. Hydrotherapies have been shown to have many health benefits, including the promotion of relaxation and sleep. Much of the evidence supporting hydrotherapies is anecdotal and historical. Hydrotherapies may be as old as human history. One centuries-old hydrotherapy effectively employed by nurses around the globe is the therapeutic footbath. As with all modalities, some hydrotherapy interventions can be practiced by licensed nurses who have knowledge of the intervention, whereas others may require further education, certification, and licensure.

RESOURCES

Aquatic Resources Network
http://www.aquaticnet.com/index.htm

Aquatic Therapy & Rehab Institute
http://www.atri.org

Watsu
http://www.watsu.com

REFERENCES

Alexandersson, O. (1997). *Living water: Viktor Schauberger and the secrets of natural energy.* Bath, England: Gateway Books.

Aydin, D., Hartiningsih, S. S., Izgi, M. G., Bay, S., Unlu, K., Tatar, M. O., ... Dane, S. (2016). Potential benefits of foot bathing on cardiac rhythm. *Clinical and Investigative Medicine*, 39(6), S48-S51.

Barbieri, M., Henrique, A. J., Chors, F. M., Maia, N. D. L., & Gabrielloni, M. C. (2013). Warm shower aspersion, perineal exercises with Swiss ball and pain in labor. *Acta Paulista de Enfermagem*, 26(5), 478-484.

Batterham, S., Heywood, S., & Keating, J. L. (2011). Systematic review and meta-analysis comparing land and aquatic exercise for people with hip or knee arthritis on function, mobility and other health outcomes. *BMC Musculoskeletal Disorders*, 12, 123.

Becker, R. (1990). *Cross currents.* Los Angeles: Jeremy P. Tarcher, Inc.

Bender, T., Karagülle, Z., Bálint, G. P., Gutenbrunner, C., Bálint, P. V., & Sukenik, S. (2005). Hydrotherapy, balneotherapy, and spa treatment in pain management. *Rheumatology International,* 25(3), 220-224.

Benfield, R. D. (2002). Hydrotherapy in labor. *Journal of Nursing Scholarship*, 34(4), 347-352.

Benfield, R. D., Herman, J., Katz, V. L., Wilson, S. P., & Davis, J. M. (2001). Hydrotherapy in labor. *Journal of Nursing Scholarship*, 24(1), 57-67.

Cal, E., Cakiroglu, B., Kurt, A. N., & Dane, S. (2016). The potential beneficial effects of hand and foot bathing on vital signs in women with caesarean section. *Clinical & Investigative Medicine*, 39(6), S86-S88.

Castro-Sánchez, A. M., Matarán-Peñarrocha, G. A., Lara-Palomo, I., Saavedra-Hernández, M., Arroyo-Morales, M., & Moreno-Lorenzo, C. (2012). Hydrotherapy for the treatment of pain in people with multiple sclerosis: A randomized controlled trial. *Evidence-Based Complementary and Alternative Medicine*, Article ID 473963, 8 pages. doi:10.1155/2012/473963

Cherian, S. (2012). The effect of footbath on sleep onset latency and relaxation among patients with cancer. *International Journal of Nursing Education*, 4(2), 188-192.

Cluett, E. R., & Burns, E. (2009). Immersion in water in labour and birth. *Cochrane Database of Systematic Reviews*, 2009(2). doi:10.1002/14651858.CD000111.pub3

Czeranko, S. (Ed.). (2013). *Philosophy of naturopathic medicine: In their own words.* Portland, OR: NCNM Press.

Dupeyron, A., Demattei, C., Kouyoumdjian, P., Missernard, O., Micallef, J. P., & Perrey, S. (2013). Neuromuscular adaptations after a rehabilitation program in patients with chronic low back pain: Case series (uncontrolled longitudinal study). *BMC Musculoskeletal Disorders*, 14, 277.

Groven, F. M. V., Zwakhalen, S. M. G., Oderkerken-Schröder, G., Joosten, E. J. T., & Hamers, J. P. H. (2017). How does washing without water perform compared to the traditional bed bath: A systematic review. *BMC Geriatrics*, 17, 31.

Harbin School of Healing Arts (n.d.) What is Watsu? http://www.harbinschoolofhealingarts.orwhat-is-watsu2.html

Harmer, B., & Henderson, V. (1939). *Textbook of the principles and practice of nursing* (4th ed.). New York, NY: Macmillan.

Harmon, R. B. (2009). Cruel or caring: Hydrotherapy in state mental hospitals in the mid-twentieth century. *Issues in Mental Health Nursing*, 30(8), 491-494.

Herrera, E., Sandoval, M. C., Camargo, D. M., & Salvini, T. F. (2010). Motor and sensory nerve conduction are affected differently by ice pack, ice massage, and cold water immersion. *Physical Therapy*, 90(4), 581-591.

Hu, Q., Zhu, W., Zhu, Y., Zheng, L., & Hughson, R. L. (2011). Acute effects of warm footbath on arterial stiffness in healthy young and older women. *European Journal of Applied Physiology*, 112(4), 1261-1268.

Inside Edition (2011, November 8). *Inside Edition investigates detox foot baths*. Retrieved from https://www.insideedition.com/investigative/3347-inside-edition-investigates-detox-foot-baths

Jefferson, T. (1944). *Letter to Doctor Vine Utley dated March 21, 1819*. In A. Koch & W. Peden (Eds.), *The Life and Selected Writings of Thomas Jefferson*. New York, NY: The Modern Library.

Karagülle, M., & Karagülle, M. Z. (2015). Effectiveness of balneotherapy and spa therapy for the treatment of chronic low back pain: A review on latest evidence. *Clinical Rheumatology*, 34(2), 207-214.

Kennedy, D. A., Cooley, K., Einarson, T. R., & Seely, D. (2012). Objective assessment of an ionic footbath (IonCleanse): Testing its ability to remove potentially toxic elements from the body. *Journal of Environmental and Public Health*, Article ID 258968, 13 pages. doi:10.1155/2012/258968

Latorre-Román, P. A., Rentero-Blanco, M., Laredo-Aguilera, J. A., & Garcia-Pinillos, F. (2015). Effect of a 12-day balneotherapy programme on pain, mood, sleep, and depression in healthy elderly people. *Psychogeriatrics*, 15(1), 14-19.

Laukkanen, T., Kunutsor, S., Kauhanen, J., & Laukkanen, J. A. (2016). Sauna bathing is inversely associated with dementia and Alzheimer's disease in middle-aged Finnish men. *Age and Ageing*, 46(2), 245-249.

Liao, W. C., Wang, L., Kuo, C. P., Chiu, M. J., & Ting, H. (2013). Effect of a warm footbath before bedtime on body temperature and sleep in older adults with good and poor sleep: An experimental crossover trial. *International Journal of Nursing Studies, 50*(12), 1607-1616.

Libster, M. (2014). *Science of energy flow: Foot reflexology with herbal stress relief*. Wauwatosa, WI: Golden Apple Publications.

Libster, M., & McNeil, B. A. (2009). *Enlightened charity: The holistic nursing care, education, and advices concerning the sick of Sister Matilda Coskery* (1799-1870). Wauwatosa, WI: Golden Apple Publications.

Lin, L., Chen, Z., Cao, Y., & Sun, G. (2017). Normal saline solution nasal-pharyngeal irrigation improves chronic cough associated with allergic rhinitis. *American Journal of Rhinology & Allergy*, 31(2), 96-104.

Lopes, J. L., Barbosa, D., Nogueira-Martins, L., & de Barros, A. L. B. L. (2015). Nursing guidance on bed baths to reduce anxiety. *Revista Brasileira de Enfermagem*, 68(3), 437-443.

McKenna, J. & Symon, A. (2014). Water VBAC: Exploring a new frontier in women's autonomy. *Midwifery*, 30, e20 – e25.

Passali, D., De Corso, E., Platzgummer, S., Streitberger, C., Cunsolo, S., Nappi, G. C., ... Bellussi, L. M. (2013). SPA therapy of upper respiratory tract inflammations. *European Archives of Otorhinolaryngology*, 270, 565-570.

Principi, N., & Esposito, S. (2017). Nasal irrigation: An imprecisely defined medical procedure. *International Journal of Environmental Research and Public Health*, 14(5), 516.

Prins, J., & Cutner, D. (1999). Aquatic therapy in the rehabilitation of athletic injuries. *Clinics in Sports Medicine*, 18(2), 447-461.

Schitter, A. M., Nedekjkovic, M., Baur, H., Fleckenstein, J., & Raio, L. (2015). Effects of passive hydrotherapy WATSU (WaterShiatsu) in the third trimester of pregnancy: Results of a controlled pilot study. *Evidence-Based Complementary and Alternative Medicine*, Article ID 437650, 10 pages. Retrieved from http://dx.doi.or10.1155/2015/437650

Silver-Isenstadt, J. (2002). *Shameless: The visionary life of Mary Gove Nichols*. Baltimore, MD: The Johns Hopkins University Press.

Sprawson, E. (2017). Pain in labour and the intrapartum use of intramuscular opioids – How effective are they? *British Journal of Midwifery*, 25(7), 418-424.

Sullivan, D. H., & McGuiness, C. (2015). Natural labor pain management. *International Journal of Childbirth Education*, 30(2), 20-25.

U.S. Consumer Product Safety Commission. (n.d.). *About the Pool Safely campaign*. Retrieved from https://www.poolsafely.gov/about-us/

Wilson, M. (2017). A review of transanal irrigation in adults. *British Journal of Nursing*, 26(15), 846-856.

World Health Organization. (1996). *Care in normal birth: A practical guide*. Geneva, Switzerland: Author.

CHAPTER 10

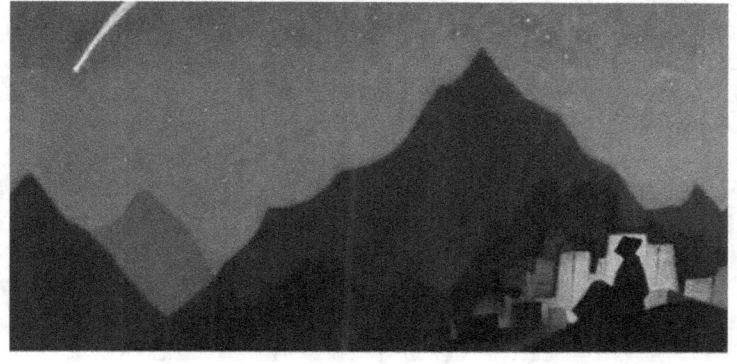

Star of the Hero, Nicholas Roerich, 1936
Courtesy, Nicholas Roerich Museum, New York, NY

AIR ELEMENT:
ESSENTIAL OILS AND AROMATHERAPY

LEARNING OUTCOME

After completing this chapter, the learner will be able to discuss essential oils and aromatherapy interventions in integrative holistic nursing practice.

CHAPTER OBJECTIVES

After completing this chapter, the learner will be able to:
1. Describe the history and science behind essential oil use and aromatherapy.
2. Explain the purpose and application of essential oils in nursing practice.
3. Identify some of the research and best practices supporting the use of essential oils and aromatherapy.
4. Discuss the professional issues associated with essential oil use and aromatherapy.

INTRODUCTION

The air element is an important focus of creating and maintaining an optimal healing environment. Florence Nightingale (1980/1859, p. 6), whose research focus was the environment, wrote that the "first rule of nursing, to keep the air within as pure as the air without." This approach suggests that the outside air was clean and "pure." Today, this notion may not be true, especially in urban areas; however, Nightingale's notion of the importance of the movement of air is still on the mark. Like water movement, air movement is essential to air quality (Nielsen, 2004). The ventilation of rooms and sickrooms in particular was the focus of health writings in the 19th century at the time that Nightingale did her work. Beecher and Stowe (2002, p. 56), famous 19th-century American women writers on domestic advice, state that the most successful mode of ventilating a house is by creating a current of warm air in a flue, into which an opening is made at both the top and the bottom of a room, while a similar opening for outside air is made at the opposite side of the room.

This basic desire to promote air quality has provided the platform for the use of fumigants (burned or smudged herbs) and incense in previous eras and essential oils today. The use of essential oil in nursing care draws attention once again to the importance of the quality of the air in a healing space. Essential oils and aromatherapy enhance the healing environment and promote health and wellbeing. This chapter discusses the use of essential oils and aromatherapy as an integrative holistic modality. Commonly used essential oils and their applications in practice are described, as well as examples of research and professional notes on best practices and cautions.

BACKGROUND

Essential oils, or "ethereal oils," are plant constituents known as volatile oils that are steam-distilled from plant parts, such as leaves and flowers. The earliest uses of aromatic plants by humans were not distillates. They included steams, fumigants, snuffs, salves, compresses, poultices, waters, baths, and perfumes. The process of distillation was first employed by the people of Egypt, Persia, and India (Guenther, 1948) in the making of waters, such as rose water. Those products were not fully distilled essential oils. Today, essential oils are typically distilled, although essential oils from some plants, such as lemon balm (*Melissa officinalis*), must be extracted through maceration or oil extraction. One of the first essential oils to be distilled in the United States was the oil of wintergreen (*Gaultheria procumbens L.*), and the first to be produced on a commercial scale was peppermint (*Mentha piperita;* Guenther, 1948).

Essential oils are the consciousness and lifeblood of the plant. They are made up of complex organic chemicals that are soluble in vegetable oil and alcohol. People can smell the aroma of essential oils from plants because these oils are chemical substances that evaporate quickly when exposed to air. The essential oils industry began with use in perfumes, foodstuffs, and beverages and later expanded to medicinal drugs and synthetic copies (Guenther, 1948). These volatile substances contain hydrogen, carbon, and oxygen. Chemically, the primary functional groups of essential oils used in aromatherapy are monoterpenes, straight-chain hydrocarbons (alcohols, aldehydes, ketones, acids, ethers, and esters), and benzene derivatives (Guenther, 1948).

The National Association for Holistic Aromatherapy (NAHA) defines *aroma-*

therapy as "the art and science of utilizing naturally extracted aromatic essences from plants to balance, harmonize, and promote the health of body, mind, and spirit" (NAHA, n.d.). This integrative holistic practice seeks to "unify physiological, psychological and spiritual processes to enhance an individual's innate healing process (NAHA, n.d.)

The origination of the term *aromatherapy* is credited to Rene-Maurice Gattefosse in 1930. He was a French chemist who was the first person to transform the practice from an anecdotal science to a well-recognized therapy. His interest in aromatherapy began when he discovered the benefits of lavender oil when it healed his burned hand without leaving any scars (Buckle, 2015). Gattefosse, along with Jean Valnet (a physician from France), and Marguerite Maury (an Austrian-born *nurse*), pioneered modern aromatherapy (Buckle, 2015) in the early 20th century.

The essential oils used in aromatherapy are found in all parts of the plant: blossoms, berries, fruits, seeds, pods, stems, leaves, needles, bark, rind, resin, wood, and roots. The plant essences, which are naturally distilled or mechanically pressed, without chemical processes, are medicinal-grade essential oils. These oils are very concentrated and volatile, meaning that they evaporate quickly when exposed to air. Essential oils from plants within the same family or genus or those that are grown or harvested in different ways or locations can demonstrate chemical differences, just as is the case with the plants from which they are distilled or extracted.

Methods of Extracting Essential Oils

Essential oils are extracted from the barks, roots, berries, flowers, stalks, leaves, and the resins of trees and plants. For an essential oil to be a true essential oil, it must be isolated by physical means. Below are some of the processes by which these essential oils can be extracted.

Steam Distillation

Steam distillation is the most common method of extracting essential oils that are contained in the glands, veins, sacs, and glandular hairs of aromatic plants. Steam extraction occurs when the cell walls of these plants are ruptured by heat. The molecules are carried in the steam through a pipe. As they cool and condense, the essential oil separates from the water.

Maceration

Maceration is a labor-intensive and costly method of extracting essential oils. Sometimes compared to the digestion of food, the process involves steeping the plant in a liquid in order to extract soluble constituents or to soften, separate, or break the molecules. It may or may not involve heat. This process is not commonly used. Examples of oils extracted by maceration are lemon balm, wintergreen, and bitter almond.

Expression

Expression is a method used exclusively to extract essential oils from the peel of citrus fruits. When the peel of such a fruit is mechanically pressed, droplets of oil and juice are squeezed out and separated. This method is also known as *cold pressing*.

Enfleurage

Enfleurage involves impregnating or soaking flowers, such as jasmine, in cold fat until they are saturated with the essential oil. This process is used when the flower oils are too delicate or short-lived to undergo distillation. It is an old extraction method that has, for the most part, been replaced by solvent extraction.

Solvent Extraction

In solvent extraction, aromatic compounds are extracted using hydrocarbon solvents. Solvent-extracted scents, or fragrances, always have a slight petroleum smell, which may or may not affect their aromas or therapeutic benefits.

Synthetics

Synthetic production uses organic chemistry to create essential oils in the laboratory that are synthetic copies of the fragrances of the original plants. Synthetics lack some of the energetic and vital healing properties of the natural products. Some people with plant allergies or reactive airway to perfumes and fragrances will react similarly to synthetic essential oils often used in potpourri, scented candles, and air fresheners.

ESSENTIAL OILS AND AROMATHERAPY IN PRACTICE

Aromatherapy is the skilled use of botanical aromatic oils for aesthetic, psychological, and therapeutic applications. A leading theory about how aromatherapy works is that when we breathe in the scents of essential oils, olfactory epithelium in the back of each nostril that contains about 5 million receptor cells (Steele, 1993) transmits chemical messages to the brain's limbic system, which affects moods and emotions. According to the former National Institutes of Health researcher Candace Pert (1997), moods and emotions are directly related to the neuropeptides that affect all aspects of the health of organs and body systems. Imaging studies in humans have shown how smells affect the limbic system and its emotional pathways (Buckle, 2015). These smell and emotion centers bypass the cognitive center. Therefore, the brain selectively responds to various emotions and senses with and without our awareness. The powerful sense of smell allows essential oils to stimulate, produce, and regulate various emotions.

Essential oils also enter the body via the skin. When essential oil molecules are massaged into the skin, they penetrate the bloodstream and act on the organs within the body, creating numerous physiological effects. This therapeutic modality helps restore harmony and energy balance between the body, mind, spirit, and the outside world – a harmony that is continually disrupted by pollution, stress, busy schedules, pathogens, diseases, and the other environmental stressors of life.

Essential oils have a variety of properties. Some classifications of these properties express the chemical and biological actions of an essential oil, such as antiseptic, antiviral, anti-inflammatory, analgesic, antidepressant, decongestant, and expectorant. Other classifications are energetic distinctions, such as stimulating, soothing, refreshing, calming, balancing, harmonizing, uplifting, sedating, rejuvenating, toning, and relaxing. Essential oils are often chosen based on their thermal energetics, such as whether they provoke a warming, cooling, or neutral experience. Rosemary essential oil, for example, is deeply warming, whereas peppermint essential oil is cold and lavender essential oil is neutral.

Each essential oil has its own special scent and healing properties. Hundreds of essential oils are available on the market today. According to the NAHA (n.d.), some of the most commonly used essential oils are classified energetically as:

- **Roman chamomile (Chamaemelum nobile):** Warming, antispasmodic, sedative, anti-inflammatory
- **Eucalyptus globulus:** Cooling, expectorant, antiviral, clearing the mind, energizing
- **Frankincense (Boswellia frereana):** Warming and cooling, soothes inflamed skin conditions, cell regenerative
- **Geranium (Pelargonium x asperum syn. graveolens):** Neutral, helpful for premenstrual syndrome, indicated for hormonal imbalance, nerve pain
- **Ginger (Zingiber officinale):** Warming, digestive, anti-inflammatory, relieves pain
- **Lavender (Lavandula angustifolia):** Neutral, calming, reduces anxiety, wound healing, burns, cell regenerative, general skin care, antispasmodic
- **Lemon (Citrus limon):** Cooling, antiviral, uplifting, detoxing
- **Lemongrass (Cymbopogon citratus):** Cooling, antiviral, insect repellant, antimicrobial
- **Neroli (Citrus aurantium var. amara):** Cooling, relieves anxiety, antidepressant
- **Peppermint (Mentha x piperita):** Cooling, nausea, analgesic, energizing, antispasmodic; do not use on children younger than 30 months of age
- **Rose (Rosa damascena):** Neutral, stress, anxiety, helpful for premenstrual syndrome
- **Rosemary (Rosmarinus officinalis):** Warming, stimulates circulation, clears the mind
- **Tea Tree (Melaleuca alternifolia):** Cooling, antibacterial, antifungal, antiviral

- **Vetiver *(Vetiveria zizanioides)*:** Cooling, grounding, astringent, calming agent (NAHA, n.d.)

Methods of Administering Essential Oils

Although almost all essential oil can be absorbed into the body via the skin (direct topical admin-istration), only certain essential oils (for example, lavender and tea tree oils) should be placed directly on the skin. Inhalation is generally considered the safest, most understood method of administering and using essential oil. In addition, inhalation via the olfactory or limbic system is considered the fastest route of administration. Aromatherapy can also be administered orally, rectally, vaginally, topically via massage, or by diffusion in the air.

Essential oils are diluted in a carrier oil for various therapeutic and clinical purposes. Some examples of carrier oils are sweet almond, grape seed, calendula, hazelnut, sesame seed, and avocado. Aromatherapy training includes content on blending. If one does not undergo specific training, it is recommended that essential oils be used one at a time. A typical dilution for a massage oil for healthy adults is a 2% solution; that is, 10 to 12 drops of essential oil per 1 ounce (30 mL) of carrier oil. For children, older adults, and the infirm, a .5% to 1% dilution or 5 drops per 1 ounce is best.

Bath Therapy

Bath therapy with essential oils can have profound effects on healing of skin disorders, alleviating muscle aches and pains, enhancing respiratory function, reducing stress levels, and increasing and supporting blood and lymph circulation. Essential oil baths, or aromatic bathing, facilitates healing on numerous levels, physiologically as well as psychologically.

In bath therapy, the water should be warm but not hot. The essential oils should be added to the bath just after or right before the individual gets into the water. The water should be swished around in order to disperse the concentration of essential oils. Note that if red blotches or irritation of the skin occurs while bathing, too much essential oil was added to the bath. In this case, a light cream without essential oils should be applied; the irritation should dissipate within 1 hour.

Aromatic baths with Epsom salts or sea salts are highly effective in aiding and supporting the body in detoxing and in wound healing. Epsom salts aid the elimination of waste material from the skin, reduce muscle aches and pains by aiding the elimination of uric acid buildup, and support and enhance the body's immune responses by stimulating lymph and blood circulation. The recommended amount is 5 to 8 drops of essential oil per cup of Epsom salts.

Foot and hand baths can be utilized for the treatment of arthritis, athlete's foot, poor circulation, low energy, stress, nail fungus, and other skin disorders of the hands and feet. For an aromatherapy foot or hand bath, add 5 to 7 drops of essential oil to a basin of warm or hot water and soak the feet or hands for 10 to 15 minutes. One-half cup of Epsom salts can be added for an additional benefit.

Inhalation Therapy

Leading perfumers and aromatherapists suggest that when engaging the air element with essential oils, all scents should be barely perceptible and never intrusive (Keville & Green, 2012; Steele, 1993). Fragrances and levels of fragrancing in a space are never held static because the sense of smell is known to habituate to a continuous onslaught of a particular odor. Continuous and excessive fragrance can be wasteful and detrimental to health.

Inhalation can be utilized as a complementary therapy or in self-care for various respiratory concerns as well as emotional states. It is most effective for relieving nasal or chest congestion or an excess or deficiency of mucus. For *steam inhalation,* bring 2 cups of water to boil, reduce the heat, and let the water cool for 5 to 10 minutes. Then, add 2 to 5 drops of essential oil (or a combination of two to three essential oils). Inhale the vapors for 5 to 10 minutes. Place a towel over the head to increase the concentration. With steam inhalation, it is critical to keep the eyes closed to avoid irritation. Inhalation can be used two to three times per day.

Inhalation therapy can also be achieved using a handkerchief or a tissue. Place 2 to 4 drops of essential oil on the tissue or cloth. Hold the cloth in the palms and take two to three deep breaths through the nose several times per day. Another variation on this theme is to place 2 to 4 drops on a pillowcase during the night. This method keeps the sinuses open throughout the night. For example, someone who is having trouble falling asleep can use eucalyptus oil and a drop of lavender oil to aid sleep.

Aerial Dispersion via Aerial Diffusers

Aerial dispersion (via electric diffusers or nebulizers) is used for respiratory ailments, sedation or stimulation, emotional upset, and as an environmental air freshener, for air purification for better quality, and also for the reduction of airborne pathogens. Aerial dispersion is best utilized in short durations; the recommended usage time is 15 minutes every 2 hours.

Christmas potpourri, clay candles, and electric pottery diffusers are other methods of aerial diffusion. Although these applications may not be considered medicinal, they do have therapeutic value. These types of diffusers are useful in the treatment of emotional upset and do provide a pleasant atmosphere for some people. They are a very simple method of environmental fragrancing. A wide variety of clay diffusers is available in retail stores. Such diffusers include clay car diffusers, clay necklaces, glass necklaces, and small-room clay diffusers. These products all are useful in creating an aromatic environment to enhance emotional well-being.

Hot or Cold Compress Therapy

Hot or cold compress therapy is a method of application best used in treating such conditions as muscular aches and pains, varicose veins, sprains, bruises, menstrual cramps, and respiratory congestion. It is also a wonderful way to relax after a long day at work. Use a cold compress for recent conditions and a hot compress for long-standing conditions or menstrual cramps. To prepare a compress, place 5 to 7 drops of essential oil in 0.5 L of water (To choose water temperature, see the water element –hydrotherapy chapter). Swish the water around, and then place a washcloth or a piece of linen or cotton fabric into the water. Wring the fabric out and then place it on the area. Allow the compress to cool or heat, as appropriate, to body temperature and then remove it.

Research

As an integrative holistic therapy, aromatherapy with medicinal-grade essential oil has both preventative and active treatment properties that can be beneficial during periods of wellness as well as during acute and chronic stages of illness or disease. Although the majority of the essential oils on the market are used for general therapeutic, culinary, or cosmetic purposes, many cultures value essential oils for their medicinal properties. Aromatherapy can be used to promote sleep, alleviate anxiety or pain, and improve mood. Many essential oils are used for their antimicrobial and antifungal properties. Dr. Jane Buckle's 2015 book lists several in vitro and clinical research studies on the antibacterial effects of essential oil.

Aromatherapy and the use of essential oils have been researched for several health concerns and diseases. For example, a quasi-experimental study of 60 participants conducted by nurses found that ginger essential oil inhalations were effective in preventing nausea and vomiting within the first 6 hours in postoperative patients who had abdominal surgery, as compared with those in the placebo group who received saline inhalations (Lee and Shin, 2017). Another clinical trial by Lua, Salihah, & Mazlan (2015) with 60 participants found 5-day aromatherapy treatment with ginger essential oil to be "encouraging" in its ability to alleviate nausea and vomiting in women with breast cancer. The aromatherapy was delivered via a necklace in the study. Participants wore the necklace day and night, which may explain the reason for the questionable results. It is a known phenomenon that people can become habituated to a scent, and therefore environmental fragrancing is typically aerosolized in "puffed" bursts (Steele, 1993).

Several studies have found essential oils such as ginger, peppermint, and citrus peel to be effective in allaying nausea and vomiting in morning sickness and nausea in labor (Buckle, Ryan & Chin, 2014). Aromatherapy footbaths and massages can reduce the need for pain medication during labor and improve postpartum mood and sleep, to name a few (Buckle, Ryan & Chin, 2014).

A systematic review of the literature, 12 studies on aromatherapy for depression, demonstrated that aromatherapy massage (more so than inhalation alone) has potential as an effective therapeutic agent in the relief of symptoms related to depression (Sánchez-Vidaña et al., 2017). This is true in children who suffer from mental health and behavioral issues as well. Pollard (2015) demonstrates (through case studies) the effectiveness of essential oils applied to specific acupuncture points, which she teaches to the children whom she treats. Because she is a practitioner of traditional Chinese medicine, she applies essential oil according to the energetics of the essential oil based on its aromatic qualities.

Aromatherapy is also used extensively in pain control in patients with cancer. One meta-analysis of randomized controlled trials on the effects of aromatherapy massage demonstrates that there was no effect on pain reduction; however, only one published study (278 participants) of 63 publications met the final inclusion criteria (Chen et al., 2016). A 3% cream with an aromatherapy blend of essential oil of marjoram, black pepper, lavender, and peppermint was applied to the necks of 60 participants with chronic pain. The findings of this randomized controlled trial suggest that this blend can be used to relieve neck pain as measured by Visual Analog Scale, pressure pain threshold test, and motion analysis system (Ou, Lee, Li, & Wu, 2014).

Another study (Bikmoradi et al., 2015), on the use of aromatherapy inhalations of lavender essential oil in postoperative patients with coronary artery bypass grafting, found no significant impact on mental stress as compared with those receiving placebo in a trial of 60 participants. Lavender essential oil inhalations did have a significant effect on systolic blood pressure, primarily on the third day postoperatively. Inhalations of lavender essential oil also have a positive effect in those with mild sleep disturbances. A review of the science on the application of essential oils in the care of surgical patients shows that studies on lavender (inhalation and topical) and orange (inhalation and massage) for anxiety, peppermint essential oil for nausea, and tea tree essential oil for infection have been effective; but studies are inconclusive about the effects of essential oil in pain control (Stea, Beraudi, & De Pasquale, 2014). A Cochrane Review of essential oils for postoperative nausea and vomiting (Hines et al., 2018) found that peppermint essential oil was not effective. This pattern supports what is well known in botanical science: Control of variables in clinical aromatherapy, as in herbalism, is a challenge.

A systematic review of quantitative studies published between 1990 and 2012 by Lillehei and Halcon (2014) yielded 11 randomized controlled trials on essential oil's effect on sleep. The total number of participants across all studies was 409. Blinding is a challenge in essential oil studies, but the studies reviewed were found to be well designed. Lavender, lavender-valerian blend, and jasmine essential oil were found to promote sleep. Peppermint, though stimulating, was also found to promote sleep.

Essential oils are also very effective for stress relief and anxiety reduction. One study found that lemongrass *(Cymbopogon citratus)* essential oil, 3 to 6 drops placed on a paper and inhaled, produced a reduction in state anxiety, tension, and heart rate in men (N = 40). Although participants were anxious about inhaling the lemongrass essential oil, the feelings passed quickly in the treatment group, whereas in the control group they did not (Goes, Ursulino, Almeida-Souza, Alves, & Teixeira-Silva, 2015). Inhalation of marijuana essential oil *(Cannabis sativa)*, a legal industrial hemp cultivar, was found to be effective in relieving anxiety, stress, and depression (Gulluni et al., 2017) in a small study of five adult participants, as measured by electroencephalogram, mood state, and autonomic nervous system parameters. An alternative for those who do not wish to engage cannabis in any form can is to consider hops instead *(Humulus lupulus)*. Hops, a member of the same plant family, contains essential oils (as does cannabis), that are known to be calming and sleep inducing (Libster, 2014). Another study of 20 female university students focused on the prefrontal cortex effects of essential oil aroma. The study found that olfactory stimulation for 90 seconds in air saturated with rose or orange essential oil induced physiological and psychological relaxation in participants, as measured by infrared spectroscopy (Igarashi, Ikei, Song, & Miyazaki, 2014).

These studies are just a few of the studies that have been done. For future research, some of the most promising leads are from the in vitro studies of essential oil in the inhibition of methicillin-resistant *Staphylococcus aureus* (MRSA). One review states that lemongrass essential oil completely inhibited all MRSA growth on the laboratory plates and lemon myrtle, mountain savory, cinnamon bark, and melissa showed a significant inhibition (Zouhir, Jridi, Nefzi, Ben Hamida, & Sebei, 2016). These data are being used for drug development.

Professional Notes

Although the U.S. Food and Drug Administration (FDA) participates in the regulation of essential oils, unless a product qualifies as a drug, the FDA can only regulate it retrospectively.

> This retrospective regulation means that FDA does not review essential oils for safety or efficacy before they can be sold and can only take action if data show them to be unsafe or the distributor makes claims that cause the product to be classified as a drug. (Mannion & Widder, 2017, e155)

There are some simple, time-honored principles of working with essential oils that the integrative holistic nurse knows when considering the use of essential oils in practice. Essential oils are a highly concentrated, single-extracted constituent of a plant and therefore pose greater risk to health when contrasted with the use of whole plants. Essential oil as a constituent in any plant can be compared with the fructose, a single constituent, in an apple. Compare what you know about the health and safety effects of extracted fructose with that of a whole apple. Although both are natural and recognized as foods, they present significantly different benefits and risks because the fructose is a concentrated sugar derived from the apple, which has hundreds of constituents in its state as an apple. Essential oils, as single constituents and highly volatile oils, present similar risks to those of apple fructose and perhaps more risks. As a rule, one should use as little as possible to achieve a healing effect. Less is best. Essential oils should not be used internally. Fragrance effects of plants can be captured in much safer forms. For example, sprinkle rose *water* on food instead of rose essential oil, boil cinnamon bark on the stove, or float whole chamomile flowers in a dish of boiled water to release its light apple-like fragrance. Fragrant whole plants are cheaper and safer to use in most cases.

The use of medicinal-grade essential oils in therapeutic applications is best carried out by knowledgeable and experienced practitioners. They use caution with people who have asthma, high blood pressure, or epilepsy. Essential oils should not be used with pregnant women. Best practice standards always include skin and sniff testing patients with oils before including them in care. In addition to the risks people may have related to allergic or reactive airway, there are psychological, emotional and spiritual concerns. Fragrances evoke memory in the brain. People carry memories that are distinctly related to their experiences, from pleasant to traumatic. Although the fragrance of a rose or lavender may be pleasing and calming to some, others may find them peculiarly disturbing because they evoke memories of someone or a time they would prefer not to remember. Therefore, those who work with essential oils typically create unique blends for their patients and test all essential oils in the patient before application. This best practice is what has led to a history of safe use. However, essential oil products mass marketed in premade blends introduce significant challenges to that safety record.

Aromatherapists and others who engage in the therapeutic use of essential oils know that certain essential oils, as there are plants, are known to induce or inhibit cytochrome P450 enzyme channels in the liver that are active in metabolizing drugs. This is especially true when these essential oils are ingested. Essential oils high in citral, such as lemongrass *(Cymbopogon citratus)* or chamazulene, such as German chamomile *(Matricaria chamomilla)*, may theoretically interact with drugs.

Essential oils should not be used on the skin undiluted (without a carrier oil), with the exception of lavender and tea tree oils. People with very sensitive skin may react to any essential oil used "neat." Essential oils that are more likely to cause contact dermatitis are those that contain large amounts of phenols (such as carvacrol and thymol) or aromatic aldehydes such as cinnamaldehyde (Buckle, 2015). Therefore, essential oil of oregano *(Origanum vulgare)*, thyme *(Thymus vulgare)*, and most particularly cinnamon *(Cinnamomum verum)*, are used with caution or perhaps not at all, as in the case of cinnamon. Know the difference between fragrance oils, which are often chemically derived, and medicinal-grade pure essential oils.

Keep all essential oils out of the reach of children. According to Keville & Green (2012), the safest essential oils for topical use in children are lavender, tangerine, mandarin, neroli, frankincense, petitgrain, and Roman chamomile. Some knowledgeable practitioners do help some parents use a very dilute rose oil for their infant's health and spiritual needs. But in general, essential oils interfere with bonding in infants, who depend on their sense of smell for identifying their parents.

Essential oils that accidently come in contact with the eyes or skin are treated as a chemical burn. Do not attempt to use water as a rinse. Essential oils do not dissolve in water. Instead, rinse the eyes or wash the skin immediately with whole milk. Milk with some fat in it is best for reducing irritation and actually removing the oil. Oil or another vegetable oil can also be used for skin reactions that may result from essential oils (e.g., a burning sensation in response to peppermint oil). If an essential oil is accidentally consumed, drink milk, eat soft bread, and go to the nearest poison control center for appropriate treatment (Buckle, 2015).

There is no required licensure to practice as an aromatherapist. However, best practice standards have been developed by the NAHA and the American Holistic Nurses Association (AHNA) in the United States and by several international aromatherapy organizations. Certification is provided through educational programs that offer training in aromatherapy. Many schools and programs exist in different states and internationally. Courses vary from school to school and state to state. These various organizations and schools strive to maintain the appropriate and required standards set forth by the NAHA and the AHNA. The NAHA aromatherapy curriculum and list of schools can be found at their website (http://www.naha.oreducation/standards).

By learning more about the proper use of essential oils, either through recognized schools or through qualified aromatherapy practitioners, nurses can explore this ancient tradition of employing a plant's fragrance in comfort and care as well as cure.

HOLISTIC TRANSFORMATION

- Reflect on your personal experience with the air element and air quality where you live and work.

- Consider the plants in the environment in which you work.

- What fragrances or essential oils (or both) do you currently use for yourself?

- And in patient care, what would you like to add to your repertoire?

SUMMARY

Employing fragrant plants in healing is as old as humanity itself. The practice continues worldwide. Knowledge of essential oils can be applied in the care of body, mind, spirit, and environment. Aromatherapy is the skilled use of botanical aromatic oils for aesthetic, psychological, and therapeutic applications. Essential oils have a variety of properties. Some classifications of these properties express the chemical and biological actions of an essential oil, such as antiseptic, antiviral, anti-inflammatory, and analgesic. Other essential oils are chosen based on their thermal energetics, such as whether they provoke a warming, cooling, or neutral experience. Research suggests that essential oils may be beneficial in the care of those who suffer nausea and vomiting postoperatively and during chemotherapy, need pain relief in labor and postpartum, or experience depression, anxiety, excessive stress, and pain. In vitro research suggests that essential oils such as lemongrass may be effective in treating people with MRSA. Those who work with essential oils create unique blends for their patients and test all essential oils with the patient before application. These and other best practices are what have led to a long history of safe use.

RESOURCES

National Center for Complementary and Integrative Health
https://nccih.nih.gov/health/aromatherapy
National Association for Holistic Aromatherapy http://www.naha.org

REFERENCES

Beecher, C. E., & Stowe, H. B. (2002). In N. Tonkavich (Ed.), *The American woman's home*. New Brunswick, NJ: Rutgers University Press.

Bikmoradi, A., Seifi, Z., Poorolajal, J., Araghchian, M., Safiaryan, R., & Oshvandi, K. (2015). Effect of inhalation aromatherapy with lavender essential oil on stress and vital signs in patients undergoing coronary artery bypass surgery: A single-blinded randomized clinical trial. *Complementary Therapies in Medicine*, 23(3), 331-338.

Buckle, J. (2015). *Clinical aromatherapy: Essential oils in healthcare* (3rd ed.). St. Louis, MO: Elsevier.

Buckle, J., Ryan, K., & Chin, K. (2014). Clinical aromatherapy for pregnancy, labor and postpartum. *International Journal of Childbirth Education*, 29(4), 21-27.

Chen, T.-H., Tung, T.-H., Chen, P.-S., Wang, S.-H., Chao, C.-M., Hsiung, N.-H., & Chi, C.-C. (2016). The clinical effects of aromatherapy massage on reducing pain for the cancer patients: Meta-analysis of randomized controlled trials. *Evidence-Based Complementary and Alternative Medicine, 2016*, Article ID 9147974, 6 pages. Retrieved from http://dx.doi.or10.1155/2016/9147974

Goes, T. C., Ursulino, F. R., Almeida-Souza, T. H., Alves, P. B., & Teixeira-Silva, F. (2015). Effect of lemongrass aroma on experimental anxiety in humans. *Journal of Alternative and Complementary Medicine, 21*(12), 766-773.

Gulluni, N., Re, T., Loiacono, I., Lanzo, G., Gori, L., Macchi, C., ... Firenzuoli, F. (2017). Cannabis essential oil: A preliminary study for the evaluation of the brain effects. *Evidence-Based Complementary and Alternative Medicine, 2018*, Article ID 1709182, 11 pages. Retrieved from https://doi.or10.1155/2018/1709182

Guenther, E. (1948). *The essential oils, vol. 1.* New York, NY: D. Van Nostrand.

Hines, S., Steels, E. Chang, A., & Gibbons, K. (2018). Aromatherapy for treatment of postoperative nausea and vomiting: a Cochrane systematic review. http://www.cochrane.orCD007598/ANAESTH_aromatherapy-treating-postoperative-nausea-and-vomiting.

Igarashi, M., Ikei, H., Song, C., & Miyazaki, Y. (2014). Effects of olfactory stimulation with rose and orange oil on prefrontal cortex activity. *Complementary Therapies in Medicine,* 22(6), 1027-1031.

Keville, K., & Green, M. (2012 -EBook). *Aromatherapy: A complete guide to the healing art.* Freedom, CA: Crossing Press.

Lee, Y. R., & Shin, H. S. (2017). Effectiveness of ginger essential oil on postoperative nausea and vomiting in abdominal surgery patients. *Journal of Alternative and Complementary Medicine*, 23(3), 196-200.

Libster, M. (2014). *Science of energy flow: Foot reflexology with herbal stress relief.* Wauwatosa, WI: Golden Apple Publications.

Lillehei, A. S., & Halcon, L. L. (2014). A systematic review of the effect of inhaled essential oils on sleep. *Journal of Alternative and Complementary Medicine, 20*(6), 441-451.

Lua, P. L., Salihah, N., & Mazlan, N. (2015). Effects of inhaled ginger aromatherapy on chemotherapy-induced nausea and vomiting and health-related quality of life in women with breast cancer. *Complementary Therapies in Medicine, 23*(3), 396-404.

Mannion, C. R., & Widder, R. M. (2017). Essentials of essential oils. *American Journal of Health-System Pharmacy, 74*(9), e153-e162.

National Association for Holistic Aromatherapy. (n.d.). [Home page]. Retrieved from http://www.naha.org

Nielsen, P. V. (2004). Computational fluid dynamics and room air movement. *Indoor Air, 14*(Suppl 7), 134-143.

Nightingale, F. (1980). *Notes on nursing: What it is, and what it is not.* New York, NY: Churchill Livingstone. First published 1859.

Ou, M. C., Lee, Y. F., Li, C. C., & Wu, S. K. (2014). The effectiveness of essential oils for patients with neck pain: A randomized controlled study. *Journal of Alternative and Complementary Medicine, 20*(10), 771-779.

Pert, C. (1997). *Molecules of emotion.* New York, NY: Scribner.

Pollard, T. (2015). Aroma acupoint therapy: A new, non-invasive healing modality perfect for children. *Journal of the American Herbalists Guild, 13*(2), 37-44.

Sánchez-Vidaña, D. I., Ngai, S. P.-C., He, W., Chow, J. K.-W., Lau, B. W.-M., & Tsang, H. W.-H. (2017). The effectiveness of aromatherapy for depressive symptoms: A systematic review. *Evidence-Based Complementary and Alternative Medicine, 2017,* Article ID 5869315, 21 pages. Retrieved from https://doi.or10.1155/2017/5869315

Stea, S., Beraudi, A., & De Pasquale, D. (2014). Essential oils for complementary treatment of surgical patients: State of the art. *Evidence-Based Complementary and Alternative Medicine, 2014*, Article ID 726341, 6 pages. Retrieved from http://dx.doi.or10.1155/2014/726341

Steele, J. (1993). The fragrant hospital: Environmental fragrancing in health care design. Transcript of presentation at AROMA '93 University of Sussex, UK. Personal library.

Zouhir, A., Jridi, T., Nefzi, A., Ben Hamida, J., & Sebei, K. (2016). Inhibition of methicillin-resistant Staphylococcus aureus (MRSA) by antimicrobial peptides (AMPs) and plant essential oils. *Pharmaceutical Biology, 54*(12), 3136-3150.

CHAPTER 11

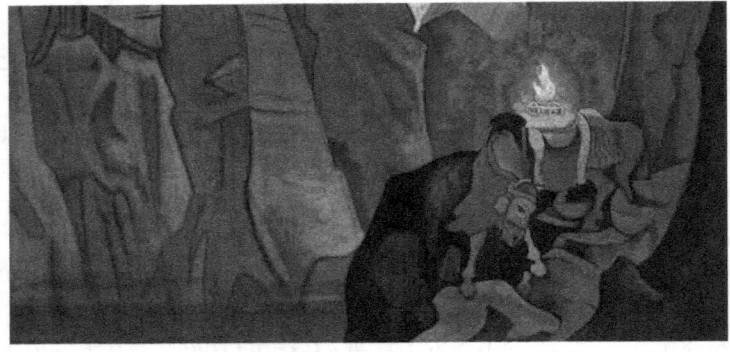

Treasure of the World, Nicholas Roerich, 1924
Courtesy, Nicholas Roerich Museum, New York, NY

FIRE ELEMENT:
RELIGIOUS AND SPIRITUAL INTERVENTIONS

LEARNING OUTCOME

After completing this chapter, the learner will be able to summarize the application of religious and spiritual interventions in integrative holistic nursing practice.

CHAPTER OBJECTIVES

After completing this chapter, the reader will be able to:

1. Describe the background of religious and spiritual care and interventions.
2. Review the role of health belief in religious and spiritual care.
3. Describe types of religious and spiritual interventions.
4. Explain some challenges with research on religious and spiritual interventions.

INTRODUCTION

"We have not yet found our consciousness – perhaps because consciousness is not something to be found ready-made, but something to kindle like a fire."

– Sri Aurobindo

In the West, consciousness is associated with thought; however, Eastern traditions have a sense of it as a much broader range of awareness that are "above and below the human range" that also include unconsciousness and "other-consciousness," such as that which is in plants, animals, atoms, and electricity (Sri Aurobindo & Satprem, 1993). Consciousness is a spiritual fire that takes many forms in the matter universe. People in medicine, nursing, and the healing arts often come to an understanding of consciousness as the Fire element by way of studying the anatomy and physiology of the body, such as the human nervous system and the elusive physiology of the brain and the mind. Descartes (1594 to 1650) postulated that the mind was the source of consciousness and that the nerves held the presence of spirits, which led him to hypothesize that the pineal gland ... was the seat of the soul, thus, controlling brain function (Porter, 1997, p. 217, 537). The root of curiosity in understanding consciousness has contributed to discoveries from the development of scientific understanding of reflex action to brain localization to today's holographic theories. Those who explore human consciousness and health as energy flow challenge those who in the past have placed restrictions on ways of knowing in science and the healing arts. Goethe said that "the extent of human knowledge has no bounds" and that "Science of nature has one goal: To find both "manyness" and whole. Nothing 'inside or 'Out there' meaning 'The outer world is all 'in here'" (Goethe & Naydler, 1996, p. 124). He was referring to the elements *within*, including the fire that is consciousness and energy flow.

BACKGROUND

Although those in the Western world were separating man from mind from nature, Eastern healing traditions continued on in the development of a centuries-old focus on energy flow and vibration as the seeds of health and longevity. As Americans focused over the years on the science of the body chemical, others in Europe were exploring the body energetic and electric (Becker, 1990). Nursing has engaged nature's reparative processes and their vital power (Nightingale, 1980/1859, p. 2) at least since the 19th century in the professional care of patients and sickroom management. Acknowledging the vital power or energy flow within and around a patient has historically represented best practice in the corporal and spiritual (e.g., integrative holistic) care of persons (Libster & McNeil, 2009). The energy for healing is recognized by some nurses as originating with the Creator/God/Divine Being (and similar names), whereas others have secularized nursing and in so doing have differentiated spirituality and religion in nursing (Blasdell, 2015; Libster, 2018), leading to broader definitions of energy-related healing.

Spirituality is defined by the American Holistic Nurses Association (2013, p. 91) as, "the feelings, thoughts, experiences, and behaviors that arise from a search for meaning ... The interconnectedness with self, others, nature, and God/Life Force/Absolute/Transcendent/Spirit not synonymous with religion." However, in addition to the distinction between spirituality and religion, there is a distinct difference between the spiritual notion of holism as "interconnectedness" and what is described in quantum physics as the implicate order that suggests holism (Bohm, 1980). Applied to nursing care, this quantum-consciousness science suggests that spiritual interconnectedness should not negate the belief that each person retains his or her own unique flame. When one's flame is enfolded together with the individual flames of others, a fire is formed.

Fire, known as *agni* in Sanskrit, is foundational to Eastern religious and spiritual traditions. For example, the first stanza of the *Rig Veda* (Sacred-texts.com, 2018), the oldest Hindu scripture, begins with an invocation or call to Agni, the Lord of Fire. Fire is a metaphor for transformative energy that is required to change consciousness from ignorance to wisdom. According to the Law of Conservation of Energy, Energy is neither created nor destroyed. It is transmuted or changed. Religious and spiritual interventions typically focus on changing energy. One simple example of changing energy can be found in Florence Nightingale's advice on the "laws of health" and the practice of nursing:

> We know nothing of the principle of health, the positive of which pathology is the negative, except from observation and experience ... It is often thought that medicine is the curative process. It is no such thing; medicine is the surgery of functions, as surgery proper is that of limbs and organs. Neither can do anything but remove obstructions; neither can cure; nature alone cures. Surgery removes the bullet out of the limb, which is an obstruction to cure, but nature heals the wound ... And what nursing has to do in either case, is to put the patient in the best condition for nature to act upon him. (1980/1859, p. 110)

Spirituality and religion both speak to health and the laws of nature. They often exist harmoniously within the same caring relationship. His Holiness, the 14th Dalai Lama of Tibet and winner of the 1989 Nobel Peace Prize, differentiates spirituality and religion this way:

> Religion I take to be concerned with belief in the claims of one faith tradition or another...Connected with this are religious teachings or dogma, ritual, prayer and so on. Spirituality I take to be concerned with those qualities of the human spirit – such as love and compassion, patience, tolerance, forgiveness, contentment, a sense of responsibility, a sense of harmony, which brings happiness to both self and others. (1999, p. 22)

People require nursing assessment and intervention for religious as well as spiritual needs. Assessment begins with seeking to understand a patient's *beliefs*. Religion and spirituality are foundational to the healing arts because all choices related to healing practices are predicated upon belief. Health beliefs are intimately woven within spiritual beliefs and religious practices. The classic Health Belief Model laid the foundation for understanding people's health choices and the variables influencing health decision making. Health behavior was determined to be dependent on the value a person places on a health goal and the person's estimate of the likelihood that an intervention will achieve their goal (Janz & Becker, 1984). It is a part of the general human experience to desire to avoid illness and hold specific beliefs about how one can avoid illness and how they participate in their own care. Understanding perceptions about health, illness, and healing interventions is foundational to the healing relationship. People who do not perceive an intervention as healing may not put forth the *energy* to participate in that intervention. Similarly, people who are committed to a goal and intervention based upon an understanding and perception of the underlying causation, be it actual or potential, are more likely to have the energy to participate in any intervention – from vaccinations to voodoo.

Belief is the cornerstone of both religious practice and interventions and spiritual life in the healing arts. They are different. *Spiritual* interventions in integrative holistic nursing can be as simple as demonstrations of inner feelings of caring and kindness, such as being present with or walking a patient to a chair. Spiritual interventions can include assisting patients to communicate their spiritual needs as they integrate their health care treatment. They may include their religious practices with support from community. Spiritual interventions may also include providing interventions that help the patient to make meaning of the health, illness, and healing experience, such as those discussed in the next sections. They can assist patients in processing their feelings, thoughts, and experiences that arise from the search for meaning. Perhaps, ultimately, such interventions can deepen their understanding of self, others, nature or environment, and the Creator/God/universal Spirit. Culture influences people's perception of an illness or disease and what they deem to be appropriate and caring treatment.

Nurses provide religious interventions with patients that assist patients in fulfilling the rituals of their faith. A faith community nurse (also referred to as parish nurse) is often designated to provide care for those of the same religious belief within a faith community (American Nurses Association & Health Ministries Association, 2017). A nurse may or may not be of the same faith tradition as a patient but can still provide religious practice support for those who are not of the same faith. For example, a nurse working in a hospital can pray with a patient or contact a religious leader in the community to provide support, guidance, and prayer for a patient of any faith. And a Muslim nurse can help a Native American patient plan for ways to complete their purification rituals (Moss, 2015).

The reintegration of the religious and spiritual, especially prayer and energy healing practices, within the dominant culture of hospitals and healthcare systems has been growing for decades (Eisenberg et al., 1998). A Gallup poll in 2016 concluded that 89% of Americans believe in God or a universal Spirit. Belief in God and a universal Spirit as well as religious practices influence a person's health beliefs and practices. People demonstrate their religious belief in many formal or informal ways. They may attend a church, temple, or mosque, worship a goddess, spend time in nature, spin prayer wheels, dance, burn tobacco, or meditate. People pray alone and in groups; read the Bible, Koran, the Torah, or other religious books; engage with spiritual and religious leaders; and participate in numerous forms of worship and fellowship within their homes, places of worship, and communities.

Religious and spiritual interventions are practiced in every culture. The American Nurses Association, American Holistic Nurses Association, and World Health Organization (WHO) all include spiritual well-being in their definitions of health. Spirituality and health are included in the National Center for Complementary and Integrative Health (NCCIH) database. Spirituality is defined by NCCIH (2022) as "an individual's sense of peace, purpose, and connection to others, and beliefs about the meaning of life. Spirituality may be found and expressed through an organized religion or in other ways." This chapter focuses on a few examples from the diverse and extensive body of religious and spiritual "interventions" that currently exist in American culture.

RELIGIOUS AND SPIRITUAL INTERVENTIONS IN PRACTICE

Energy is life. Movement, or flow, of energy is health. The focus of the Fire element as religious and spiritual intervention is energy flow. There is flow of energy between nurses and patients as they engage everyday practices and interventions designed to conserve energy, build energy, and restore energy. The focus of this work is building physical, emotional, mental, and spiritual strength needed for the adaptation, change, and restoration inevitable in the healing process. All nursing interventions are energy therapies. All interventions described throughout the text – from hydrotherapies to communication strategies – involve energy and therefore could be classified as energy therapies. The NCCIH (2022) classifies most interventions in its catchall classification of "mind and body practices." The official use of mind and body, however, does not include the religious or spiritual. Neither does the NCCIH or the WHO's (2013) classification of indigenous and traditional medicine practices, in which the religious, spiritual, or energetic domain (or all of these) is fundamental to their historical and cultural existence in community. Instead, those who present general information to the public in these venues all but marginalize the religious and spiritual while focusing on the tasks, treatments, and therapist credentials. The sociocultural and political debate about the separation of the religious and spiritual from the body and mind – and now the body mind – is a centuries-old phenomenon in the history of medicine (Starr, 1982). Attention is given here to a few examples of religious and spiritual interventions that are foundational to the role of integrative holistic nurses who would support the religious and spiritual beliefs of patients as they seek to conserve, build, or restore energy flow.

Prayer and Faith Healing

According to Ameling (2000, p. 42), prayer is an ancient healing act of "turning our minds and our hearts to the sacred" that has historically been a central part of daily life. Tuck, Pullen, and Wallace (2001) state that prayer is a holistic religious and spiritual intervention based on the belief in harmonious connectedness within the universe. Of all the religious and spiritual interventions practices, prayer is the one of the most commonly used. One definition of prayer is the "healing intentions or appeals directed toward a higher being, force, or power" (Ameling, 2000). Prayer can be offered in public or in private. Prayer can be both passive and active, with the most private part of prayer as meditation. Ameling (2000) identifies at least seven traditional categories of prayer: petition, intercession, confession, lamentation, adoration, invocation, and thanksgiving. Buddhist prayer incorporates meditation, mantra or chants, and the use of a prayer wheel. The prayer wheel, an apparatus used mainly by Buddhists in Tibet, consists of a wheel to which a written prayer is attached. Each revolution of the wheel counts as an utterance of the prayer.

Ameling (2000) notes that, although the American public generally believes that prayers can cure, prayer is rarely used purposefully in practice for curing in biomedical institutions today. Prayer is not unique to one religion; it is practiced by most of the world's major religions, including Christianity, Judaism, Islam, Hinduism, and Buddhism. Prayer with focused dedication is thought to help a person achieve moments of transcendence from their physical experience, which in times of great discomfort can bring tremendous relief.

Historically, spirituality and religious practices, such as prayers, have served as personal and communal sources of liberation, solace, hope, meaning, forgiveness, and healing for many people. For example, spirituality and religion are prominent components of African American culture (Newlin, Knafl, & Melkus, 2002). Spirituality is demonstrated in individual, family, and communal relationships and is expressed not only by going to church but also in prayer, song, music, dance, drumming, art, literature, and health beliefs and practices. When Africans and African Americans are faced with stressful events, such as illness, they often turn to prayer to help them cope. Religion and spirituality are also used to cope with social, political, and economic injustices. Drumming, dance therapy, holy water, visual imagery, and prayer are among some of the religious and spiritual practices used among African Americans as part of faith healing (Morrison & Thornton, 1999).

Indigenous peoples in Africa and countries around the globe continue to engage in their traditional healing practices that include religious and spiritual interventions (WHO, 2013). Faith-based organizations that mindfully practice prayer are major health providers in developing countries, providing an average of about 40% of services in sub-Saharan Africa (WHO, 2008). Many developing countries have traditional faith healers who are fully incorporated into health systems in which different religious and spiritual practices, such as prayer, are integrated with biomedical treatments and nursing care. Faith healers are deeply respected people who are typically chosen through community-recognized cultural and spiritual processes. Nurses also have their own faith and spiritual traditions that compel them to explore the role of prayer and contemplative caregiving in 21st century nursing (O'Brien, 2018).

Imagery

When people close their eyes in prayer, meditation, or contemplation, what are they thinking about? People often hold an image in their minds. This is one way of many ways that imagery can be useful. The power of the mind expressed in the movement of images can be accessed for use in supporting the healing process of self and others. Imagination engages the energy of vision as the fuel for all creative processes, including the process of healing and the promotion of health in all patient populations and across the life span.

Dr. Martin Rossman (1987, p. 14), identified as a pioneer in the field of imagery work, describes imagery as the

> flow of thoughts you can see, hear, feel, smell, or a taste. An image is an inner representation of your experience or your fantasies – a way your mind codes, stores, and expresses information. Imagery is the currency of dreams and daydreams; memories and reminiscence; plans, projections, and possibilities. It is the language of the arts, the emotions and most important, of the deeper self.

Imagery is a spiritual therapeutic modality that can be used as a tool for helping patients to make meaning of their health and illness experiences through connection with the unlimited capabilities of the body and mind. Barbara Dossey, a leader in holistic nursing, published one of her first papers in 1991 on "awakening the inner healer through imagery." Imagery, she wrote, can be "thought of as a bridge between the conscious processing of information and physiologic change, since images can influence both the voluntary (peripheral) and involuntary (autonomic) nervous systems" (p. 31). As a nursing intervention, imagery work is a powerful, noninvasive, cost-effective relaxation tool that can be performed by the patient themselves or directly in their work with a nurse or therapist. Integrative holistic nursing interventions support a person as they move through changes that they often first imagine. If a person cannot imagine their healing, one might question if that healing process can actually take place. This is the nature of the questions in imagery science. Ancient healing traditions in many cultures, however, provide some guidance. They identify health as movement and death as stagnation. Movement first begins in the mind, when a person imagines that health and healing, however they define it, are possible.

There are different types of imagery work. First, imagery work is not the same as daydreaming, dreaming, and therapeutic dream work. Daydreaming involves fantasizing about an abstract or concrete visionary fantasy, usually spontaneously while awake. In contrast, dreaming involves subconscious awareness of images, visions, and thoughts during sleep. During imagery work, a person uses his or her imagination, thought to be a function of the right brain, which, according to the Nobel prize-winning work of Roger Sperry, processes or thinks in pictures, sounds, and feelings. The left-brain processes logically and is oriented around names and words (NobelPrize.org, 2018).

Imagery is effective in health promotion and disease prevention work because it can provide the space for the deliberate and intentional focus on any symptom that rises to the level of conscious awareness, perhaps long before it becomes part of the disease process. Arnold Mindell (2004) likens a body symptom to a "telephone call from the universe" asking a person to "pick up" (p. 135). But, he says that people may not have any room on their desk for the phone and make no room for the ringing. "Marginalizing imaginary time is not just a scientific problem but a public health issue … a symptom is worthy of consideration only when it bothers you ... your body flirts and flickers are unimportant" (p. 136) in the biomedical world that engages in what he refers to as "consensus reality" (p. 135). Imaginary time, according to quantum physicist Stephen Hawking, ruled the beginning of the universe as we know it before there was space, time, or matter as we know it (Mindell, 2004, p. 11).

A primary decision point in imagery work is whether it is to be practiced as a "guided" or unguided intervention. *Guided imagery* typically involves the inclusion of specific directions from a nurse or nurse-psychotherapist. For example, in one study of women in preterm labor, a recorded female voice was used to instruct women in the study via an MP3 player. The women heard a 13-minute recording that said to close their eyes, feel their body sensations, and do head-to-toe muscle relaxation and meditation on a "peaceful" scene (Chuang Liu, Chen, & Lin, 2015). The findings suggested that women with a high risk for preterm birth and greater perceived stress showed higher adherence to and positive effect by relaxation guided imagery. The investigators concluded that the women who did not "adhere" to the prescribed relaxation guided imagery required relaxation techniques that were adapted to their "individual preferences" (p. 567). This idea makes sense. Any attempts to control the imagination of another with a prescribed image would be rejected if it is not in some way meaningful. Many people who work with imagery use different techniques to individualize the imagery work experience for the unique client. In general, the nondirective imagery guidance or counseling given is designed to *facilitate and record* the patient's own imagery work. For example, I typically ask a patient to describe a safe place using their imagination from which they can do their imagery work. As the patient becomes quiet and relaxed, often with eyes closed, they start by describing their safe place using image, color, sounds, tastes, smells, and sensations.

There are counseling and coaching techniques that nurses can utilize to assist the patient in recognizing the meaning that they assign to their imagery experiences. After the session, the nurse or therapist, who has been listening deeply to the patient's imagery, provides the patient a reflection on the nurse's recording of the session so that the patient can then process the experience and set goals based on what he or she has learned. Nurses can also help the patient to monitor changes in heart rate, blood pressure, respiratory and gastrointestinal patterns, and immune system function known to be positively affected by imagery work.

One research institution that incorporates imagery work in self-help stress reduction techniques is the HeartMath Institute in northern California. Their techniques, such as the Freeze-Frame technique (Childre, 1998), blend guided imagery techniques with space for personalized imaginary time. Those who are new to imagery work are provided more structure at the beginning through this approach. HeartMath science based on over 26 years of research was first published in the cardiology literature and is now a full body of work utilized in many branches of health care. HeartMath has discovered that our heart rhythm patterns are the best reflection of our inner state. Some of their research is now focused on the study of synchronization of the human autonomic nervous system with solar and geomagnetic activity (McCraty, et al., 2017).

Effort-Shape Movement

The Fire element as human consciousness is expressed in movement. Movement is the vehicle that a person, starting at birth, uses for communicating thoughts, feelings, beliefs, and experiences. Movement is the foundational communication science of demonstrating care in nursing (Libster, 2001). *How* a nurse approaches exemplifies the spirit of their caring communication. Florence Nightingale (1980/1859, p. 34) addresses this issue of nursing practice saying, "A firm light quick step, a steady quick hand are the desiderata; not the slow, lingering shuffling foot, the timid uncertain touch. Slowness is not gentleness, though it is often mistaken for such." Nurses today can learn to incorporate the science and art of movement in the development of their repertoire of ways to express their "fire" of caring for patients. Movement expresses meaning through rhythm, frequency, and vibration. *Rhythm* is a "movement or fluctuation marked by the regular recurrence or natural flow of related elements" (Rhythm, 1999). *Frequency* is "the number of repetitions of a periodic process; the number of complete oscillations per second of energy in the form of waves" (Frequency, 1999). *Vibration* is "oscillation...a characteristic emanation that infuses or vitalizes someone or something and that can be instinctively sensed" (Vibration, 1999). Rhythm, frequency, and vibration, instruments of nonverbal communication, demonstrate the relationships between persons and their environment.

A German movement scientist, analyst, and founding father of expressionist dance named Rudolf Laban, created one of the most historically significant forms of dance and movement notation that is used in many fields. Laban was able to successfully organize human movement into four components so that it could be studied and used to develop the movement repertoire, or a collection of movement skills and behaviors. Movement styles, like personalities, attract; but new facets of movement, like personality, can be learned. One way to expand one's expression of self as energy flow is to work on one's movement and exertion patterns, particularly what Laban referred to as the effort-shape of movement. "Movement quality is an aspect of behavior and can be considered a product of learning, metabolism, perception of the environment, whatever your particular bias is about what produces differences in behavior" (Dell, 1977, p. 12). The four components of the Laban system of effort-shape are flow, weight, time, and space (direction).

- ***Flow:*** The qualities of flow appear on a scale from bound to free. They represent the degree of tension in a movement. Bound flow is more tense, and free flow is more relaxed. One example of inappropriate free flow is the proverbial bull in a china shop. Carefully carrying a pot of hot water is an example of appropriate use of bound flow.
- ***Weight:*** The scale of qualities of weight spans from strong to light. Dell says, "As you observe changes in the quality of weight in people around you, you may find that people sometimes deal with themselves, with one another, or with many objects as if they were either large pieces of furniture or delicate paper flowers" (Dell, 1977, p. 21).

- **Time:** The range of the quality of time is from quick to sustained movement. These qualities are not used to measure rate of speed in movement but are descriptive of the qualitative changes toward sustained or quick movement. "The qualities of quickness and sustainment can occur and be observed when 'speed' is irrelevant and/or impossible to measure" (Dell, 1977, p. 26). Engaging the movement quality of time is observed when a nurse matches the pace of a patient who is walking with him down a hallway. Movement can be used as a nonverbal intervention for modeling a patient's world.

- **Space (Direction):** Attention to space can be indicated by visual contact or attention to the physical space. Indirect and direct are the qualities of the space component. "Movement in which spatial attention consists of overlapping shifts in the body among a number of foci, we call indirect. Movement in which spatial attention in the body is pinpointed, channeled, single focused, we called direct (Dell, 1977, p. 29). All four components can be put together in a variety of combinations with different intensities and presentations used in demonstrating the energy and consciousness of caring as well as the thoughts, feelings, and beliefs about caring. The way that these efforts are used in movement repertoire can inform nursing practice. An expanded repertoire prepares nurses for the energy and effort of patients who communicate through behaviors and movement styles that are different from their own. The nurse is more fully equipped within his or her own body to respond to the energy flow between themselves and the patients for whom they care.

PROFESSIONAL NOTES

Research on consciousness and energy as they relate to healing can be a challenge for health professionals in the biomedical culture, who seek randomized controlled trials (RCTs) for assurance of truth, safety, and effectiveness. Those who require RCTs on religious and spiritual interventions, a scientific construct easily applied to exploring the physiological effects of single-constituent pharmaceutical drugs, may be left wanting. Researching religious and spiritual interventions and energy healing (for lack of a better term) with the RCT is equivalent to attempting to fit a square peg in a round hole. When RCTs are attempted, scientists often conclude that the research is flawed or the findings inconclusive (Astin, Harkness, & Ernst, 2000), when it is often the original research question and the choice of the RCT as a method that was flawed from the beginning (Dossey, 1998). Many of the global leaders in subtle energy research have contributed to raising significant questions about the foundational flaws of the valued biomedical methods when trying to scientifically understand consciousness and energy.

There is another elusive professional issue related to the Fire element, and that is the issue of educational preparation and certification. Whether or not people attend a house of religious practice or subscribe to a doctrine, they can provide spiritual care to others. One need not be a religious leader or healthcare provider to be able to administer or recommend religious or spiritual care or energetically support another human being. In fact, it is often considered inhumane to not lend one's energetic support to someone in need. In the history of nursing, kindness is the epitome of energetic and spiritual support and has been known as the "remedy of remedies" in professional practice since the 17th century work of the French Daughters of Charity of Vincent de Paul (Libster & McNeil, 2009, p. 241).

Certification is not required to provide basic spiritual interventions. However, before using any religious and spiritual interventions practice or activity as an intervention to promote client healing, a nurse must be comfortable with his or her own spiritual well-being (Tuck et al., 2001). Although certification is not needed to provide certain spiritual care and advice, ethically and legally, nurses collaborate with patients before implementing any such practice.

Early faith community nurses, such as the Sisters and Daughters of Charity of Vincent de Paul, were given specific training on how to provide care that did not impose the nurse's religious or spiritual concerns upon the vulnerable patient. Contrary to popular belief, religious sister-nurses had strict guidelines against "interfering religiously" or proselytizing when providing care (Libster & McNeil, 2009, p. 123). Today, the secularization of care has not removed the opportunities for religious and spiritual interference with vulnerable patients. It is possible to pray for or direct energy toward someone without their permission or knowledge when serving in a professional capacity as a nurse, raising concern about the spiritual and religious ethics. Some patients might never know, and although some might benefit, others may not. There are sensitive people, especially infants and children, who are aware when others are encroaching on their energy field and experience that person's energy as a disturbance and unwelcome force. Energy therapies, faith healing interventions, and prayer can pose challenges when there are few techniques, movements, or efforts that can be analyzed (spiritually, emotionally, mentally, or physically) for congruence with patient patterns and needs in light of the dynamics of ever-changing consciousness. This area, while highly respected and developed for centuries in Asian countries, for example, has room for further development in the West in relation to application in clinical practice. For example, assessments that have been published could be used to establish need for prayer support (Taylor, 2003).

Faith community nursing certification was offered by the American Nurses Association for a time but is currently unavailable. It has also been referred to as "parish nursing." There is a *Faith Community Nursing: Scope and Standards of Practice* publication (American Nurses Association & Health Ministries Association, 2017) that does address religious and spiritual practice and ethics. In general, a nurse does not need formal religious training to meet the needs of a patient in spiritual distress. Being an advocate for patients experiencing spiritual distress rewires presence, compassion, and empathy. Some organizations require anyone who is interested in offering religious and spiritual interventions to seek counsel with a spiritual leader/elder. In assessing spiritual need, the nurse must determine whether he or she is comfortable providing the spiritual care or whether referral should be made to a formally trained minister of the patient's denomination. Tuck and colleagues (2001) note that as nurses become an integral part of faith communities, they serve as liaisons with hospitals and provide a bridge within a healthcare system for those seeking the incorporation of the spiritual in nursing care.

HOLISTIC TRANSFORMATION

- *Reflect on your personal experience with the Fire element and how your beliefs (health, spiritual, religious) influence your nursing practice.*

- *Reflect on the movement efforts that you use in patient care. Are there any that you do not use?*

SUMMARY

Religious and spiritual interventions that contribute to a caring dimension for the foundation of nursing are found in every culture around the globe. Consciousness is a spiritual fire that takes many forms in the matter universe. Spirituality and religion both speak to health and the laws of nature. They often exist harmoniously within the same caring relationship. According to the Dalai Lama, religion is concerned with belief in the claims of one faith tradition or another, its religious teachings or dogma, rituals, and prayers. Spirituality is concerned with qualities of the human spirit – such as love and compassion, patience, tolerance, and forgiveness. Spirituality comprises the feelings, thoughts, experiences, and behaviors that arise from a search for meaning. Belief is the cornerstone of both religious practice and interventions and spiritual life in the healing arts. Prayer is one example of a religious and spiritual intervention. It is the most commonly used religious and spiritual intervention in practice and can be offered as a component of spiritual care. Imagery and effort-shape movement are spiritual interventions that can conserve, build, and restore energy flow. Spiritual and religious interventions can provide the fire for healing.

RESOURCES

Dance Notation Bureau (Labanotation)
http://www.dancenotation.org

The Healing Mind (healing and the mind, imagery and the mind, Martin Rossman and other Pioneers) https://thehealingmind.org

Henry S. Olcott Memorial Library (one of the largest religious, spiritual, and philosophical collections) https://www.theosophical.orlibrary

HeartMath Institute www.heartmath.org

Institute of Noetic Sciences   http://noetic.orabout/overview

Subtle Energies & Energy Medicine Journal – ISSSEEM (free access archive)
http://journals.sfu.ca/seemj/index.php/seemj

Westberg Institute for Faith Community
 Nursing https://westberginstitute.org

REFERENCES

Ameling, A. (2000). Prayer: An ancient healing practice becomes new again. *Holistic Nursing Practice,* 14(3), 40-48.

American Holistic Nurses Association. (2013). *Holistic nursing: Scope and standards of practice.* Silver Spring, MD: American Nurses Association and American Holistic Nurses Association.

American Nurses Association and Health Ministries Association, Inc. (2017). *Faith community nursing: Scope and standards of practice* (3rd ed.) Silver Spring, MD: American Nurses Association.

Astin, J. A., Harkness, E., & Ernst, E. (2000). The efficacy of "distant healing": A systematic review of randomized trials. *Annals of Internal Medicine*, 132, 903-910.

Becker, R. O. (1990). *Cross currents: The perils of electromedicine.* Los Angeles, CA: Tarcher.

Blasdell, N. D. (2015). The evolution of spirituality in the nursing literature. *International Journal of Caring Sciences*, 8(3), 756-764.

Bohm, D. (1980). *Wholeness and the implicate order.* New York, NY: Routledge.

Childre, D. (1998). *Freeze-frame* (2nd ed.). Boulder Creek, CA: Planetary Publications.

Chuang, L., Liu, S. C., Chen, Y. H., & Lin, L. C. (2015). Predictors of adherence to relaxation guided imagery during pregnancy in women with preterm labor. *Journal of Alternative and Complementary Medicine,* 21(9), 563-568.

Dalai Lama. (1999). *Ethics for the new millennium.* New York, NY: Riverhead Books.

Dell, C. (1977). *A primer for movement description using effort-shape and supplementary concepts.* New York, NY: Dance Notation Bureau.

Dossey, B. (1991). Awakening the inner healer. *American Journal of Nursing,* 91(8), 30-32.

Dossey, L. (1998). The right man syndrome: Skepticism and alternative medicine. *Alternative Therapies,* 4(3), 12-19, 109-114.

Eisenberg, D. M., Davis, R. B., Ettner, S. L., Appel, S., Wilkey, S., Van Rompay, M., & Kessler, R. C. (1998). Trends in alternative medicine use in the United States, 1990-1997: Results of a follow-up national survey. *Journal of the American Medical Association, 280*(18), 1569-1575.

Frequency. (1999). In *Merriam-Webster's collegiate dictionary.* Springfield, MA: Author.

Gallup, (2016, June 29). *Most Americans still believe in God.* Retrieved from http://news.gallup.com/poll/193271/americans-believe-god.aspx.

Goethe, J., & Naydler, J. (Ed.). (1996). *Goethe on science: An anthology of Goethe's scientific writings.* Edinburgh, Scotland: Floris Books.

Janz, N. K., & Becker, M. H. (1984). The Health Belief Model: A decade later. *Health Education Quarterly*, 11(1), 1-47.

Libster, M. (2001). *Demonstrating care: The art of integrative nursing.* Albany, NY: Delmar.

Libster, M. M. (2018). Spiritual formation, secularization, and reform of professional nursing in antebellum America. *Journal of Professional Nursing*, 34(1), 47-53.

Libster, M., & McNeil, B. (2009). *Enlightened charity: The holistic nursing care, education, and "Advices Concerning the Sick" of Sister Matilda Coskery (1799-1870).* Wauwatosa, WI: Golden Apple Publications.

McCraty, R., Atkinson, M., Stolc, V., Alabdulgader, A., Vainoras, A., & Ragulskis, M. (2017). Synchronization of human autonomic nervous system rhythms with geomagnetic activity in human subjects. *International Journal of Environmental Research and Public Health,* 14(7), 770.

Mindell, A. (2004). *The quantum mind and healing: How to listen and respond to your body's symptoms.* Charlottesville, VA: Hampton Roads Publishing Company.

Morrison, E. F., & Thornton, K. A. (1999). Influence of southern spiritual beliefs on perceptions of mental illness. *Issues in Mental Health Nursing,* 20(5), 443-458.

Moss, M. P. (Ed.). (2015). *American Indian health and nursing.* New York, NY: Springer.

National Center for Complementary and Integrative Health. (2022). *Complementary, alternative, or integrative health: What's in a name?* Retrieved from https://nccih.nih.gov/health/integrative-health

Newlin, K., Knafl, K., & Melkus, G. D. (2002). African-American spirituality: A concept analysis. *Advances in Nursing Science,* 25(2), 57-70.

Nightingale, F. (1980). *Notes on nursing: What it is, and what it is not.* New York, NY: Churchill Livingstone. First published 1859.

NobelPrize.org. Official website of the Nobel Prize. *The Split Brain Experiments.* https://www.nobelprize.oreducational/medicine/split-brain/background.html

O'Brien, M. E. (2018). *Spirituality in nursing: Standing on holy ground.* Burlington, MA: Jones & Bartlett.

Porter, R. (1997). *The greatest benefit to mankind: A medical history of humanity.* New York, NY: W. W. Norton & Company.

Rhythm. (1999). In *Merriam-Webster's collegiate dictionary.* Springfield, MA: Author.

Rossman, M. L. (1987). *Healing yourself: A step-by-step program for better health through imagery.* New York, NY: Pocket Books.

Sri Aurobindo & Satprem (1993). *Sri Aurobindo or the adventure of consciousness.* Mount Vernon, WA: Institute for Evolutionary Research.

Starr, P. (1982). *The social transformation of American medicine.* New York, NY: Basic Books.

Taylor, E. J. (2003). Prayer's clinical issues and implications. *Holistic Nursing Practice, 17*(4), 179-188.

Tuck, I., Pullen, L., & Wallace, D. (2001). A comparative study of the spiritual perspectives and interventions of mental health and parish nurses. *Issues in Mental Health Nursing, 22*(6), 593-605.

Vibration. (1999). In *Merriam-Webster's collegiate dictionary*. Springfield, MA: Author.

Sacred-texts.com (2018). The Rig Veda. http://www.sacred-texts.com/hin/rigveda/index.htm

World Health Organization (2008). *Building from common foundations: The World Health Organization and faith-based organizations in primary healthcare*. Geneva, Switzerland: Author.

World Health Organization (2013). *WHO traditional medicine strategy, 2014-2023*. Geneva, Switzerland: Author.

CHAPTER 12

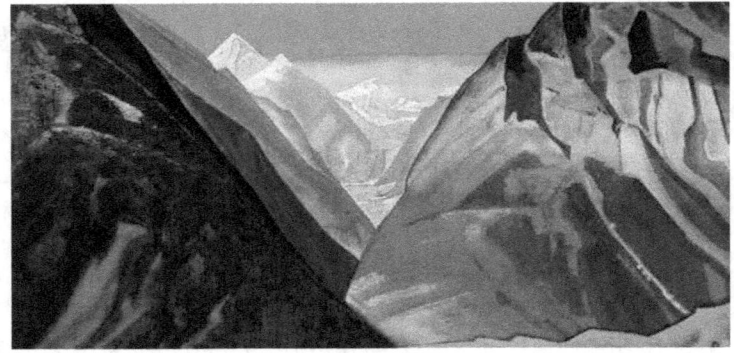

Lahul, Nicholas Roerich, 1932
Courtesy, Nicholas Roerich Museum, New York, NY

EARTH ELEMENT: NUTRITION INTERVENTIONS

LEARNING OUTCOME

After completing this chapter, the learner will be able to discuss the use of nutrition interventions in integrative holistic nursing practice.

CHAPTER OBJECTIVES

After completing this chapter, the learner will be able to:

1. Describe the role of taste in nutrition interventions.
2. Discuss the background of the use of broth and porridge in nutrition interventions.
3. Define macrobiotic diet, a popular nutrition intervention program.
4. Discuss one concern related to the macrobiotic diet as a nutrition intervention.

INTRODUCTION

"The heavenly energy descends and the earthly energy ascends ... the result is a balance of sunshine and rain, wind and frost, and the four seasons."

– The Yellow Emperor's Classic of Medicine

The Earth element is represented in all things of the material world. This chapter focuses on food as the representative of Earth in the Elements of Care®. Much of the Western literature on nutrition interventions focuses on the constituents of foods that originate from plants. As people's bodies respond to climate change, population health experts and those in the health food industry respond to increased public interest in the relationship between foods and the body's reactivity to the environment. People refer to their experiences in terms such as food allergy, reactivity, intolerance, and sensitivity. Some concerns people have center on the foods that are known to commonly trigger these reactions to environment, such as wheat and dairy products.

As with all areas of scientific research, there are conflicting studies as to the benefits and risks of restricting certain foods, such as wheat and dairy, from the diet. For example, one review of the nutritional studies literature reaches this conclusion:

> It is therefore unlikely that the health of more than a small proportion of the population will be improved by eliminating wheat or gluten from the diet. In fact, the opposite may occur as wheat is an important source of protein, B vitamins, minerals and bioactive components (Shewry & Hey, 2016).

However, these studies typically investigate only the effects (benefits and risks) of the constituents of the foods on human health and behavior. The energetics of foods is not explored. For example, wheat and dairy are classified in classical traditional Chinese medicine (TCM) as "tonifying" foods, which means that they are tonifying and damp. When children are experiencing a growth spurt, they may need tonifying food, such as dairy and wheat. But when a child or an adult has a damp condition, such as excessive phlegm or cysts, they may no longer be able to tolerate tonifying, damp foods. The spleen, which likes dryness, will become sluggish. People then feel the effects of this imbalance as extreme fatigue, loose bowels, and digestive problems, which are known effects of spleen dampness in TCM. According to energetics pattern knowledge, practitioners would suggest restricting these foods despite literature reviews of the lack of scientific correlation between the foods and symptoms. The focus of this chapter is the energetics of nutrition science of the whole food as is prominent in Eastern tradition.

BACKGROUND

According to the World Health Organization (WHO, 2021), obesity has reached epidemic proportions globally. Obesity, which has been linked to excessive stress and a sedentary lifestyle, also increases the risk and prevalence of health problems such as diabetes, cardiovascular disease, renal disease, bone fractures, some cancers, anxiety, breathing problems, and depression in rural, urban, industrialized, and agrarian countries (WHO, 2021). One of the oldest biomedical nutritional interventions is a simple formula for creating balance between the number of calories a person puts into his or her body versus the number of calories that the person burns during daily activity. A *calorie* is a unit of heat expressing energy potential from food when digested. For example:

- Protein produces 4 kilocalories per 1 g.
- Carbohydrates produce 4 kilocalories per 1 g.
- Fat produces 9 kilocalories per 1 g.
- Alcohol produces 7 kilocalories per 1 g.
- Water, fiber, vitamins, and minerals do not produce any kilocalories.

To gain weight, a person would increase caloric intake, decrease activity (calorie burning), or both. To lose weight, a person would increase exercise, decrease unnecessary caloric or food intake, or both. Striking a proper balance requires behavioral and lifestyle change and therefore is not easy. Although water, fiber, vitamins, and minerals do not contribute to caloric intake, their roles in metabolism and cell function are important. Calories from fat and carbohydrates are needed for energy, and protein is needed for repairing injured tissue. When the body (such as the brain) does not receive the fats and carbohydrates it needs to produce energy, these roles can reverse and create a state of metabolic imbalance that leads to fatigue and illness. One other consideration is that food scientists have also developed products with "zero calories" that people who are counting calories can then feel free to eat in massive amounts. This idea might seem to be a good one, but it is true that highly processed foods often lack nutrients, particularly micronutrients, that come from whole foods made from plants grown in the healthy soil of the earth.

The depth of food science knowledge from a Western perspective is beyond the scope of this chapter, where the focus is the Earth element as the energetics contribution of whole foods to integrative holistic health care. When the focus is the constituents of foods, such as occurs in Western nutrition, patient education, and the functional food industry, the outcome is a sense that all people can benefit from a one-size-fits-all model of care and that there is a specific number of a particular nutrient that all people need for health. However, dietary therapies from enduring ancient wisdom traditions do not have this focus on constituents. People's health improves when their nutritional needs are addressed as individuals.

Western reductionistic philosophy of nutrition that emphasizes the importance of knowing and measuring the constituents of foods is best complemented by an understanding of the Eastern philosophy of the energetics of foods that match the *precise* energetics needs of people. Although many prelicensure nursing programs continue to include a Western-based nutrition course in their curriculum, the focus of this text is the Eastern perspective of the energetics of foods that is congruent with an integrative holistic and person-centered philosophy of care. The energetics of foods begins with the five tastes.

Energetics First with Eight Principle Patterns

As discussed previously, the energetics qualities used to describe health patterns and in designing interventions that restore harmony and balance to those patterns include heat/cold, excess/deficiency, interior/exterior, and yin/yang. These Eight Principle Patterns that are the foundational theory of classical TCM, and sometimes summarized and referred to as "yin-yang theory," were discussed in the *Yellow Emperor's Classic of Medicine* (Ni, 2011) written at the end of the Western Han dynasty. This approach continues to be used by practitioners and the public today.

Many acupuncturists and TCM practitioners utilize the Five-Element theory in their assessment diagnosis and treatment of patients. However, the Five-Element theory is "deemphasized (Zhou, 2009, p. 9) because the terms were not discussed in the Nei Jing," one of the most revered medical texts in China and is not used to describe complex phenomena (Zhou, 2009) so often seen today.

In TCM, the five seasons include autumn, winter, spring, summer, and late summer. Nurses do incorporate the energetics of the five seasons and tastes with the Eight Principle Patterns theory when working with foods and diet therapies (see Figure 12-1). Using the Eight Principle Patterns, seasons, and tastes approach to nutritional interventions is the foundation for precision nutritional care. Two people with the same biomedical diagnosis can receive completely different nutritional intervention based on an Elements of Care® integrative holistic nursing energetics assessment and diagnosis. For example, two people may be diagnosed with dementia – one exhibits the symptom/sign pattern for heat (thirst for cold drinks, red face, dark urine, rapid pulse, and combative behavior), whereas the other exhibits a cold or cool pattern (thirst for warm drinks, pale urine, and slow movement). Warm, spicy food, although the "hot" patient may like it, is contraindicated because it may make the patient's behaviors (symptom-sign patterns) worse because the hot food is adding heat to the existing hot condition.

An understanding of the different energetics qualities and the relationships between the Eight Principle Patterns can be foundational to effectively applying the Elements of Care® integrative holistic nutrition interventions in nursing care. The goal of a nurse's energetics assessment is to develop plans of care that create balance and harmony. "Harmonious and creative adaptability is the hallmark of correctly applied yin-yang theory" (Pitchford, 2002). In general, according to the Eight Principle Patterns, if there is too much of one quality, the nurse introduces or suggests the opposite manifest in a chosen care such as food, but only to the point of creating balance. Too much of the opposing quality can then create an imbalance as well.

One experiment a nurse can use to train his or her sense to keenly observe energetics patterns is to taste foods. To experience bitter taste, eat leafy greens or herbs or the rind of a grapefruit. The bitter principles of the plants can be tasted immediately, but then, as you continue to chew, a sweet taste typically emerges. For sour taste, try the fruit of citrus, such as a lime or a lemon. Notice the body's reaction to the sour taste. To experience sweet taste, eat a baked sweet potato or drink some cow's milk. To experience pungent taste, taste a small amount of cayenne pepper or ginger powder. Taste different kinds of salts to experience the flavor of salt. Sea vegetables, such as kelp, also have a salty taste from the ocean.

FIGURE 12-1:
FIVE SEASONS AND TASTES IN CLASSICAL TRADITIONAL CHINESE MEDICINE

	Fire	Wood (Ether)	Earth	Metal (Air)	Water
Organ	Heart	Liver	Spleen	Lungs	Kidneys
Taste	Bitter	Sour	Sweet	Pungent	Salty
Season	Summer	Spring	Late summer	Autumn	Winter

According to Indian Ayurveda tradition, each taste is composed of two of the five elements. Bitter is Air and Ether; sour is Earth and Fire; sweet is Earth and Water; pungent is Fire and Air; and salty is Water and Fire. Ayurveda recognizes a sixth taste as well: astringent. Certain plants, such as the tea plant *(Camellia sinensis)*, which contain constituents known as tannins, are very astringent or drying to the mouth. Some berries, such as cranberries *(Vaccinium macrocarpon)*, also are astringent.

The Sanskrit word for taste is rasa, which means "essence." Taste directly affects the nervous system through the vital energy in the mouth. Chewing is very important to healthy nervous system function. Also, Frawley & Lad (2010) stated the effects of stimulating *prana*, or life force, through the mouth when tasting and stimulating gastric nerves:

> taste affects *agni* and enhances the power of digestion. For this reason, bland food may not be nourishing in spite of its vitamin or mineral content ... To improve *agni* and eliminate disease, it is necessary to improve our sense of taste. (p. 24)

In classical TCM, digestion is a twofold process: xiao, the dispersion of substances to be retained by the body, and *hua*, the transformation of impure substances to be excreted (Flaws, 2013). Digestion is understood in terms of the functions of the spleen and the stomach. The stomach is thought of as a pot on a stove, where warmth is required for all transformations to occur. The spleen is the fire and the mechanism for distillation of pure substances from foods that become qi within the lungs and blood within the heart. "The sending up of the pure part of the foods and liquids by the spleen is called ascension of the clear" (Flaws, 2013, p. 10). The stomach then sends the impure substances to the large intestine to be transformed by the large and small intestines. The primary purpose and starting point for all digestion health and the subsequent nourishment of all other body systems with energy is the maintenance of the 100°F "soup" in the "cooking pot" of the stomach. Therefore, in ancient traditions, the warmth of the stomach is maintained through cooking of food and the use of herbs and spices that are typically warming to the stomach. Nutrition interventions using this centuries-old theoretical foundation include commonsense applications such as reminding those with digestive problems to avoid iced beverages with meals (a common practice in the United States) and eating raw foods, such as salad.

This enduring understanding of the importance of the stomach and the spleen's needs for warmth and experiencing tastes explains why nursing care that begins with setting up an environment for the preparation and serving of food is foundational to digestion and overall health and well-being. For example, children who always sit in front of a television to eat – where their senses are distracted while tasting their food – may develop nervous systems, sensory systems, that become numb to taste. In addition, the ability to detect subtle tastes can be hampered in those who eat prepared foods replete with flavor enhancers and preservatives. Nursing care that addresses simple lifestyle changes, such as mindfully tasting and chewing food, has the potential for significant impact on changes to the nervous and gastrointestinal systems in particular. Review and application of these energetics principles lays the groundwork for a greater chance of success of nutritional interventions.

NUTRITION INTERVENTIONS IN PRACTICE

The background information provided in the preceding sections included general principles of nutrition intervention that bring a focus on the Earth element in caring practice. Integrative holistic nurses can include numerous dimensions to nutritional interventions in practice – from mindfulness eating strategies to coaching or counseling approaches using prescriptive dietary instructions. This section focuses on a sample of two nursing interventions. The first is "broth and porridge," a historic focus of sickroom diet in nursing. The second is an example of a prescribed diet rooted in the Eight Principle Patterns and the Five-Element theory called the "macrobiotic diet."

Broth and Porridge

Some of the foods considered to be the most easy-to-digest come in a bowl. They include broth and porridge. Some of the earliest professional nurses, such as the French Daughters of Charity of Vincent de Paul formed in 1633, included the art and science of broth, called "bouillon" in French, in their *Orders of the Day in the Hospital* instructions for nurses (Libster & McNeil, 2009). Broths were chosen as a nutrition intervention when the nurses wanted to strengthen a patient. They were made from different combinations of meat, vegetables, herbs such as sorrel, chicory, and caraway, and occasionally from grains, such as barley. The Daughters of Charity foundress, Louise de Marillac, said that it was the "exactitude" by which she prepared the broth rather than the "quantity of meat" that made the broth "pleasing to patients" (Libster & McNeil, 2009, p. 176). For centuries, nurses have openly and "lovingly" shared their recipes and remedies for healing (Libster, 2004), to include even what appears to be the simplest of foods: namely, broth. Today that trend continues as "bone broth," which is simmered for 12 to 24 hours and has become popular once again for health concerns from inflammation to digestive weakness (*Harvard Women's Health Watch,* 2015). Serving broth before a meal can also aid in weight loss because people tend to eat less food overall when feeling full after consuming broth. This practice was common among early faith community nurses, whose mission it was to feed thousands of poor people.

Porridge is also a centuries-old nutrition intervention used by nurses in strengthening those who are sick. For example, one of the nurses of the early Church of Jesus Christ of Latter-day Saints, Mary Ann Pratt, is credited with saving many lives with the administration of "porridge" during pioneer treks to Utah. Most of the women pioneers had contracted "the cholera," and the warm porridge helped them to recover (Libster, 2004, p. 174). Foods nurses use in treating the sick are often so common that the ingredients and recipes may not be recorded; but generally, porridge is made from some type of grain, such as barley or rice.

Rice porridge, also known as "congee" or "jook," is considered a food for nourishing young and old alike (Flaws, 1995). It is called *shi fan* in Mandarin, or "rice water." Although it may not sound appetizing, it can, if prepared with exactitude (as was the broth of the Daughters of Charity), result in a sweet, bland food that "results in the five flavors automatically supplementing the five viscera" (Flaws, 1995, p. 20). Oats also make a good porridge, particularly for those who have a dry cough, because the energetics qualities of oats lead to moistening of the lungs. For Westerners who eat much more dairy, fruit juice, and fats and are categorically more moist or "damp" (and therefore may be obese), porridge is made with rice rather than oats, and it has beans, vegetables, a small amount of animal protein, and medicinal herbs. Most of the time, Chinese jook is made with rice. Rice fortifies the spleen, harmonizes the stomach, and drains dampness.

The focus of TCM is longevity. One renowned book on longevity states that, "Old people who eat gruel all day, not sticking to fixed times, are also able to keep their body strong and fortified and enjoy great longevity" (as cited in Flaws, 1995, p. 24). Rice congee is beneficial for anyone with weak digestion, such as infants and older adults, and anyone who is ill or recuperating from prolonged illness. Many parents know this and provide rice porridge for their infants as the first food while weaning from breast milk.

To cook rice congee, use 1 part rice to 5 to 8 parts water instead of the usual 2 parts water. The congee can be cooked for 2 to 4 hours on the stove or overnight in a slow cooker. "Almost anyone who is sick can benefit from a simple rice congee" (Flaws, 1995, p. 31). Rice is a diuretic; therefore, eating a lot of rice congee is contraindicated in those with frequent urination. Many "diets" recommended for weight loss and general health stress eating protein foods and a diminished use of carbohydrates. The discussion of protein and carbohydrate is part of the reductionist system and, although it may contribute helpful information, stands lacking without attention to the energetics of foods, as demonstrated in the centuries-old tradition of using broths and porridge. Some diets attend to both energetics and food constituents. One example is the macrobiotic diet.

The Macrobiotic Diet

Macrobiotics is a predominantly vegetarian, whole-foods diet based on a "philosophy, cultural movement, and eating pattern" (Kushi, Cunningham, & Teas, 2001, p. 3057S). The use of the term "macrobiotics" was popularized by Japanese philosopher Georges Ohsawa (1893 to 1966) and his student Michio Kushi to describe the Chinese view of the science and medicine of achieving happiness utilizing the Eight Principle Patterns, specifically yin-yang. Ohsawa writes the following in his classic little book, *Zen Macrobiotics: The Art of Rejuvenation and Longevity* (1965, p. 25):

> Macrobiotics, the medicine of longevity and rejuvenation, is very simple, extraordinarily practical and economical. One can apply it at any time, on any level of life and under any circumstance. It is more educational than curative and depends entirely on your comprehension and will. It is, in truth, the study of the way to SATORI – realization of self and liberation – and you must achieve it yourself.

Macrobiotics, like Eastern philosophies of health and longevity, is based on the science and art of energy balance. For example, if a person is hot, they need to be cooled. If a person is dry, they need moisture. There are specific terms that describe energetics differences, such as hot and cold. Yin and yang are the two principle patterns of the Eight Principle Patterns that Ohsawa made the primary focus of his macrobiotic diet. This diet has been taught to thousands of students around the world. The diet is used in self-care practices but is taught within the context of learning how to assess one's own energetics patterns. People who live within the macrobiotic culture, as do many Asian peoples, first view the world energetically. For example, if a person's stomach is bloated from overeating, they know that to be an "excess" condition for which there are lifestyle changes, foods, or both that balance or drain the excess. One example would be to drink bancha, toasted green tea, in lieu of a meal to let the body rest. Bancha also drains excess, energetically speaking.

Yin is energetically cold and dark, whereas yang is characterized by heat and light (Ohsawa, 1965). Ohsawa discusses yang as a contracting energetic force and yin as an expansive force. The example of overeating given in the previous paragraph would be termed a "yin" condition in macrobiotics. Macro-biotic science discusses the classification of foods and the patient's health patterns in these simple dualistic terms of *yin* versus *yang* (Wicke, 1992; Libster, 2012). In contrast, in TCM, yin and yang are incorporated as part of the overarching Eight Principle Patterns analysis of people and foods. The example of overeating is not just a yin situation in which the solution that would create balance is to eat a yang food. Overeating and bloating is also an excess situation that can be addressed by draining excess to create balance.

Ohsawa (1965, p. 40) correctly states that "There is Yin and Yang in everything." Although macrobiotics can at times be operationalized as a dualistic or oppositional philosophy of yin versus yang, its original roots are in the Eight Principle Patterns detailed in the *Yellow Emperor's Classic of Medicine* in which the have shown that the macrobiotic diet plan outlined in the Kushi Institute's Way to Health has a greater anti-inflammatory nutritional profile than the Mediterranean or "average" American diet and that some nutrients such as vitamin D, vitamin B12, and calcium tend to be low in the diet (Harmon, et al., 2015).

Studies by Goldin et al. (as cited in Kushi et al., 2001) suggest a lower risk for breast cancer for the women eating macrobiotically. Women consuming a macrobiotic diet have "modestly lower circulating estrogen levels, suggesting a lower risk of breast cancer. This may be due in part to the high phytoestrogen content of the macrobiotic diet" (Kushi et al., 2001, p. 3056S). Theoretically, the high level of phytoestrogens (plant hormones – not human estrogen) from the soy-based foods may not be appropriate for some women with certain cancer-tumor sensitivities; however, the benefits to those with familial risks of certain cancers in terms of cancer prevention may be improved with the macrobiotic diet (Kushi et al., 2001).

Some studies have also examined concerns about developmental problems related to cobalamin (vitamin B) deficiency in adolescents who have eaten a macrobiotic diet since early childhood. Although some studies have found no correlation, the findings of one study indicate that the adverse effects of cobalamin deficiency in the macrobiotic community may not be restricted to just early childhood: It may also cause symptoms related to impaired cobalamin status in later life, such as neurological and psychiatric disease, even after the person eats dairy and some meat for some time (van Dusseldorp et al., 1999).

PROFESSIONAL NOTES

The scope of practice of registered nursing includes nutrition interventions. The Earth element of integrative holistic nursing care includes the energetics of foods in assessment, diagnosis, inter-vention, and evaluation. Nurses interested in basic energetics can incorporate theories, such as the Eight Principle Patterns, with nursing theory (Libster, 2012; Libster, 2022). Although there are dieticians and nutritionists, including some who are involved in integrative and functional medicine, whose focus is the holistic nutrition needs of clients, their approach is often reductionistic. Their focus, as is demonstrated in the *U.S. Dietary Guidelines 2015-2020* (see the Resources section), is to measure intake of specific constituents, such as vitamin C. Their worldview includes exchange lists and measurement of food intake. An energetics first approach is person-centered precision nursing science.

Nurses who wish to include an energetics first approach start by studying the energetics of foods beginning with the *Yellow Emperor's Classic of Medicine* and taking continuing education courses on nutrition intervention from functional medicine to macrobiotics and Chinese diet therapy. Refer to your state's Board of Nursing website and the *Nurse Practice Act* for further details about the nurses' role in nurturing patients with nutrition interventions.

Eight Principle Patterns demonstrate the relationship of seemingly opposing patterns or energies. The symbol of the yin-yang (see Figure 12-2) depicts the circular nature of the relationship between yin and yang. It suggests that the energy of yin becomes yang and yang becomes yin. For example, salt (which is warm and therefore yang) when ingested by a person in large amounts, can cause a person to retain water (which is yin). Yang *becomes* yin.

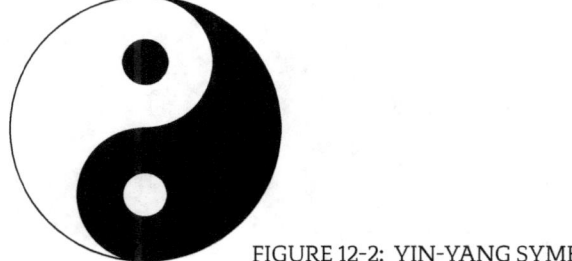

FIGURE 12-2: YIN-YANG SYMBOL

The foods consumed by those on the macrobiotic diet consist primarily of cereal grains. The sages who wrote the *Upanishads*, ancient spiritual treatises written in Sanskrit between 800 and 400 B.C., translated to mean "sitting at the feet of a master" (Mascaró, 1965, p. 7), wrote that grain represented the Creator (Ohsawa, 1965, p. 32). In many cultures, rice is considered sacred and used as food and as medicine. Early on in the history of Ohsawa's Zen macrobiotics, the American Medical Association condemned the diet based on a mistaken perception that the diet promoted the achievement of a 100% grain-only diet (Kushi et al., 2001). This is not the case. Vegetables are equally important. Flesh from wild birds, fish, and shellfish are preferable. In addition, all preservatives, chemical additives, industrialized foods and drinks, and coffee are prohibited for those eating the macrobiotic way. Bancha (toasted green tea) tea is preferable. People are encouraged to drink less in general so as to place less stress on the kidneys (Ohsawa, 1965, p. 29), so that a woman typically urinates twice and a man three times in a 24-hour period. Chewing each bite of food at least 50 times is also a foundational part of the macrobiotic diet culture to place less stress on the digestive organs.

Macrobiotics Research

A search of the published scientific literature suggests that there has been little to no clinical research published on the macrobiotic diet as a whole nutritional intervention program since its development in the 1920s. However, many people can attest to its health benefits. The diet continues as one of the most popular therapeutic diets in America (National Center for Complementary and Integrative Health, 2022). Much of the research on the macrobiotic diet has focused on examining the constituents of the foods recommended in the diet. These studies

HOLISTIC TRANSFORMATION

- *Reflect on your personal experience with the Earth element and your relationship to the five tastes of foods.*

- *How does your family's cultural food traditions influence your health?*

SUMMARY

Nutrition interventions (such as the preparation of strengthening broths) have been a foundational part of nursing practice and sickroom diet for centuries. Porridge or congee is an easily digestible healing food that supports spleen and stomach energy and is used especially for the young, older adults, and the infirm recuperating from illness. Traditional Chinese diet therapy and the macrobiotic diet are examples of nutrition interventions that are based on the energetics of foods. Although little clinical trial evidence supports the use of the macrobiotic diet, there are decades of studies conducted on the constituents of the foods or lack thereof (such as B vitamins) and anecdotal support for the use of this diet in people with cancer and inflammation.

RESOURCES

Centers for Disease Control and Prevention (CDC). Nutrition.
https://www.cdc.gov/nutrition

U. S. Department of Agriculture. Choose My Plate.
http://www.choosemyplate.gov

U.S. Department of Agriculture (USDA) – Food and Nutrition Information Center
https://www.nal.usda.gov/fnic/diet-and-health-0

U.S. Department of Health and Human Services & U.S. Department of Agriculture. 2015-2020 Guidelines–"Diet, Nutrition & Eating Right"
http://www.health.gov/DietaryGuidelines

U. S. Food and Drug Administration (FDA) – Food.
https://www.fda.gov/Food/default.htm

Kushi Institute. What is macrobiotic diet?
https://www.kushiinstitute.orwhat-is-macrobiotics/

Kushi, Michio. Spirals of everlasting change. [YouTube video].
https://www.youtube.com/watch?v=71swvmrZ8dQ

REFERENCES

"Bone Broth." (2015, September). *Harvard Women's Health Watch*. Retrieved from https://www.health.harvard.edu/nutrition/whats-the-scoop-on-bone-soup

Flaws, B. (1995). *The book of jook: A healthy alternative to the typical Western breakfast.* Boulder, CO: Blue Poppy Press.

Flaws, B. (2013). *The Tao of healthy eating: Dietary wisdom according to Chinese medicine*. Boulder, CO: Blue Poppy Press.

Frawley, D., & Lad, V. (2010). *The yoga of herbs: An Ayurvedic guide to herbal medicine.* Twin Lakes, WI: Lotus Press.

Harmon, B. E., Carter, M., Hurley, T. G., Shivappa, N., Teas, J., & Hébert, J. R. (2015). Nutrient composition and anti-inflammatory potential of a prescribed macrobiotic diet. *Nutrition and Cancer, 67*(6), 933-940.

Kushi, L. H., Cunningham, J. E., & Teas, J. (2001). The macrobiotic diet in cancer. Journal of *Nutrition, 131*(11 Suppl), 3056S-3064S.

Libster, M. M. (2004). *Herbal diplomats: The contribution of early American nurses (1830-1860) to nineteenth-century health care reform and the Botanical Medical Movement.* Wauwatosa, WI: Golden Apple Publications.

Libster, M. M. (2012). *The nurse-herbalist: Integrative insights for holistic practice.* Wauwatosa, WI: Golden Apple Publications.

Libster, M. M. (2022). The Tao of Integrative Nursing Assessment (TINA) An East-West Model for Precision, Complementarity, and Inclusion in Relationship-Centered Care. *Holistic Nursing Practice* (In press).

Libster, M., & McNeil, B. A. (2009). *Enlightened charity: The holistic nursing care, education and "Advices Concerning the Sick" of Sister Matilda Coskery* (1799-1870). Wauwatosa, WI: Golden Apple Publications.

Mascaró, J. (1965). *The Upanishads*. New York, NY: Penguin Books.

National Center for Complementary and Integrative Health. (2022). Statistics on Complementary and Integrative Health Approaches. Retrieved from https://nccih.nih.gov/research/statistics/2007/camsurvey_fs1.htm#therapy

Ni, M. (2011). *The yellow emperor's classic of medicine.* Boston, MA: Shambhala.

Ohsawa, G. (1965). *Zen macrobiotics: The art of rejuvenation and longevity (The philosophy of oriental medicine, Vol. 1)*. Los Angeles, CA: Ohsawa Foundation.

Pitchford, P. (2002). *Healing with whole foods: Asian traditions and modern nutrition.* Berkeley, CA: North Atlantic Books.

Shewry, P. R., & Hey, S. J. (2016). Do we need to worry about eating wheat? *Nutrition Bulletin, 41*(1), 6-13.

van Dusseldorp, M., Schneede, J., Refsum, H., Ueland, P. M., Thomas, C. M. G., de Boer, E., & van Staveren, W. A. (1999). Risk of persistent cobalamin deficiency in adolescents fed a macrobiotic diet in early life. *American Journal of Clinical Nutrition, 69*(4), 664-671.

Wicke, R. W. (1992). *Clinical handbook of herbal medicine: Vol. 1.* Hot Springs, MT: Rocky Mountain Herbal Institute.

World Health Organization (WHO, 2021). Obesity and overweight. Retrieved from http://www.who.int/mediacentre/factsheets/fs311/en/

Zhou, J. (2009). New understanding of the basic theory of traditional Chinese medicine. *Chinese Journal of Integrative Medicine, 15*(1), 7-12.

CHAPTER 13

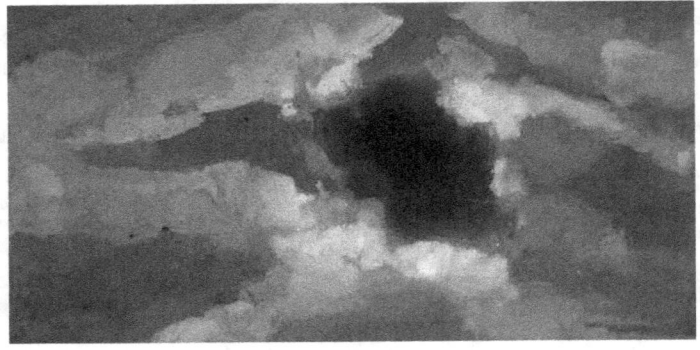

Study Of Clouds, Nicholas Roerich, 1936 - 1942
Courtesy, Nicholas Roerich Museum, New York, NY

ETHER ELEMENT: HERBAL INTERVENTIONS

LEARNING OUTCOME

After completing this chapter, the learner will be able to describe herbal interventions used in integrative holistic nursing practice.

CHAPTER OBJECTIVES

After completing this chapter, the learner will be able to:
1. Describe approaches to nurse-herbalism.
2. Explain the regulation of herbal dietary supplements.
3. Cite at least one oral, topical, and environmental herbal intervention.
4. Summarize nursing responsibilities associated with herbal interventions.

INTRODUCTION

The Ether element is perhaps the most elusive of the five elements. The term *ether*, as it is used in this final chapter, should not be confused with the substance used as an anesthetic agent. Ether, the element defined in ancient texts as "infinite substance," (Blavatsky, 1888, p. 671), is also defined as "quintessence" (Hauck, 1999), or that which binds together the other four elements. The quintessence of the Elements of Care® is that which binds together and encompasses all of the elements of integrative holistic nursing care. The example of Ether intervention that is the focus for this chapter is nurse-herbalism. The examples given in the practice section will show how nurse-herbalism incorporates all five elements.

Herbalism, or partnering with plants in care and comfort, is essential nursing practice. It has more recently been defined in nursing as a "complementary therapy" to biomedical care and may be used by holistic nurses as such (American Holistic Nurses Association & American Nurses Association, 2018). However, research demonstrates that nurses have helped the public use herbal remedies in safe and effective self-care and in the comfort and care of others for centuries (Libster, 2004). Nurses who partner with plants in care and comfort follow a tradition of an integrative holistic repertoire of interventions rooted in centuries of scientific experimentation, creative caring practice development, and recorded demonstrations of the spirit and essence of nursing as a call to healing. "Herbal remedies – like touch, compassionate communication, diet therapies, and creating a healing environment – are essential elements of nursing and midwifery care" (Libster, 2012, p. 1). They are a part of health systems in developed, technologically focused countries as well as in developing nations. Nurse-herbalism practiced according to the energetics first Elements of Care® approach is precision nursing science.

According to the last global survey by the World Health Organization and published by Farnsworth, Akerele, Bingel, Soejarto, & Guo in 1985 on the subject, 80% of the world's population continues to use their traditional methods of healing, including the use of medicinal plants and traditional medicines that are the "mainstay of health care" across the world (WHO, 2014. This chapter advances the registered and advanced practice registered nurse's (APRNs) knowledge of nurses' historical leadership in the precision science and art of nurse-herbalism.

As a healing modality, herbal interventions have been shown through scientific study and hundreds of years of traditional use to be quite safe. According to Dr. Norman Farnsworth (1930 to 2011), a renowned pharmacognosist, researcher, and global health expert on herb safety, "Based on published reports, side effects or toxic reactions associated with herbal medicines in any form are rare" (1993, pp. 36C-36D). That safety is related, however, to the type of medicinal plant and the part used, the application of the plant, and the knowledge base of the user. There are *potential* risks associated with using any plant as food or medicine. People die each year from ingesting common foods, such as ordinary nuts, for example. Pre-licensure nursing programs typically focus on the risks associated with ingesting herbal dietary *supplements*. The examples of nurse-herbalism interventions provided in this chapter reflect nursing's safe history of knowledgeable application of whole herbs in comfort and care. In addition to the examples of whole-plant oral, topical, and environmental interventions and research, this chapter includes a brief introduction to herbal dietary supplements and their regulation in the United States.

BACKGROUND

Today's pharmaceutical drugs have their "roots" in the early production of herbal remedies now referred to as "dietary supplements." It is the herbal medicine production and international herb company of the early Shaker nurses and their community brothers and sisters that in the 19th century laid the foundation for what ultimately became the American pharmaceutical industry (Libster, 2004). The Shaker nurses made and marketed herbal pills, syrups, tinctures, teas, and floral waters (Libster, 2004). They tested their remedies in their community infirmaries while caring for patients and documented their efficacy. Knowledge of safe practice was passed from nurse to nurse through receipt (or recipe) books, infirmary records, and oral reports. Today, the American Holistic Nurses Association's *Holistic Nursing: Scope and Standards of Practice* (American Holistic Nurses Association, 2018) clearly delineates a role for nurses and APRNs in counseling and coaching patients in their choices of dietary supplements, such as herbal remedies.

Approaches to Nurse-Herbalism

Although many nurses realize the importance of integrating their biomedical knowledge of health care with healing traditions, actually integrating the two, such as applying herbal remedies with conventional high tech nursing care, can be challenging. Integrative holistic nursing is the creation of evolving, collaborative healing relationships with patients (Libster, 2001) that respect personal and sociocultural differences. Nurses and APRNs take numerous approaches in demonstrating best practice with herbal remedies:

1. Respect the patient: Identify and demonstrate respect for the patient's cultural beliefs and practices related to medicinal plants. Listen and ask clarifying questions to best understand what, if any, help the patient needs in decision making regarding herbal remedies.
2. Provide information, resources, and referral: Patients may require information and resources about herbal remedies. Nurses can educate and inform patients about herbs without having the knowledge to provide nurse-herbalist assessment and care. First, identify what plant or plant constituent the patient is asking about. Second, ask about the application the patient is considering, such as a supplement (tablet, capsule, or standardized extract) or traditional application, such as a liniment or compress. Use the medical, nursing, pharmacy, and botanical science literature to answer questions. Consumers may request assistance in evaluating the literature and making appropriate choices with regard to the uses, dosing, adverse effects, interactions, and product quality of these supplements. Nurses are accessible to their communities and, when knowledgeable about herbal supplements, can assist patients in the appropriate use of these products to achieve better health. Common medicinal plants typically have multiple uses. Nurses can incorporate several forms of evidence in the care of patients considering the use of herbal remedies and supplements in self-care and nursing care: traditional and indigenous

knowledge, patient experience, and qualitative and quantitative research studies, including clinical trials. Nurses can also make referrals to knowledgeable herbal practitioners (Libster, 1999).

3. Use a "simples" focus: This approach is similar to the previous one, except that the nurse has studied the medicinal plants in question and may recommend "simples," or single-herb interventions, to the patient, such as the centuries-old nursing remedy of a hops *(Humulus lupulus)* poultice for pain (Coskery, 1840, as cited in Libster & McNeil, 2009; Harmer, 1924; Libster, 2012).

4. Use a nurse-herbalism focus: Nurses are educated in the practice of nurse-herbalism with its associated assessment strategies, scientific theories, herbal formulations, benefits and risks, and plans of care (Libster, 2012).

Herbs Versus Drugs

Herbal remedies include teas, liquid extracts, poultices, syrups, soups, juices, compresses, baths, and steams. A more modern use of plant medicines is in the form of a standardized extract, a plant preparation typically in capsule or tablet in which the active constituent has been standardized or made uniform from individual product to individual product. This method is seen as beneficial by those practitioners who work within a biomedical worldview because the belief is that the active constituents in a plant can be identified, extracted, purified, and standardized. This approach makes the remedy more like a pharmaceutical drug and thereby easier to dose than any other plant preparation. A plant remedy being standardized means that the practitioner can discuss a specific dose of a "known" active constituent. The benefit is that the constituent is in a "natural" form compared with synthetic drugs. Many practitioners and patients prefer drugs that are from a natural source and therefore prefer herbal supplements that are standardized extracts.

The ability to produce a standardized herbal medicine rests on the ability of researchers to identify the active constituent of a plant. In some plants, such as senna *(Cassia senna L.)*, a plant that has been traditionally used for constipation, an active constituent has been identified. In senna, the active constituents that seem to have a bowel irritant or stimulant effect are identified as *sennosides*. Standardization of sennosides means, for the consumer, that taking a certain amount of herbal product should have a laxative effect. Because the sennosides are identifiable, they can be researched in much the same way a pharmaceutical drug would be. However, sennosides are a plant constituent, not the whole plant. The history of relatively safe use of senna has to do with the traditional use of the whole leaf, not the constituent sennosides. Identifying a single active constituent as the "mechanism of action" in a single plant, such as the commonly used herb Echinacea, has not been feasible in many cases. Herbs, unlike pharmaceutical drugs with known mechanisms of action related to a single constituent, contain hundreds of constituents. The mechanism of action could be assigned to any number of those constituents, and often the constituents have opposing actions – further complicating our understanding of how a plant actually exerts its effect.

Herb Safety

Nurses have a social mandate to provide the best care possible, and there are many reasons for including medicinal plants in that care. Herbs are accessible; people can even grow their own medicine in window boxes in apartments and backyard gardens. Herbs, such as dried plants used in teas, are much less expensive than pharmaceutical drugs, although standardized extracts (supplements) can be as expensive as some drugs. Whole-herb applications also have a history of few to no adverse effects when used according to tradition.

One reason for the long history of safe use of herbal remedies is that plants are made up of hundreds of different biochemical constituents. When herbs are used in whole form, whether decocted as tea or used as an extract or salve, the action of whole-plant therapies is complex when looking at them through a reductionist lens. The chemical constituents in plants occur in very small amounts. Herbs, although they have healing properties and the ability to create change and even chemical reactions in the body, are not pharmaceutical drugs typically produced from one substance. They are much more complex. When people ingest, apply, or inhale herbs, they are taking in very small "doses" of particular substances that are in a natural, not synthetic, state and are in formulation, so to speak, as they occur in nature.

The historical safe use of whole plants is related to the use of the plant in its complex natural state. However, when people decide to use a standardized extract of a single constituent of an herb (much like a drug) or use an herb in a form that departs from traditional use, the historical safety record is no longer applicable. For example, if the safety record of traditional medicinal use of garlic is related to eating the fresh, chopped bulb in food or as an infused oil, new safety data will have to be collected for the use of powdered garlic tablets taken as a medication every day for hypertension. Whereas safety information related to traditional use of herbs is shared through oral tradition – where/when to harvest, how to gather and prepare and apply, how much to take and when, and so on – biomedical use of herbs compels research and further gathering of population safety information about new forms of herbal remedies and applications. When herbs are used in the treatment of biomedically defined diseases, the same safety standards are followed as are used with drugs.

In a similar manner as when they use drugs, people experience a wide range of biological responses to herbs. For example, factors that influence individual expression of the cytochrome P450 system, the pathway in the liver where drug metabolism occurs, include gender, age, race, genetics, and hepatic condition. Research on the mechanism of action of certain medicinal plants may discuss metabolic pathways, such as cytochrome P450. The challenge is that plants comprise hundreds of constituents with seemingly conflicting actions. St. John's wort may induce the cytochrome P450 system (inducing cytochrome P450 3A4 in hepatocyte cells), but it also contains the bioflavonoid quercetin, which is a cytochrome P450 3A4 inhibitor (J. Duke, personal communication, April 2001). This juxtaposition occurs in the body when both inhibitors and inducers are present in the same herb.

As medicinal plants are being studied further, there is consideration that because of their complexity, it may be possible that there are no clinical sequelae all when taking certain herbs with certain drugs in combination or formulation. In Asia, drugs and herbs are knowledgably combined in formulation as a means of increasing the benefits of both. Studies are being conducted on the "entourage effects" within certain plants that suggest that complex whole-plant preparation may be a "better drug"; that is, a more safe and effective substance than the single-constituent natural products isolated from them (Russo, 2011, p. 1345).

Herbs as Dietary Supplements

The National Health Interview Survey (NHIS) is a nationally representative, cross-sectional household interview survey conducted by the Centers for Disease Control and Prevention's National Center for Health Statistics. It provides estimates of the health of the U.S. population. According to the 2012 NHIS, the most commonly used complementary therapy (in 17.7% of adults and 4.9% of children) was the use of dietary supplements other than vitamin/mineral supplements, primarily herbs (Black, Clarke, Barnes, Stussman, & Nahin, 2015; Clarke, Black, Stussman, Barnes, & Nahin, 2015).

The U.S. Congress passed the Dietary Supplement Health and Education Act (DSHEA) in 1994. The primary purpose of this act was to reclassify vitamins, minerals, and herbs as dietary supplements. This reclassification reduced the amount of control the U.S. Food and Drug Administration (FDA) has on monitoring and regulating the use of these products by the public. As a result, the FDA must prove that an herbal preparation is unsafe before the product can be forced off the market. This regulation, which no longer subjects herbs to the strict safety standards of conventional pharmaceutical (single-constituent) drugs, has made it possible for people other than herbalists, pharmacists, and physicians to be involved with the sale and recommendation of herbal therapies and preparations.

When advertising herbs in their whole form (bulk herbs) or as dietary supplements, manufacturers and sellers are allowed to make three types of claims without clinical trial data as evidence: health claims, structure/function claims, and nutrient content claims. These claims can link culinary (food) or medicinal herbs to a disease or health-related conditions and discuss the product's potential health benefits. Claims about a product's efficacy must have supportive data, which often comes from its history of safe and effective traditional use. Although some medical herbs can be eaten, they are traditionally extracted, decocted, infused, or applied rather than ingested as a whole plant ground up in a capsule. Historical evidence provides background data for evaluating the soundness of the use of supplements as well as oral, topical, and environmental traditional remedies. Labels that cite claims about how an herbal dietary supplement affects the structure or function of the body must be followed by the words, "This statement has not been evaluated by the U.S. Food and Drug Administration (FDA). This product is not intended to diagnose, treat, cure, or prevent any disease" (FDA, 2018).

Until the 1950s, the FDA had regulated herbs as drugs, and most drugs used in conventional medicine originate from herbs. For example, the drug digitalis (cardiac glycosides), made from the foxglove plant, is used to treat congestive heart failure, and the drug aspirin, which derives from willow bark, is well known for its analgesic, anti-inflammatory, antipyretic, and anticoagulant-antiplatelet properties. These drugs go through the full process of FDA review and approval.

HERBAL INTERVENTIONS IN PRACTICE

The focus of nurse-herbalism is the application of plant-based remedies in comfort and care. The medicinal constituents of plants and plant parts (Earth element) are mindfully (Air element) extracted through water (Water element) and heat (Fire element) and applied orally (tea, extract, syrup, soup) or topically (compress, poultice, salve, liniment) or through the environment, such as in a steam or inhalation (Air element). The nurse assesses the patient's health pattern and chooses herbal applications according to the energetics of the Elements of Care® and eight principle patterns that will promote greater balance in body and peace of mind. A basic example of this is from first aid. When a person has an acute injury with swelling and heat (inflammation), the nurse routinely chooses to recommend a cold application to ease the heat and contract the swollen area. Using knowledge of energetics, ice packs are used to create balance in body. The same energetics first approach is used in precision nurse-herbalism. The following are examples.

Oral Intervention: Tea

Teas, also called tisanes, are water extractions of herbs. Fresh or dried plant material can be used for a tea. For 1 cup of tea with dried plant, use 1 teaspoon (3 to 5 g). For fresh herb teas, use 3 teaspoons (9 to 15 g). More plant is used for fresh herb teas because of the water content in the fresh herbs. There are two types of basic preparation: an infusion and a decoction. *Infusion* is used with delicate plant parts, such as flowers and leaves. The procedure for an infusion is to place the herb into a cup or small pot with a lid. Pour 1 cup (240 mL) of boiled water over the herb and cover and steep (let it sit) for 3 to 5 minutes, depending on the type of herb used. The decoction method is used for hard plant materials such as barks (i.e., cinnamon) or roots (i.e., burdock). For *decoction*, use 1 ounce (30 g) of dried herb per 3 cups (750 mL) of water. Cover the pot and bring the water to a boil. Turn off the heat and let the decoction stand for at least 4 hours or overnight. (Skip this step if using fresh roots or barks.) After the presoak, simmer the herbs for 20 to 30 minutes (do not bring to a rolling boil), and strain.

Peppermint (*Mentha piperita*) is a common culinary herb that is also used as a medicinal tea. In the Chinese *Materia Medica* (i.e., herbal formulary), peppermint is classified as "cool herb that releases the exterior wind heat" (Bensky & Gamble, 1993). This classification is translated to biomedical conditions such as heat or fever (particularly in the head), red eyes, and headache. Peppermint tea clears the heat in the head. This action is so well known and common that there are typically no clinical trials seeking to "prove" its action. Conducting clinical trials on traditional teas, which would cost millions of dollars, may not be considered the best use of tax dollars when, as is emphasized by the World Health Organization Traditional Medicine Collaborating Centers (2014), there are hundreds of years of traditional evidence for their safe and effective use.

However, studies are conducted and published on the home remedies, also referred to as "folk remedies," "domestic medicines," and "self-care," for which common culinary and medicinal herbs are used (Arcury, Preisser, Gesler, & Sherman, 2004). One review of the medical literature found that peppermint tea was extremely common and effective in relieving pain in those diagnosed with tension and migraine headache (Malone & Tsai, 2018).

Topical Intervention: Compress

A compress is a quintessential nursing intervention. A compress, also referred to as a "stupe" or "fomentation," particularly when used with larger parts of the body, is a folded piece of material applied moist to the body. Herbal compresses are hydrotherapy plus herbal intervention: a cloth soaked in an herbal infusion or decoction. Compresses differ from poultices in that a poultice cloth holds a slurry of softened herbs or plant paste. The compress is dipped in a strained infusion or decoction and applied either cold or warm. When applied cold, the compress is turned or replaced when it becomes warm from absorbing the heat of the body. When applied warm, the compress is replaced with another hot compress. The new compress is placed on top of the old compress and then flipped over so as to avoid exposure of the skin to the air. The cooled compress is removed and resoaked in the herbal infusion or decoction.

One example is a witch hazel (*Hamamelis virginiana*) distillate cool compress applied externally to puffy eyes or to the swollen perineum of a women who has given birth. Topical applications of herbs, such as those in compresses, are excellent topics for nursing research. Ginger (*Zingiber officinale*) compresses, for example, have been the focus of several nursing studies including action research, phenomenology, and randomized controlled trial (Libster, 2008; Therkleson, 2010, 2014). To make a ginger compress, grate 4 ounces of fresh gingerroot and place it in a small cloth bag in 1 gallon of simmering hot water. Allow the ginger to steep, but not boil, for 5 minutes. Dip the central portion of a small hand towel into the ginger decoction while holding both ends. Remove it from the decoction and then wring out the towel. Be careful when touching the compress to the body so as to apply it as hot as is tolerable without harming the skin. Gingerroot moves qi and blood stagnation and is anti-inflammatory. Ginger compresses are often applied to the back over the kidneys area or on joints. They should not be used on the abdomen of a pregnant woman or used on infants or older adults whose peripheral circulation is impaired. They should also not be used when fever is present (too hot).

Environmental Intervention: Herbal Baths

Hippocrates, a founding father of modern medicine, is commonly cited as saying that a daily aromatic bath and scented massage were keys to good health. Herbal full-body baths, sitz baths, and footbaths can be used in the care of patients. As discussed in Chapter 9, water and baths have their own healing properties. The combination of hydrotherapy and herbal intervention can effect powerful change and healing.

Baths utilize the infusions and decoctions of whole fresh or dried plants or plant parts. The infusion or decoction is strained when it is the right strength, as may be measured by smell, color, and taste, and then poured into the bath. Some herb companies make prepared herbal bath oils from single herbs or a formula of herbs. These herbs are concentrated and are used according to the recommendations on the label.

One example of integrative holistic herbal bath intervention is in the care of postpartum women. Herbal sitz baths are used to heal swollen and torn tissues as well as hemorrhoids related to pregnancy and labor. Herbs commonly infused for sitz baths are nettles (Urtica dioica), yarrow (*Achillea millefolium*), and chamomile (*Matricaria recutita*). Herbal teas and sitz baths are included in the services of traditional birth attendants (TBAs) and nurses around the world. For example, one study of Guatemalan TBAs and nurses was conducted with 39 local experts in the field of maternal-child health. The nurses were included in the study because of their knowledge of both traditional birth practices and nursing. The biggest contribution of traditional herbalism in postpartum care is the promotion of postpartum uterine involution using the *chuj*, or traditional wood-fired Mayan sauna-bath, and herbal baths and teas. The sauna-bath is used on a weekly basis to "normalise, heal, and warm the uterus. The concept of 'warming' the uterus is based on their cultural belief of 'hot-cold balance" (Radoff, Thompson, Bly, & Romero, 2013, p. 228).

Spanish-speaking (Ladina) women do not use the chuj, but they use a bath containing herbs to expel clots from the uterus after birth. Herbs are also used to prepare a woman's breast milk. Example of herbs that are used to warm the uterus are marjoram, chicajol (snakeroot – *Ageratina ligustriana*), chilca (Barkley's ragwort – *Senecio salignus*), and apple and peach leaf (Radoff et. al, 2013).

PROFESSIONAL NOTES

As with all nursing interventions, nurses and APRNs are minimally required by state statute to have knowledge of and training in any modality or practice that they engage in, and they must also follow any practice guidelines for the application of herbal interventions set down by an employer for whom they might work. Some states may have other requirements for the recommendation of herbal dietary supplements. According to safe practice in traditional nurse-herbalism, it is also customary for a nurse to be properly "introduced" to each plant that she or he is planning to partner with in practice before doing so. Simply reading about a plant is not sufficient. Experience of the plant is essential for knowledge of the plant's medicinal properties and safety issues.

Because nurses are public servants with access to large numbers of people, they have the additional responsibility of protecting plant populations, particularly wild plant populations from overharvesting should they plan to teach the benefits of an herb. For example, the root of a cultivated Echinacea plant (*Echinacea spp.*) can take 5 to 10 years to mature for harvest and production. In the past, when nurses and other trusted health professionals have advised Americans to take Echinacea for the common cold, the demand for Echinacea increased and the supply of the root dropped quickly. This result may have led to some Echinacea supplement products being adulterated with the root of a similar but different plant called *Parthenium integrifolium* (Foster & Tyler, 1999). Part of the problem was that people were overusing the herb. They were taking the root as a daily regimen when its immune stimulating action is best used sporadically or as needed. In addition, they were taking the root in capsules, when the root should be tasted rather than ingested encapsulated because it is known that Echinacea's immune system response begins with the stimulation of lymphatic tissue in the mouth (Foster & Tyler, 1999).

HOLISTIC TRANSFORMATION

- *Reflect on your personal experience with the Ether element and your relationship to the plant world.*

- *What are some of your family's cultural traditions that include green plants, flowers, trees, herbs, and grasses?*

SUMMARY

Herbal interventions have been part of nursing care for centuries. Herbs are used as food and medicine. People around the world continue to partner with plants in self-care and healing traditions. Nurses apply them orally as in teas, soups, and syrups, topically as in compresses, poultices and salves, and environmentally as in baths and steams. Herbs are regulated as dietary supplements by the federal government. Like drugs, herbs can be classified according to their physiological effects on the body. However, manufacturers of herbal dietary supplements cannot claim that an herb has medicinal properties unless the herb undergoes a rigorous FDA approval process. In addition, manufacturers must ensure that the labels are not misleading to consumers. Nurses conduct research, teach, and coach their patients about health choices involving the applications of culinary and medicinal plants. Like touch, compassionate communication, diet therapies, and creating a healing environment, nurse-herbalism is essential nursing care and is a prime example of a way that nurses can integrate the Elements of Care® including the elusive ether element in the practice of person-centered, precision nursing science.

RESOURCES

American Botanical Council
   http://www.herbalgram.org

American Herbal Products Association
   http://www.ahpa.org

Herb Research Foundation
   http://www.herbs.orherbnews/

National Institutes of Health (NIH), U.S. National Library of Medicine, Medline Plus.
   Herbal medicine.
   http://www.nlm.nih.gov/medlineplus/herbalmedicine.html#cat57

Natural Medicines Comprehensive Database
   https://naturalmedicines.therapeuticresearch.com

The Nurse-Herbalist Institute
   https://www.goldenapplehealingarts.com/nurse-herbalist-institute

United Plant Savers
   https://unitedplantsavers.org

REFERENCES

Arcury, T. A., Preisser, J. S., Gesler, W. M., & Sherman, J. E. (2004). Complementary and alternative medicine use among rural residents in western North Carolina. *Complementary Health Practice Review*, 9(2), 93-102.

American Holistic Nurses Association. (2018). *Holistic nursing: Scope and standards of practice* (3rd ed.). Silver Spring, MD: American Nurses Association Press.

Bensky, D., & Gamble, A. (Comp. & Trans.). (1993). *Chinese herbal medicine: Materia medica – Volume I* (Rev. ed.). Seattle, WA: Eastland Press.

Black, L. I., Clarke, T. C., Barnes, P. M., Stussman, B. J., & Nahin, R. L. (2015). Use of complementary health approaches among children aged 4-17 years in the United States. *National Health Statistics Reports*, 78, 1-19.

Blavatsky, H. (1888). *The secret doctrine: The synthesis of science, religion, and philosophy.* London, England: The Theosophical Publishing Company.

Clarke, T. C., Black, L. I., Stussman, B. J., Barnes, P. M., & Nahin, R. L. (2015). Trends in the use of complementary health approaches among adults: United States, 2002-2012. *National Health Statistics Reports, 79,* 1-16.

Farnsworth, N. R. (1993). Relative safety of herbal medicines. *HerbalGram*, 29, 36A-H.

Farnsworth, N. R., Akerele, O., Bingel, A. S., Soejarto, D. D., & Guo, Z. (1985). Medicinal plants in therapy. *Bulletin of the World Health Organization, 63*(6), 965-981.

Foster, S., & Tyler, V. E. (1999). *Tyler's honest herbal: A sensible guide to the use of herbs and related remedies* (4th ed.). Binghamton, NY: Haworth Herbal Press.

Harmer, B. (1924). *Text-book of the principles and practice of nursing.* New York, NY: MacMillan.

Hauck, D. W. (1999). *The emerald tablet: Alchemy for personal transformation.* New York, NY: Penguin Putnam.

Libster, M. (1999). Guidelines for selecting a medical herbalist for consultation and referral: Consulting a medical herbalist. *Journal of Alternative and Complementary Medicine, 5*(5), 457-462.

Libster, M. (2001). *Demonstrating care: The art of integrative nursing.* Albany, NY: Delmar Cengage Learning.

Libster, M. (2004). *Herbal diplomats: The contribution of early American nurses (1830-1860) to 19th century health care reform and the Botanical Medical Movement.* Wauwatosa, WI: Golden Apple Publications.

Libster, M. (2008). Documentary. "Healing Journeys." Teaching herbal medicine making and healing traditions to health science students at Northside High School. https://www.goldenapplehealingarts.com/free-resources

Libster, M. (2012). *The nurse-herbalist: Integrative insights for holistic practice.* Wauwatosa, WI: Golden Apple Publications.

Libster, M., & McNeil, B. A. (2009). *Enlightened charity: The holistic care, education and "Advices Concerning the Sick" of Sister Matilda Coskery (1799-1870)*. Wauwatosa, WI: Golden Apple Publications.

Malone, M., & Tsai, G. (2018). The evidence for herbal and botanical remedies, Part 1. *Journal of Family Practice*, 67(1), 10-16.

Radoff, K. A., Thompson, L. M., Bly, K. C., & Romero, C. (2013). Practices related to postpartum uterine involution in the Western Highlands of Guatemala. *Midwifery, 29*(3), 225-232.

Russo, E. B. (2011). Taming THC: Potential cannabis synergy and phytocannabinoid-terpenoid entourage effects. *British Journal of Pharmacology, 163*(7), 1344-1364.

Therkleson, T. (2010). Ginger compress therapy for adults with osteoarthritis. *Journal of Advanced Nursing, 66*(10), 2225-2233.

Therkleson, T. (2014). Topical ginger treatment with a compress or patch for osteoarthritis symptoms. *Journal of Holistic Nursing, 32*(3), 173-182.

U. S. Food and Drug Administration. (2018). *Structure/function claims.* Retrieved from https://www.fda.gov/Food/LabelingNutrition/ucm2006881.htm

World Health Organization. (2014). *WHO Traditional medicine strategy: 2014-2023*. Geneva, Switzerland: World Health Organization.

CONCLUSION

Nursing and nurses exist to care and comfort others. The integrative holistic nursing approach prepares nurses to provide diplomatic care to the people who are actively engaged in their culture's healing heritage. Integrative holistic nurses initiate the nursing process with an assessment and modeling the unique *energetic health patterns* and needs of an individual, family, or community. The nursing process is then used in role-modeling, that is designing and providing nursing care that integrates modalities, which are precisely matched to address those identified needs that consider energetic patterns first.

Integration of the five elements in creating healing environments of care and comfort within and without is foundational to the application of the science of energetics in nursing practice. For centuries, the five Elements of Care® – ether, fire, air, water, and earth – have provided a structural focus for sickroom management, creating healing environments, and the holistic care of patients. When in balance, the five elements are considered a full measure of health. Integrative holistic nursing care and comfort that includes the actual presence or representation of the five elements during the nursing process is energetic science. The patient's underlying energetic pattern is the foundation for precision nursing science.

The goal of *precision* integrative holistic nursing is to provide care that addresses the unique energetic needs for healing the whole person and promoting health. That care includes engaging in touch, energy flow, and communication, providing counsel in diet and nutrition, and creating healing environments within and without. An integrative holistic nursing approach is the ethical and clinical foundation for precision nursing science that applies the five Elements of Care® in the design of person-centered relationship-centered care and healing environments.

Nurses are often the most accessible professional supporters for many individuals' life transitions resulting from personal, family, and community change. Integrative holistic nursing addresses healing crises and illnesses that are evolutionary in that they are a period of change, transition, and transformation for the patient. Integrative holistic nursing skills that are used in supporting people in transition employ nursing scientific theory and follow the nursing process informed by the five Elements of Care® to assist the patient in the meaningful re-creation of internal and external environments. It is the consultation with the five elements of nature within each person and permeating the environment without that has been the foundation of the healing arts and nursing for centuries.

NEXT STEPS

This text, *Precision Nursing Science*, has detailed the elements of integrative holistic nursing care philosophy and practice and described how advanced practice and registered nurses demonstrate precision nursing science utilizing the Elements of Care®. The following are suggested resources for those who would like to continue to learn and engage with a community of nurses, who also are furthering the energetics first philosophy of precision nursing science.

Join the Self-care and Nurse-Herbalist Institutes at
www.GoldenAppleHealingArts.com

Dr. Martha's educational programs:
Certified Nurse-Herbalist
Certified Science of Energy Flow® Foot Reflexology
Elements of Care® Certification Program

Books by Dr. Martha
www.GoldenAppleHealingArts.com/store

Follow Dr. Martha:
www.DrMarthaLibster.com

You Tube Channel:
https://www.youtube.com/user/GoldenAppleHealing

PUBLICATIONS BY DR. MARTHA

BOOKS
Libster, M.M. (2022). *Precision self-care for nurses: The Elements of Care® program for beating burnout.* Wauwatosa, WI: Golden Apple Publications.

Libster, M.M. (2015). *The Science of Energy Flow® foot reflexology with herbal stress relief.* Wauwatosa, WI: Golden Apple Publications.

Libster, M.M. (2012). *The nurse-herbalist: Integrative insights for holistic practice.* Wauwatosa, WI: Golden Apple Publications.

Libster, M., & McNeil, B. A. (2009). *Enlightened charity: The holistic nursing care, education and "Advices Concerning the Sick" of Sister Matilda Coskery (1799-1870).* Wauwatosa, WI: Golden Apple Publications.

Libster, M.M. (2004). *Herbal diplomats: The contribution of early American nurses (1830-1860) to nineteenth-century health care reform and the Botanical Medical Movement.* Wauwatosa, WI: Golden Apple Publications.

Libster, M.M. (2002). *The Integrative herb guide for nurses.* Albany, NY: Delmar Thomson Learning. Available for download www.GoldenApplePublications.com

Libster, M.M.. (2001). *Demonstrating care; The art of integrative nursing.* Albany, NY: Delmar Thomson Learning. Available for download www.GoldenApplePublications.com

Guest Editorials
Libster, M. (2010). Guest Editorial - From Flame to Bonfire: A Call for Companions. *Curationis: Journal of South African Nurses Assn.,* 33(1),3.

Libster, M. (2009). Guest Editorial - Behind the Shield: A Perspective on H1N1 from the Inner Terrain. *Journal of Holistic Nursing,* 27(4), 218-22

Libster, M. (2003). Guest Editorial – "Integrative Care Product and Process – Considering the three T's of Timing, Type, and Tuning." *Complementary Therapies in Nursing and Midwifery.* 9(1): 1-4.

Policy

ANA and AHNA. (2018). *American Holistic Nurses Assn. Scope and Standards* 3rd Ed. **Contributing Author** Core Values, Standards and Content on Herbs, Healing Environment, Nursing History, APRN practice, Self-care, Faith Community, and Culturally Congruent Practice.

Articles and Monographs

Libster, M. (2022). The Tao of integrative nursing assessment (TINA): An East-West model for precision, complementarity, and inclusion in relationship-centered care. *Holistic Nursing Practice.* (In Press).

Libster, M. (2021). Kindness as the remedy of remedies: A History of psychiatric mental health nursing. Wauwatosa, WI: Golden Apple Publications Monographs. Available for download www.GoldenApplePublications.com

Libster, M. (2021). *Medicinal Marijuana.* Wauwatosa, WI: Golden Apple Publications Monographs. Available for download www.GoldenApplePublications.com

Libster, M. (2019). Gentle Remedies: Restoring faith in the first step of nonpharmacological infant mental health care for the prevention and treatment of "disruptive behavior." *Archives of Psychiatric Nursing.* 33, 299 – 306. *Special Issue Infant Mental Health.*

Libster, M. (2018). Spiritual formation, Secularization, and Reform of Professional Nursing in Antebellum America. *Journal of Professional Nursing,* 34, 47-53.

Libster, M. (2015). Editorial- Enlightenment in the Circle of Culture In *Perspectives on Cultural Diplomacy*, Vol. 1 Nursing. Wauwatosa, WI: Golden Apple Publications. Available for download www.GoldenApplePublications.com

Libster, M. (2015). Cultural Diplomacy: Demonstrating Person-Centered Care and Coaching. *Perspectives on Cultural Diplomacy*. Vol. 1 Nursing. Wauwatosa, WI: Golden Apple Publications. Available for download www.GoldenApplePublications.com

Libster, M., Phillips, S., Smith Taylor, J., Southard, M., and Bryant, S. (2015). The Cultural Diplomacy Model™ for Demonstrating Person-Centered Care and Coaching. *Perspectives on Cultural Diplomacy.* Vol. 1 Nursing. Wauwatosa, WI: Golden Apple Publications. Available for download www.GoldenApplePublications.com

Libster, M. (2014). APRNVoices: Holes in the historical fabric of American nursing. Wauwatosa, WI: Golden Apple Publications Monographs. Available for download www.GoldenApplePublications.com

Libster, M. (2009). *Healing journeys.* Northside High School Documentary - short. Wauwatosa, WI: Golden Apple Publications. View on You Tube: https://www.youtube.com/channel/UC-PXSslk9Gp9U2wzH4Lir_A

Libster, M. (2011) Lessons Learned from a History of Perseverance and Innovation in Academic-Practice Partnerships. *Journal of Professional Nursing.* 27(6), e76-e81.

Libster, M. (2011). Nursing's Heritage of Forming Innovative Academic-Practice Partnerships. *American Association of Colleges of Nursing Task Force on Academic Practice Partnerships.* http://www.aacn.nche.edu/downloads/academic-practice-partnerships-task-force/NursingHeritageForgingPartnerships.pdf

Libster, M., Mulaudzi, M., Collins, S., Liang, O., Southworth, J., & Long, M. (2010). Tradition Meets Technology: Building Caring Community Online. ANS: *Advances in Nursing Science*, 33(4), 362-375.

Libster, M. (2009). A History of Shaker Nurse-herbalism, health reform, and the American Botanical Medical Movement (1830-1860). *Journal of Holistic Nursing*, 27(4), 222-231.

Mulaudzi, F. M., **Libster, M.**, & Phiri, S. (2009). Suggestions for creating a welcoming nursing community: Ubuntu, cultural diplomacy, and mentoring. *International Journal of Human Caring*, 13(2), 45-51.

Libster, M. (2008). Perspectives on the History of Self Care. *Self-Care, Dependent-Care and, Nursing*, 16 (2), 8-1.

Libster, M. (2008). Commentary and Plant Perspective on Hypericum and Nurses: A Comprehensive Literature Review on the Efficacy of St. John's Wort in the treatment of depression. *Journal of Holistic Nursing*, 26 (3), 208-211.

Libster, M. (2008). Elements of Care: Nursing Environmental Theory in Historical Context. *Holistic Nursing Practice*, 22(3), 160-170.

Libster, M. (1999). "Guidelines for selecting a medical herbalist for consultation and referral." *Journal of Alternative and Complementary Medicine*, 5(5): 457-462.

Libster, M. (2011). Nursing's Heritage of Forming Innovative Academic-Practice Partnerships. *American Association of Colleges of Nursing Task Force on Academic Practice Partnerships.* http://www.aacn.nche.edu/downloads/academic-practice-partnerships-task-force/NursingHeritageForgingPartnerships.pdf

Libster, M., Mulaudzi, M., Collins, S., Liang, O., Southworth, J., & Long, M. (2010). Tradition Meets Technology: Building Caring Community Online. ANS: *Advances in Nursing Science*, 33(4), 362-375.

Libster, M. (2009). A History of Shaker Nurse-herbalism, health reform, and the American Botanical Medical Movement (1830-1860). *Journal of Holistic Nursing*, 27(4), 222-231.

Mulaudzi, F. M., **Libster, M.**, & Phiri, S. (2009). Suggestions for creating a welcoming nursing community: Ubuntu, cultural diplomacy, and mentoring. *International Journal of Human Caring*, 13(2), 45-51.

Libster, M. (2008). Perspectives on the History of Self Care. *Self-Care, Dependent-Care and, Nursing*, 16 (2), 8-1.

Libster, M. (2008). Commentary and Plant Perspective on Hypericum and Nurses: A Comprehensive Literature Review on the Efficacy of St. John's Wort in the treatment of depression. *Journal of Holistic Nursing*, 26 (3), 208-211.

Libster, M. (2008). Elements of Care: Nursing Environmental Theory in Historical Context. *Holistic Nursing Practice*, 22(3), 160-170.

Libster, M. (1999). "Guidelines for selecting a medical herbalist for consultation and referral." *Journal of Alternative and Complementary Medicine*, 5(5): 457-462.

Index

A

AAT (Animal-assisted therapy), 134, 141, 144–46, 148

Accreditation Commission for Acupuncture and Oriental Medicine (ACAOM), 56, 59

acupuncture, 21, 54–55, 57, 59, 61–62

adaptation, 29–30, 65, 81, 83, 94, 140, 190

advanced practice registered nurse. *See* APRNs

advocacy, 22, 42

African Healing Traditions, 4, 50

agni, 55, 104, 188, 206

AHNA (American Holistic Nurses Association), 19, 21, 24, 65–66, 70, 76, 181–82, 187, 190, 199, 229, 234

air element, 5, 7, 33–34, 88, 171, 177, 182, 222

Alaska Native American Indian, 32, 46

alchemy, 15, 39, 229

allopathic, 26, 79

allostasis, 29, 33, 81, 83

alternative medicine, 19, 21, 45, 60, 62, 133, 168, 170, 184–85, 199

American Holistic Nurses Association. *See* AHNA

American Nurses Association. *See* ANA

ANA (American Nurses Association), 18–19, 21, 24, 41, 72, 76, 149, 190, 196, 199, 234

anger, 51, 55, 139

Animal-assisted therapy. *See* AAT

animals, 35, 47, 134, 144–46, 149, 187

antidotes, 81, 102

antimicrobial, 175, 178

antipyretic, 222

antiseptic, 175, 183

anxiety, 50, 55, 89, 92, 117, 119, 138, 142–43, 145, 158–59, 175, 178–79, 183

APRNs (advanced practice registered nurse), 67–68, 94–95, 217–18, 224

APRNVoices, 234

aquatic exercise, 7, 162, 168

archetypes, 32, 48, 60

aromatherapists, 177, 181

aromatherapy, 7–8, 11, 125, 171–74, 176, 178–79, 182–85

aromatherapy massage, 178–79, 184

Aromatic baths, 115, 176

assessment, 27–28, 30–31, 36, 52, 57, 65–69, 74–75, 91–92, 94, 188, 196

astringent, 176, 206

Ayurveda, 4, 21, 55–56, 61, 161, 206

B

Bach, 105, 111–12

balance, 18, 22, 45–48, 52–53, 55, 65, 93, 96, 122, 126, 202, 204–5, 209

balneotherapy, 7, 152, 157, 163, 168–69

baths, 33–34, 70, 154–55, 157–58, 162, 168, 172, 176, 219, 224, 227

bed baths, traditional, 158, 169

beliefs, 14–15, 22, 33, 41–46, 48, 66, 71–72, 79–80, 91, 102–5, 139, 141, 188–90, 194–95, 197–98

  spiritual, 188, 190

Benner, 27–28, 39, 41–42, 60

Bingen, 35, 40, 47, 61

biofeedback, 5, 88–89, 98

biomedical culture, 20, 22, 43–44, 57, 66, 79, 195

biomedicine, 14, 22, 45

blood pressure, 6, 88, 126–27, 193

body mind, 22, 190

bodywork, 6, 114–16, 119, 130

Bohm, 15, 24, 34, 39, 125, 131, 188, 199

Botanical Medical Movement, 24, 39, 61, 214, 229, 233

bouillon, 207

bowels, 162, 203, 219

brain, 80, 137, 142, 163–64, 174, 181, 187, 204

breathe, 93, 106, 174

breathing, 55, 88, 94, 106–7, 153, 162–63

  conscious, 5, 93–94, 105

broth and porridge, 9, 202, 207–8

Buckle, 173–74, 178, 181, 184

Buddhism, 32, 191

burns, 54, 81, 90, 93, 168, 175

C

cannabis, 179, 184
Caraka Samhita, 55–56, 60
care
  biomedical, 43–44, 56–57, 71, 74, 78–79, 217
  plan, 58, 85, 135
Careful Nursing, 17
Careful Nursing system, 22
care plans, 33, 69, 146
caring, 14, 28, 33, 38–40, 42–43, 65, 69, 73, 93, 189, 194–95
caring modalities, 22, 31, 65, 74
caring relationship, 188, 198
Case Study, 3–7, 36, 57, 94, 109, 128, 146
causation, 140, 189
caution, 51, 143, 164, 166, 181
certification, 57, 89, 127, 144, 148, 165, 167, 181, 195–96
certification programs, 146, 165
change, 16, 18, 20, 29–32, 35, 38–39, 52, 69–71, 81–83, 88, 92, 125, 139, 150–51, 153–54
  behavior, 136, 139
change process, 139
chaos, 34, 184
chemotherapy, 57–58, 74, 119, 143, 183
Childre, 92–93, 98, 137, 149, 193, 199
children, 85, 91, 117, 119–20, 133, 142, 144–45, 176, 178, 181, 185, 203, 207
Chinese herbal medicine, 61, 229
Chinese medicine
  classic traditional, 34
  traditional, 21, 32, 106, 116, 178, 215
Christian healing churches, 50
Christianity, 32, 50, 153, 191
Christian religions, 50
chronic illnesses, 139
cinnamon, 181, 222
Classical Traditional Chinese Medicine, 4, 42, 51, 203, 206
classifications, 175, 183, 190, 209, 222
Clinical Vignette, 4–5, 67–74, 91
coaching, 42, 45, 61, 136, 139–40, 207, 234
coaching techniques, 7, 139–40, 193

comfort, 3, 5, 11–12, 14, 16, 20, 22, 27–33, 36–38, 77–79, 83–85, 88–90, 96–98, 217, 231
Common Rules, 16
communication, 20, 34, 42–43, 72, 120, 122, 134, 137, 141–42, 146, 148–49
communication interventions, 6, 11, 134–35, 141, 143–44, 148
communication skills, 7, 66, 68, 88, 135–36, 146
community building, 93–94, 97
compassion, 22, 36, 91, 100–101, 109, 112, 188, 196, 198
competencies, 19, 65, 67–68, 149
  entry-level, 57
complementarity, 45, 61, 214, 234
complexities, 28, 138, 221
compresses, 9, 87, 90, 165, 172, 178, 218–19, 222–23, 227, 230
  cool-water, 18
concentration, 155, 162, 176–77
concept, major, 30–31, 138
conditions, best, 17, 27, 33, 188
conflicts, 98, 105, 138
  internal, 92
confrontation, 140
Confucius, 51
congee, 208, 213
congruent, 11, 65, 70, 204
connective tissue manipulation, 126, 131
consciousness, 22, 33, 35, 52, 55, 100–101, 103–5, 111–12, 186–87, 195, 198
  expanding, 25, 40, 76
constituents, 86, 180, 203–4, 206, 210–11, 213, 219–20
consumers, 20, 218–19, 227
contentment, 22, 188
control, 68, 93, 109, 179, 193, 221
cortisol, 117–18, 131
counsel, 73, 196
counseling, 136, 139–40, 150–51, 193, 218
  nondirective, 140, 149
counseling techniques, 134, 138
courtesy, 152, 171, 186, 202, 216
Cowling, Richard 66, 76

creativity, 102, 107, 155, 165
crisis, 44, 75, 83
cultural diplomacy, 42, 46, 57, 61, 66, 234–35
Cultural Diplomacy Model, 10, 42–43, 61, 234
cultural skill, 4, 57–58
cytochrome P450, 181, 220

D

dampness, 52, 203, 208
death, 29, 31, 48, 68, 92, 165, 192
decisions, shared, 86, 140
deficiency, 30, 57, 177, 211
dementia, 34, 142, 145, 151, 169, 205
Demonstrating care, 24, 35, 39, 64, 76, 98, 194, 200, 229, 233
depression, 6, 84, 92, 107–8, 117–19, 127, 163, 169, 178–79, 203, 235
design, 18, 22, 32, 38, 231
detoxing, 175–76
diabetes, 139, 163, 203
diagnose, 69, 135, 222
diagnosis
  pulse, 53
  tongue, 53
diet, sickroom, 207, 213
Dietary Supplement Health and Education Act (DSHEA), 221
dietary supplements, 9, 20–21, 25, 217–18, 221, 224, 227
digestion, 55, 157, 173, 206–7
dignity, 91, 138
dimension, 6, 28, 83, 91, 93, 116, 122, 207
discernment, 4, 64, 72–75, 78, 101
discernment process, 73–74
disciplines, 41, 43, 52
discomfort, 29, 78, 81, 85, 89, 97, 107, 116, 126, 191
diseases
  self-limited, 27, 39, 80
  treatment of, 152–53
dissociation, 103, 105
distance, 82, 114, 146
distillation, 172, 174, 206

distress, spiritual, 92, 196
diversity, 46, 98
Dix, Dorothea, 17
dogma, 22, 91, 188, 198
dosage, 118, 132
Dossey, Barbara, 192
dreams, 101, 104, 192
drug treatments, 71, 83, 95
DSHEA (Dietary Supplement Health and Education Act), 221

E

earth, 11, 18, 22–23, 32–33, 35, 37–38, 46–47, 60–61, 64, 141, 202, 204, 206
earth element, 5, 8, 35, 85, 202, 204, 212, 222
Eastern philosophies, 204, 209
Eastern traditions, 187, 203
East-West Model, 61, 214, 234
effectiveness, 86, 132, 140, 142, 185, 195
efficacy, 54, 89, 151, 180, 199, 218, 235
effort-shape movement, 8, 194, 198
EFT (equine facilitated therapy), 145–46
elders, 44, 61, 85
elements, five, 11, 18, 26–27, 31–38, 42, 53, 55, 78, 84, 141, 144, 216–17, 231
emergency situations, 44, 75
emotional states, 92, 177
empathy, 7, 136–37, 139, 150, 196
energetic patterns, 3, 15, 27, 35, 205, 209, 231
energetics, 11, 16, 178, 203–5, 208, 211, 217, 222, 232
  thermal, 175, 183
Energetics First, 9, 11, 15-16, 204, 211, 217, 222, 232
energetics qualities, 33, 52, 204–5, 208
energy, 50, 52, 72, 74, 89, 105–6, 116, 122, 124, 187–90, 192, 194–95, 202, 204, 210
energy balance, 124, 174, 209
energy centers, 122
energy fields, 30–31, 122, 125, 196
energy flow, 6, 10, 52, 123, 125, 132, 184, 187, 190, 194–95, 231, 233
Enlightened Charity, 24, 39, 76,

98, 170, 200, 214, 230, 233
entourage effects, 221
  phytocannabinoid-terpenoid, 230
entrainment, 143
environment, 18, 22, 26–30, 34–36, 69, 72, 131, 134–35, 143, 145, 182–83, 194, 203
environmental intervention, 9, 217, 224
epsom salts, 70, 159, 176
equine facilitated therapy. *See* EFT
Erickson, 34, 37, 39, 72, 76
Eriksson, 28, 30, 39, 142–43, 149
essence, 18, 28, 33, 35, 39, 42, 52, 61, 81, 141, 206
essential oils, 12, 70, 171–85
  application of, 171, 179
essential oils and aromatherapy, 7, 11, 172
  use of, 171–72
ether, 11, 18, 22–23, 32–33, 35, 37–38, 53, 55, 64, 94–95, 135, 141, 206
ethics, 24, 72, 76, 98, 127, 132, 144, 196, 199
evaluation, 4, 28, 31, 65, 71, 74, 86, 138, 184, 211
evidence, 73, 146, 158, 160, 167, 169, 218, 221, 230
  anecdotal, 89, 160
evidence base, 99
evolution, 25, 111, 142, 199
evolutionary research, 112, 200
expanding consciousness theory, 37, 69
expertise, 19, 27, 43, 50
extract, 173–74, 220, 222
eyes, 28, 55, 92, 177, 181, 191, 193

F

faith community, 94, 189, 197–98, 234
faith healers, 191
faith healing, 8, 190–91
faith tradition, 22, 91, 188–89, 198
familiarity, 30–31, 102, 136
Farnsworth, Norman, 217
fathers, 51, 115, 121
Father Sebastian Kneipp, 156
Fawaz, 16, 24
Fawcett, 30, 39, 99, 149

feedback, 69, 86, 88
fever reduction, 67–68
First Nation, 46
Five Element herbal footbath ablution, 125
five elements approach, 54
five Elements of Care, 3, 11–12, 14, 18, 22–23, 26, 30, 36–38, 77–78, 94, 97, 231
five elements position, 78
five elements thought, 18
Five-Element theory, 53, 205, 207
Flaws, Bob, 52, 60, 206, 208, 214
flowers, 159, 172–73, 194, 222, 226
fluids, 52, 73, 116, 155
focus, 14–15, 18, 20, 27–29, 31, 33, 83, 106–7, 121–22, 140–41, 190, 203–4, 207–8, 211, 217
Food & Drug Administration, 20, 25, 55
foods
  constituents of, 202, 204, 208
  energetics of, 203–4, 208, 211, 213
  tonifying, 203
foot, 122, 124, 126
foot and hand baths, 176
foot bathing, 159, 168
footbaths, 7, 70, 125, 153, 157, 159, 165, 168, 224
foot reflexology, 6, 114–16, 122–27, 130–32, 169, 184, 233
  effects of, 126, 132
Foot Reflexology Chart, 10, 123
forgiveness, 22, 46, 55, 91, 188, 191, 198
formation, 41–42, 44–45
freedom, 160, 184
Freeze frame, 98, 149, 199
frequency, 74, 118, 194, 199
fundamental processes, 53

G

ginger, 86–87, 175, 178, 184, 223
ginger compresses, 10, 87, 94–95, 223
goals, patient's health, 71
God, 16, 47, 50–51, 69, 73, 91, 189, 199
Goethe, 34, 39, 187, 199

grief, 68, 142, 145
guidance, 158, 189, 192
guilt, 91–93, 99, 140

H

habits, 102, 139–40, 160
handouts, 67–68, 95
happiness, 22, 65, 91, 111, 188, 209
Harmer, 39, 149, 154, 169, 219, 229
Harmer & Henderson, 137, 154
harmonious, 34, 205
harmonious connectedness, 190
harmony, 22, 46, 48, 52, 55–56,
  64–65, 101, 142, 149, 175, 188
headaches, 18, 89, 91, 94–95, 109, 157, 161, 223
healers, 32, 47–48, 50, 56, 60
  folk, 50
  indigenous, 21, 44
  inner, 72, 192, 199
  traditional, 22, 44–45, 50–51
healing crises, 35, 38, 135, 231
healing modalities, 43, 125, 217
healing relationship, 14, 22, 64–66,
  71, 74, 139–40, 146, 148, 189
Healing Relationship Model, 10, 82
healing touch, 21, 120
healing traditions, 28, 38, 46–47,
  66, 81, 85, 159, 163, 218, 227, 229
health and healing, 22, 30, 60, 80, 111, 115, 192
health behavior, 61, 140, 188
Health Belief Model, 200
health beliefs, 11, 14, 41, 44, 46,
  49, 72–74, 79, 188, 191
  person's, 189
  role of, 44, 186
health care, 14, 24, 36, 42, 45,
  57, 61, 92, 99, 135, 139, 184
healthcare cultures, 85
health patterns, 2, 31, 65, 68–69,
  75, 78, 135, 141, 204
  unique energetic, 27, 65, 231
health professionals, 43, 122, 195

health promotion, 89, 112, 156, 192
HeartMath Institute, 92, 97, 136–37, 193, 198
heat, 52, 54, 70, 87, 90, 157–58, 161, 173,
  177–78, 203, 205, 209, 222–23
helix, 82, 236
  double, 82
  expanded, 83
Henderson, 24, 39, 149, 154, 169
herbal, 50, 125, 216–17, 221, 224, 227, 230
herbal diplomats, 24, 39, 61, 214, 229, 233
herbal formulas, 52, 58
herbal interventions, 9, 11–12,
  216–17, 222–24, 227
herbalism, 179, 217
herbal medicines, 46, 50, 62, 214–15, 217, 228–29
herbal remedies, 44, 50, 53–54, 86, 217–20
herbal stress relief, 132, 169, 184, 233
herbal supplements, 218–19
herbs, 9, 48, 53–54, 57–58, 60, 70–72,
  156, 159, 205, 207, 214, 217–27, 234
  use of, 2, 206, 229
herb safety, 9, 217, 220
Hildegard Peplau, 135
Hippocrates, 115, 152, 224
history, medical, 40, 200
history, self care, 235
holism, 3, 11–12, 14–15, 22–23, 30–31, 38, 77, 188
holistic approach, 28, 31
  integrative, 31, 36
holistic care, 15–17, 19, 23, 27, 35, 76, 97, 230–31
holistic nursing, 3, 14, 18–21, 24, 28, 39, 98, 149,
  151, 170, 192, 199-200, 214, 229–30, 233, 235
holistic nursing philosophy,
  integrative, 11–12, 14, 57, 64
holistic philosophy, 15, 35, 66, 68
holistic practice, 24, 39, 76, 83, 214, 229, 233
  integrative, 78, 173
Holistic Transformation, 3–9, 37, 58,
  75, 96, 110, 129, 147, 166, 182, 197
hologram, 122, 125
homeostasis, 81
home remedies, 43, 48, 67–68, 223
hops, 179, 219

horses, 102, 144–45
hospitalizations, 66, 84, 146
hospitals, 16–17, 19, 35, 42, 86, 90, 120, 124, 128, 142, 147, 154, 189
hot baths and packs, 154
hot springs, 62, 215
hot-water bottles, 5, 34, 37, 89–91, 94–95, 98, 161
HRV (heart rate variability), 92, 121–22, 137
hug, 5, 90–91
human beings, 18, 47, 81–82, 136
human caring, 150, 235
human experience, 65, 85, 109, 188
humanity, 16, 28, 33, 40, 48, 93, 183, 200
Humulus lupulus, 179, 219
hydrotherapies, 7, 11, 70, 116, 125, 152–54, 156–58, 160–61, 164–69, 190, 223–24
hydrotherapy interventions, 12, 152, 167
hydrotherapy methods, 153
hypothalamic-pituitary-adrenal-cortical axis, 118

I

illness
  acute, 84, 119, 130
  mental, 45, 50–51, 142, 200
imagery, 8, 50, 71, 191–92, 198, 200
  guided, 21, 130, 193, 199
imagery science, 192
imagination, 192–93
imbalance, 203, 205
immersion, 159, 164, 168
immersion baths, 7, 158–59
implementation, 4, 65, 69
implicate order, 24, 125, 131, 188, 199
improvement, 45, 80, 86, 116, 119, 159
inclusion, 2, 61, 84, 117, 193, 214, 234
indigenous healing systems, 11, 44, 56, 59
infant, 84–85, 87, 119–22, 133, 181, 196, 208, 223
  infant behavior, 85, 131
  infant massage, 6, 115, 119–21, 128, 132
  infant massage instructors, 74, 120, 122
infection, 55, 146, 161, 164, 179

inflammation, 86–87, 160–61, 164, 207, 213, 222
infusion, 70, 222–24
Ingham Method, 124
inhalation therapy, 8, 177
injuries, 21, 51, 117, 119–20, 153
inner terrain, 233
innovation, 234
integration, 15, 19, 22–23, 31, 74, 92, 146, 231
integrative holistic nurses, 22–23, 64, 69, 71–75, 81, 85, 111, 120, 125, 135–36, 139
integrative holistic nursing, 3–4, 11, 14, 16–18, 21–22, 27–29, 31, 36, 42–45, 64–66, 68, 74–75, 78–79, 134, 231
integrative holistic nursing assessment, 67–68
integrative nursing, 12, 22, 24, 39, 65–66, 75–76, 98, 200, 229, 233
intention, 45–46, 69, 85
interconnectedness, 187–88
interdependence, 30
interior/exterior, 52, 205
Interpersonal Relations, 76, 135, 150
interventions, nonpharmacological, 77, 79, 84, 91, 165
invention, 18, 102, 153
ionic footbaths, 160, 169

J

Jefferson, Thomas, 93, 160, 169
joints, 163, 223
jook, 208, 214
Judaism, 153, 191

K

Kabat-Zinn, 100–101, 103–4, 111–12
kindness, 17, 28, 70, 101, 189, 196, 234
kindness training, 109
Kushi Institute, 213

L

Laban, Rudolf, 194
Labanotation, 198

Laban system, 194
Langer, Ellen, 100, 102
Latter-day Saints, 48, 208
lavender, 175–76, 179, 181, 184
laws, 46, 141, 165
Leininger, Madeleine, 28, 39, 42, 61
lemongrass, 175, 179–81, 183
Libster, Martha 17–18, 20, 22, 24, 28–31, 39, 41–43, 48, 61, 65–66, 76, 125, 169–70, 200, 207–9, 211, 214, 217–19, 229–30, 233–35
licensure, 19, 21, 56, 74, 78, 127, 135, 144, 165, 167
lifestyle, 16, 30, 46, 52–54, 95, 153
lifestyle changes, 204, 209
limbic system, 174, 176
listening, 34, 68, 101, 136, 138, 142, 193
living water, productive, 155
loneliness, 84, 114, 138, 145
longevity, 52, 60, 107, 187, 208–9, 214
loss, 69, 81, 84, 93, 142
loving kindness, 100–101

M

macrobiotic diet, 9, 202, 207–11, 213–15
macrobiotics, 209, 211
Macrobiotics, Zen, 209, 214
management, 29, 84
massage, 45, 50, 56, 74, 78, 115–22, 126, 128–30, 163, 176, 178–79
massage therapy, 21, 114, 116–19, 121–22, 130–32
MBSR (mindfulness-based stress reduction), 100–101, 103, 107–8, 112
medical acupuncture, 54–55, 57, 59–60, 62
medicine
  functional, 211
  traditional, 22, 45, 217
medicine wheel, 47, 62
meditation, 17, 21, 52, 100–105, 107–8, 110, 191, 193
meditation practice, 17, 52, 101, 108
Meleis, Afaf 29, 40
memories, 31, 33, 55, 103, 107, 125, 141, 143, 150, 181, 192

mental health, 16, 93, 133, 142, 178, 201
mental health nursing, 136, 169, 200–201, 234
mercy nurses, 17
meridians, 52, 54
metabolism, 15, 55, 194, 204
metabolites, 156, 163
methicillin-resistant Staphylococcus aureus (MRSA), 180, 183, 185
MI (Motivational interviewing), 39, 61, 139–40, 149, 151
mind, 18, 21, 23, 33–34, 46, 50, 53–55, 101–5, 140–41, 157, 173–75, 187, 190–92, 198
mindful learning, 102, 112
mindfulness, 5, 42–43, 100–107, 111–13, 145
mindfulness-based stress reduction. See MBSR
mindfulness meditation, 102, 105, 107–9, 112, 130
mindlessness, 5, 100–102, 104
mind-set, 102
minerals, 20–21, 35, 47, 203–4, 221
mobility, 126, 168
modeling, 34–35, 38–39, 66–68, 72, 74, 76–77, 85–86, 95, 128, 135–36, 148
modeling and role-modeling, 39, 76, 85
Modeling and Role-Modeling theory, 34
modes, 30, 143, 172
moods, 117, 142–43, 157, 163, 165, 169, 174, 178
morphic resonance, 82, 99, 125, 132
music, use of, 142–43
music therapists, 141–42, 144
music therapy, 7, 134, 141–44, 148–49, 151

N

National Center for Complementary and Alternative Medicine (NCCAM), 19, 118
National Center for Complementary and Integrative Health. See NCCIH
National Institutes of Health (NIH), 19, 79, 99, 118, 174, 228
nations, 15, 43, 46, 60, 78
natural products, 3, 11, 20, 23, 141, 174
nature, 17–18, 26–27, 29, 33–35, 46–48, 77,

80–81, 84–85, 88–89, 91, 93, 155, 187–89, 192
  five elements of, 27, 231
  human, 22, 102
  laws of, 156, 188, 198
nature care, 27–28
nature cure, 11, 18, 153, 156
naturopathic medicine, 168
naturopathic medicine movement, 156
naturopathy, 154
Navajos, 46
NCCAM (National Center for Complementary and Alternative Medicine), 19, 118
NCCIH (National Center for Complementary and Integrative Health), 19–21, 24–25, 55, 61, 77, 79, 119, 141, 183, 190, 210, 214
nerves, 88, 116, 157, 187
  stimulating gastric, 206
nervous systems, 70, 88, 125, 153–54, 192, 206–7
  autonomic, 137
neuropeptides, 30, 174
neuroplasticity, 142
neurotransmitter, 86
Newman, 15, 25, 30–31, 37, 40, 76
Nicholas Roerich Museum, 152, 171, 186, 202, 216
Nightingale, Florence, 16-17, 25, 27, 32, 39-40, 171-172, 185, 187, 188, 194, 200
NIH. *See* National Institutes of Health
nondirective counseling and coaching, 136, 140
nonjudgment, 103, 109, 136
nonjudgmental acceptance, 72, 143
nonjudgmental attitude, 137
nonpharmacological, 20, 77–78, 84, 164
nurse-herbalism, 9, 216–19, 222, 227
nurse-herbalist, 24, 39, 214, 229, 233
Nurse-Herbalist Institute, 228, 232
Nurse Practice Act, 211
nurses
  advanced practice, 54, 57
  parish, 189, 201
Nurse's Answers, 3–7, 36, 57, 95, 109, 128, 146
Nurses' understanding of patient

health behaviors and choices, 20
nursing, history of, 14, 16, 25, 131, 196, 234
nursing care, 11, 16–18, 20, 23, 28, 31, 36–37, 40, 82, 84, 114–15, 188, 191, 205, 207
nursing interventions, 150, 190, 192, 207, 224
nursing process, 4, 18–19, 23–24, 27–28, 30–33, 44, 64–67, 75, 85, 135, 231
  five-phase, 67
nursing research, 40, 85, 132, 223
nursing science, 2, 24, 27, 40, 43, 76, 82, 154, 200, 235
nursing theory, 3, 28, 30–31, 72, 211
nutrition, 20, 55, 72, 204, 213–14, 231
nutrition interventions, 8, 11–12, 74, 202, 206–7, 211, 213

O

oats, 208
obesity, 6, 107–8, 163, 203, 215
observation, 36, 65, 109, 118, 135, 137, 145, 188
  keen, 42
  psychotherapeutic, 145
observation skill, 6, 36, 109
Ohsawa, 209–10, 214
oils
  aromatic bath, 159
  botanical aromatic, 174, 183
  volatile, 172, 180
opiates, 66, 78–79, 164–65

P

pacing, 68–69, 74
pain, 54–55, 77–79, 81–92, 94–95, 97–99, 107–8, 111–13, 116–17, 119, 131–32, 142, 157–58, 161–65, 168–70, 175–78
  chronic, 20, 77, 79, 97, 99, 153, 162, 179
  emotional, 5, 89, 92
  physical, 5, 83, 85–86
  psychological, 5, 88
pain management, 98, 168
pain measures, 5, 86
pain medicine, 133

pain relief, 54, 68, 77, 84, 86, 89, 92, 97, 158, 161, 164

pain scales, 86, 95

Paracelsus, 32, 35

paradigms, biomedical, 19

parents, 74, 112, 120–22, 128, 138, 146, 181

patient care, 30, 44, 69, 152–53, 158, 166, 182, 197

patterns, 15, 30–31, 52–53, 66, 69, 82, 86, 91, 102, 107, 155, 205, 210

  symptom/sign, 205

  symptom-sign, 205

peace, 43, 46–47, 62, 65, 93, 103, 105, 111, 125, 190, 222

Peacemaker, 46

Peacemaking, 43

Peplau, Hildegard, 64–66, 76, 135–37, 150

peppermint, 172, 175, 178–79, 222

perception, 29, 31, 33, 82–83, 88, 91, 94, 97, 103, 110, 115, 189, 194

personality, 64–65, 88, 98, 194

person-centered care, 42, 61

perspectives, 34, 62, 102, 136, 233, 235

  acting from a single, 102

  cognitive, 112

  historical, 131

  integrative, 74

  spiritual, 17, 201

pharmaceutical drugs, 85, 218–20

philosophy, 11, 15, 18, 24, 40, 53–54, 60, 66, 78–79, 209, 214

placebo effect, 5, 77, 79–81, 90, 98

plants, 47, 70–71, 134, 139, 172–74, 180–82, 185, 187, 202, 204–6, 217–22, 224–25, 227

  medicinal, 17, 71, 217–21, 227

pneuma, 3, 18, 35

poisons, 101, 153

  perceived, 153

populations, 22, 89, 108, 145, 203, 221

porridge, 9, 202, 207–8, 213

positive effect, 118, 121–22, 142, 158–59, 179, 193

poultices, 172, 219, 222–23, 227

power, 27, 33, 46, 51, 60, 72, 104, 112, 136, 141, 191

political, 14

protective, 50

spiritual, 48

vital, 30, 187

Practice Acts, 21

pray, 73, 189, 196

prayer, 8, 16–17, 33, 50, 91–92, 159, 188–91, 196, 198–99, 201

prayer wheel, 191

precision, 3, 15, 26–27, 35, 38, 61, 214, 231, 234

precision health, 15, 24

precision nursing science, 3–4, 11–16, 18, 21–23, 27, 53, 63–66, 125, 217, 227, 231–32

precision self-care, 139, 233

pregnancy, 87, 117, 146, 161, 164–66, 170, 184, 199, 224

prevention, 21, 45, 156, 162–63, 165, 213, 234

Principle Patterns, 9, 52–53, 204–5, 207, 209–11, 222

Principle Patterns and Five Elements approach, 54

principle patterns and fundamental processes, 53

principle patterns theory, 205

Professional Notes, 6–9, 119, 122, 127, 143, 146, 165, 180

protein, 203–4, 208

psychotherapy, 136, 140–41, 149

Q

qi, 52, 116, 132, 156, 161, 206, 223

quality of life, 11, 107, 142

quintessence, 216–17

R

races, 114, 143, 220

randomized controlled trials (RCTs), 80, 127, 132, 151, 168, 179, 184, 195, 223

reactivity, 203

readiness, 73–74, 128

realization, 209

Recipe for Ginger Compress for Pain, 10

recipes, 2, 48, 87, 129, 207–8, 218

recognition, 20, 92
recovery, 66, 140
reflexology, 124–27, 131
rehabilitation, 66, 154, 163, 170
relatedness, 15, 137
relationship-building, 68
relationship-centered care, 38, 42, 45, 61, 69, 214, 234
  person-centered, 18, 231
relationships, 15, 30, 50, 52, 65–66, 103, 105, 134, 136–37, 139–40, 142, 144, 203, 205, 210
  nurse-patient, 138
relationship skills, 146
relax, 159, 162, 177
relaxation, 117, 125, 130, 142–43, 152–53, 156, 158, 164, 167–68, 193, 199
religion, 16, 22, 46, 60, 91, 143, 187–88, 191, 198, 229
religion and spirituality, 91, 188, 191
religious and spiritual interventions, 8, 11, 188, 190, 198
religious and spiritual pain, 5, 91
religious pain, 91–92
religious teachings, 22, 91, 188, 198
research, 5–8, 43–44, 91, 107, 115, 120–22, 124–25, 136–37, 145–46, 158–59, 171–72, 193, 195, 217, 220
resistance, 81, 83, 139, 155, 163–64
respect, 2, 41, 56–57, 64, 137–38, 218
  mutual, 138
response, 36, 57, 80, 86, 88, 90, 117, 130, 137, 140, 181
restoration, 51, 190
rhythms, 35, 137, 143, 194, 200
risk factors, 93, 116, 121
rituals, 31, 50, 91, 136, 153, 188–89, 198
Roerich, 33, 40
  Nicholas, 152, 171, 186, 202, 216
Rogerian Nursing Science, 149
Rogers, Martha, 30, 40
role-modeling, 34, 39, 72, 76–77, 85, 231
role-modeling theory, 34, 37
rosemary, 70, 175
rosemary footbath, 70–71

Roy, Sr. Callista, 39, 82, 99
Roy Adaptation Model, 30, 39, 99
Rush, Benjamin, 79

S

sacred dances, 46
sacred scriptures, 55
safety, 54, 74–75, 164, 180, 195, 217
safety record, 54, 181, 220
salts, 205, 210
Satprem, 104–5, 112
sauna, 153, 157, 163–64
school nurse, 5, 18, 91
science, emerging, 22, 28, 125
Scope and standards, 65, 76, 234
Scope and standards of practice, 19, 24, 135, 149, 196, 199, 218, 229
SEF foot reflexology, 125
self, 22, 28, 32–33, 35, 66, 91, 94, 103–4, 187–89, 192, 194
  inner, 52
  physical, 68
self-awareness, 7, 136–37, 139
self-care, 12, 15, 42–45, 65–66, 68, 80, 85, 94–95, 156, 158, 223, 235, 227, 234–35
Self-care Institute, 139, 148
self-care remedies, 94, 97
Selye, Hans, 81, 83, 88, 99
senna, 219
Shaker nurses, 218
shamans, 50
Sheldrake, Rupert, 99, 125, 132
Shiatsu, Zen, 163
sickroom management, 11, 17–18, 23, 27, 187, 231
silence, 105, 139, 151
Sister Mary Xavier Clark, 16
Sister Matilda Coskery, 24, 27, 39, 76, 98, 170, 200, 214, 230, 233
Sisters of Charity in America, 17
sitz baths, 7, 157, 159, 161, 224
sleep, 53, 101, 109, 126, 131, 159, 167, 169, 178–80, 184, 192

sleep disturbances, 107, 179
sleeplessness, 53, 157
smell, 70, 106, 120, 172, 174, 192–93, 224
Solution-focused brief therapy (SFBT), 140, 150
Solution-Focused Therapy, 140, 148, 150
solutions, 53, 66, 69, 76–78, 83, 93–95, 97, 138, 140, 150, 162
song, 127, 133, 180, 184, 191
songwriting, 143
soul's purpose, 111
Southard, Mary Elaine, 61, 140, 149, 151, 234
space
  physical, 35, 114, 135, 195
  psychological-emotional-spiritual, 71
spas, 153–54, 160, 165
spine, 89–90, 126, 129
spiritual interventions, 8, 11–12, 186, 188–91, 195–96, 198
spirituality, 22–23, 91, 99, 141, 187–88, 190–91, 198–200
spirituality and religion, 187–88, 191, 198
spiritual pain, 5, 91–93, 99
spiritual practices, 101, 191, 196
spleen, 203, 206–8, 213
sprouting, 10, 49
sprouting lids, 49
sprouting *seeds*, 49
sprouts, 49
Sri Aurobindo, 104, 112, 186, 200
Sri Aurobindo & Satprem, 187, 200
stagnation, 89, 116, 192
standardized extracts, 218–20
standards, best practice, 180–81
State Boards, 21, 25, 138, 150
steam baths, 7, 163–64
steam distillation, 8, 173
steams, 173, 219, 222, 227
St. John's Wort, 220, 235
stress, psychological, 84, 89, 98, 108
stress conditions, 81, 118
stress reduction, 32, 83, 89, 137, 143
mindfulness-based, 100, 112
stress relief, 5, 77, 81, 125–26, 130, 153, 179
stress response, 30–32, 40, 81, 83, 99
suffering, 5, 21, 79, 83, 85–86, 97, 99, 105, 111, 117, 139
sun, 46, 116, 133, 162, 170
symbol, 50, 153, 210
sympathetic nervous system activity, 158
synchronization, 193, 200
synchronize, 92
synergistic effect, 54
syrups, 218–19, 222, 227
Systems Model, 64
systems theory, 30
system wholeness, 82

T

Tadodaho Chief Leon Shenandoah, 62
Tao, 52, 61
Taoism, 32, 52
Tao of integrative nursing assessment, 61, 214, 234
Tao of Integrative Nursing Assessment. *See* TINA
tapping, 116–17
tastes, sour, 205
tasting, 206–7
TCM (traditional Chinese medicine), 4, 10, 32, 34, 42, 51–58, 116, 203, 205–6, 208–9, 215
teas, fresh herb, 222
techniques, 20–21, 87, 89, 114, 116, 120, 124, 127, 130, 149, 151, 193, 196
  counseling and coaching, 7, 139–40, 193
temperature, 15, 67, 70–71, 87, 154, 159, 166
tension, muscle, 89, 163
theory, 81, 114, 116, 122, 124–25, 149, 153
  basic, 215
  emerging middle-range, 40
  scientific prescriptive, 54
therapeutic footbaths, 159, 167
therapeutic herbal baths, 70

therapeutic modalities, 2, 23, 70, 143, 174
therapeutic relationships, 134–38, 141
   cultivating, 7, 134–36
therapeutic use, 66, 181
therapies
   cold compress, 8, 177
   expressive arts, 7, 141
   pet, 144–45
therapists, 95, 136, 142–43, 145, 158, 167, 192–93
therapy sessions, 144, 146
thermal springs, 160
Thich Nhat Hanh, 100–101, 105–7, 109, 111, 113
Thich Nhat Hanh's breathing exercises, 105
Thomsonianism, 48
Thorne, Sally, 44, 62
thoughts
   habitual, 104
   judgmental, 110
   limiting, 103
TINA (Tao of Integrative Nursing Assessment), 61, 214, 234
tolerance, 22, 81, 188, 198
tone, 56, 66, 143
tongue, 53, 56
tongue tissue, 53
topical, 179, 216–17, 221
topical intervention, 9, 223
touch, 34, 37, 40, 70, 72, 74, 78, 87–88, 114–20, 122, 128, 131–32, 134
Touch Skills, 6, 128
touch therapies, 11–12, 54, 114, 116, 120, 129–30, 138
toxic reactions, 217
toxins, 101, 160, 164
traditional birth attendants, 51, 224
traditional Chinese medicine. *See* TCM
traditional healing, 22, 44–45, 56, 60
Traditional/Indigenous Healing Systems, 4, 41, 45
Tradition Meets Technology, 235
training, 16, 54, 56, 67, 78, 101, 106, 119–21, 138, 176, 182

tranquility, 83
Transcultural Nursing Society, 59
transformation, 26, 29, 38, 41, 65, 69, 71, 73, 82–83, 85, 92, 206, 231
   large-group, 93
   measure, 142
   personal, 39, 229
   social, 62, 99, 200
transition, 26, 29–30, 35, 38, 40, 44, 65, 69–71, 73, 82–83, 92, 97, 231
transmutation, 33
treatment, 70, 72–73, 75, 122, 125–26, 142, 160–61, 163, 168–69, 176–77, 181, 184, 234–35
tridosha, 55
trust, 71, 74, 138, 140
truth, 102, 195, 209
Turtle Island, 46

U

Ubuntu, 235
uncertainty, 102, 137–39
unitary-transformative philosophies, 30
unity, 23, 93, 105, 156
universe, 14–15, 33, 52–53, 102, 190, 193
Upanishads, 210, 214

V

Vedas, 55
vegetables, 207–8, 210
   sea, 205
viewpoints, 138
violence, 93, 117, 131
visions, 39, 56, 92, 149, 192
Visual Analog Scale, 86, 165, 179
vitamins, 20–21, 203–4, 206, 211, 213
vomiting, 178–79, 183–85
vulnerability, 81, 158

W

Wallace, Paul, 46, 62, 190, 201
warming, 175, 224

warmth, 18, 33, 71, 74, 88, 156, 161, 206–7
warm water immersion baths, 159
water birth, 7, 164
watercourse, 155
water cure, 48, 153
water element, 5, 7, 34, 89, 152, 166, 178, 222
water element application, 70, 159
water immersion, 164
water movement, 155–56, 172
water therapy, 7, 89, 152, 162, 167
Watson, Jean, 28, 30, 40
Watsu, 162–63, 165, 167, 169
weight, 128, 194, 204
weightlessness, 154, 162
weight loss, 208
Welcoming Integrative Insights, 4, 66
wellness, 68, 136, 178
Western reductionistic philosophy, 204
Western world, 114, 187
WHO (World Health Organization), 22, 25, 45, 56, 59, 62, 164, 190–91, 201, 203, 215, 217, 229–30
WHO Fact Sheets, 99
WHO Traditional medicine strategy, 62, 230
Wigmore, Ann, 48–49
withholding judgment, 74
women, pregnant, 146, 164, 180
world community, 120
worldviews, 14, 78, 211
  biomedical, 219
worries, 53, 214
worship, 189
wounds, 55, 71, 139, 188

Y

yang, 52, 116, 119, 132–33, 209–10
Yellow Emperor's Classic, 53, 202, 205, 209, 211
yin-yang, 10, 52, 116, 209–10
yin-yang theory, 205
  applied, 205
yoga, 21, 107, 214
  hatha, 108

Z

Zen, 104, 112
Zingiber officinale, 86–87, 175, 223
zones
  reflex, 126
  vertical, 122

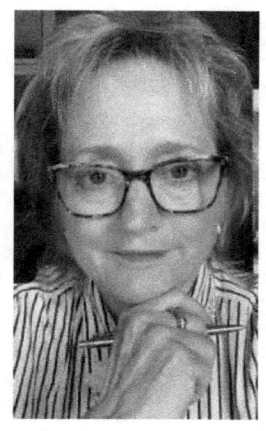

MARTHA MATHEWS LIBSTER.

Martha Mathews Libster, PhD, MSN, APRN-PMHCNS, APHN-BC, FAAN, is Founder and Executive Director of Golden Apple Healing Arts, an education and consultation company. Since 2006, she has led the Bamboo Bridge Global Tea House and the Nurse-Herbalist and Self-Care Institutes, innovative teaching and learning communities and forums for dialogue in health culture diplomacy. Dr. Libster is the author of ten books including: *The Nurse-Herbalist, Integrative Herb Guide for Nurses, Demonstrating Care: The Art of Integrative Nursing, Enlightened Charity,* and *Herbal Diplomats.* She is an inspirational speaker whose practice models are used by nurses on five continents. Dr. Libster is a professor and award-winning historian of nursing. She is an educational program designer, board-certified holistic Psychiatric Mental Health Clinical Nurse Specialist, and Herbal Diplomat® with 30 years' experience in the integration of traditional Chinese herbal medicine and nursing practice. She lives in Wisconsin, USA and can be reached at www.drmarthalibster.com and www.goldenapple-healingarts.com.

HELIX IS A VISUAL EXPRESSION OF HOW PATIENTS AND THEIR CAREGIVERS GROW AND EVOLVE IN UNDERSTANDING EACH PERSON'S UNIQUE PERCEPTIONS OF STRESS, CHANGE, TRANSITION, AND TRANSFORMATION THAT IS FOUNDATIONAL TO THE PROCESS OF HEALING.

Martha Libster, 2001

www.ingramcontent.com/pod-product-compliance
Lightning Source LLC
LaVergne TN
LVHW010314070526
838199LV00065B/5560